ANNUAL PROGRESS IN CHILD PSYCHIATRY AND CHILD DEVELOPMENT 1983

Edited by

STELLA CHESS, M.D.

Professor of Child Psychiatry
New York University Medical Center

and

ALEXANDER THOMAS, M.D.

Professor of Psychiatry
New York University Medical Center

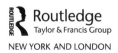

Routledge
Taylor & Francis Group

NEW YORK AND LONDON

First published 1984 by BRUNNER/MAZEL Philadelphia and London

This edition published 2015 by Routledge
711 Third Avenue, New York, NY 10017, USA
27 Church Road, Hove, East Sussex BN3 2FA

Routledge is an imprint of the Taylor & Francis Group, an informa business

Library of Congress Catalog Card No. 68-23452

ISBN: 9-78087-630-343-6 (hbk)

ISSN 0066-4030

CONTENTS

ANNUAL PROGRESS IN CHILD PSYCHIATRY AND CHILD DEVELOPMENT 1983

Part I

DEVELOPMENTAL THEORY

In last year's Annual Progress we pointed out that "the explosion of new knowledge in child development and child psychiatry in the past 10-15 years has of necessity demanded a reevaluation, modification, and even radical change in long-established and influential theoretical formulations." The first two papers in this section, by distinguished and highly influential developmental theorists, the psychiatrist John Bowlby and the psychologist Jerome Kagan, highlight this exciting trend.

Kagan reviews the data from his own studies and the work of others bearing on the explanations for the emergence of a concept of self in the young child, indeed one of the fundamental aspects of human psychological characteristics. He reveals that he and his colleagues began by assuming "the reality and theoretical utility of abstract constructs like passivity, sociability, hostility, achievement, reflectivity, and identification," and made their observations accommodate to these ideas. As he began to challenge these established formulations, he reversed his research strategy to give primary evidence to the empirical observation of the young child's behavior, instead of accommodating these observations to a priori theory. With this shift, he was able to develop a body of research data which, together with related findings by other investigators, led him to challenge accepted concepts on the emergence of self-awareness and to formulate an alternative approach, which he spells out in this contribution.

Bowlby's paper traces the personal history of his studies which led to his well-known and influential concepts of maternal deprivation, attachment and loss. In conducting this research, he had to challenge a number of the hallowed tenets of the psychoanalytic establishment, with which he had been identified, and for which he was chided by Anna Freud and other lesser lights in the psychoanalytic movement. Like Kagan (though his theoretical revisions preceded Kagan's by many years), he found it necessary to give primary consideration to data derived from actual observations of children instead of fitting such data into some

3

Procrustean bed of established concepts. Considering the broad scope of Bowlby's studies and their significance for developmental theory, individual workers may disagree with one or another of his formulations. Bowlby himself would be the last to take exception to this basic scientific tradition of scrutiny of theory and data, considering his own willingness to reexamine and modify certain of his own conclusions in the light of new empirical findings.

The remaining papers of this section constitute critical evaluations of new variations on old themes. First are the recently popular statements on the developmental significance of parent-infant bonding and attachment, a new version of the recurrent theme of the decisive importance of the mother for the child's development. Second is Kohlberg's theory of moral development, which affirms the concept of invariant stage sequences in development, a prominent theoretical theme in this and past centuries.

The past two issues of the Annual Progress reprinted several specific studies which challenged the view that the initial postpartum mother-infant interaction could have the profound developmental influence asserted in the concept of infant "bonding." In this section, the papers by Chess and Thomas and by Herbert and the Sluckins provide systematic overviews of the infant bonding literature, and agree in their judgments that the concept rests on insufficient contradictory data, that it has undesirable theoretical and practical implications, and that it should be abandoned. Chess and Thomas also extend their critical review to a consideration of the relaxed formulation of infant attachment.

As to Kohlberg's theory of invariant stages of moral development, Dien's paper points up its limitations when applied to Chinese culture, and Gilligan offers impressive data as to the fallacies which derive from Kohlberg's ignoring of different moral developmental pathways of boys versus girls. These papers emphasize anew the lesson that generalizations are dangerous if based on data from white middle-class males from highly industrialized Western cultural backgrounds.

The papers in this section highlight the truth that the growth of any science rests on the critical examination and reevaluation of established ideas. But this does not justify the eagerness of some to take potshots at respected theories which rest on substantial bodies of research data, potshots which all too often pick away at presumed methodological weaknesses in the name of "hard science," while ignoring the substantive issues which are central to the body of work under attack.

PART I: DEVELOPMENTAL THEORY

1

The Emergence of Self

Jerome Kagan

Harvard University

INTRODUCTION

The products of every scholarly mission gain clarity if viewed against two reference sources—the dominant ideology of the period and the idiosyncratic intellectual history of the investigator. This evening's talk on the emergence of self-awareness is no exception to that generalization. Since the end of World War I most observers of human development, especially those in England and the United States, have awarded major formative power to material social experience and have been loyal to the principles of gradual and connected growth. The young child's first word, first cry at maternal departure, and first sign of self-consciousness were assumed to be the visible result of a long and cumulative history of underground constructions built in small units from the many social interactions with family members. This was not the view of nineteenth century scholars like Preyer or Stern, who believed that the early appearing human qualities were more autochthonous and inevitable as long as the child met the minimal conditions of living in a world of objects and people. The data to be presented seem to be in closer accord with these century-old views than with beliefs held by contemporary theorists.

The phenomena to be discussed should also be viewed as a continuation of a strategy I began to adopt about half a dozen years ago. In

Reprinted with permission from the *Journal of Child Psychology and Psychiatry*, 1982, Vol. 23, No. 4, 363–381. Copyright 1982 by the Association for Child Psychology and Psychiatry. Psychology and Psychiatry.

Presented as the 9th Emanuel Miller Lecture to the Association for Child Psychology and Psychiatry, London, 6 January 1982.

earlier work my colleagues and I assumed the reality and theoretical utility of abstract constructs like passivity, sociability, hostility, achievement, reflectivity, and identification, and made our observations accommodate to those ideas (Kagan and Moss, 1962; Kagan, 1971). Although these concepts seemed useful in integrating both naturalistic and experimental observations with older children, they were less appropriate to the behavioral repertoire of the infant. Gradually, almost unconsciously, I began to shift my empirical strategy and accommodate to the typical surface behaviors of the young child. During the first year, infants look, smile, and babble to stimuli, play with objects, and show imitation or distress at the unexpected and the unfamiliar. I noted the developmental course of these behaviors to varied incentives and, after discovering regularities, invented constructs like inhibition and enhanced retrieval capacity, consciously resisting the use of constructs that implied a theoretical similarity to the behaviors of older children or adults (Kagan et al., 1978).

It seemed reasonable to extend this Baconian attitude to the second year of life. I began these studies without an overarching theoretical conception of the major milestones between 12 and 24 months of age. Piagetian theory is not a particularly useful guide to this era, and systematic research on this period is still sparse. But no investigator begins his work without prejudice. The selection of variables is the first demand of science, and selection always implies a priori ideas. The tasks we chose and the behaviors we selected for quantification were influenced by a central supposition about early development: namely, the emergence of cognitive competences resulting from the maturation of the central nervous system in children living with people and objects is essential to understanding the changing profile of behavior during the early years.

The history of developmental psychology contains a guide for the choice of procedures. The study of behaviors that dominate the repertoire during a particular phase of development often leads to inferences about processes that are occasionally concealed when the reactions to experimental procedures are assessed, especially if the situations require responses less natural to that stage.

Young children are uncertain in most experimental situations, and this state is often a major cause of their reactions. Thus we devoted a great deal of time to observing behaviors that are prominent during the second year in the familiar home setting with the mother present. These included symbolic play with toys, imitation, speech, and reciprocal social interaction. The explicit assumption was that these are universal behaviors whose time of appearance reflects the rate of maturation of more basic psychological functions, as the age of appearance of pubic and axillary hair indexes the times when important changes are occurring in the hypothalamus, pituitary, and gonads. Indeed, the changes of puberty provide a useful model for our work. As reproductive fertility is established, there are surface changes in the distribution of hair, size of the genitals, pitch of voice in males, and breast size in females. It is not obvious that these diverse phenomena have their origin in an endocrine mechanism that is triggered by an alteration in hypothalamic sensitivity to circulating sex hormone.

METHOD

We evaluated five classes of behavior that emerged during the second year: intelligible speech, concern with parental prohibitions and violations of parental standards, avoidance of tasks that are difficult to implement, patterns of social interaction with adults and children, and, finally, symbolic play.

The research passed through three stages. During the first, we followed two cohorts of children for about 10 months. The younger cohort of 14 children was observed twice a month every month from 13 to 22 months of age. The older cohort of 16 children was observed on the same schedule from 20 to 29 months and again at 30, 32, and 34 months. All the children were Caucasian, from middle-class families, and all the observations took place in our laboratory. The investigation revealed two facts of importance. First, there was a major change in cognitive performance around the second birthday. Second, and of more significance, obvious distress appeared in the months before the second birthday when the child saw an examiner model some acts in front of the attentive youngster. The need to understand this phenomenon more deeply led to the second phase of the project, which involved more study of two cross-sectional samples of children in order to eliminate alternative interpretations of the anxiety we noted. Reflection on these results suggested a need for a richer corpus and led to the final set of studies. One was a detailed examination of the growth of six children who were observed in their homes longitudinally every three weeks for close to 10 months. A second was a comparable investigation of 67 Fijian children growing up on isolated atolls in the Pacific (Katz, 1981). A third was a longitudinal study of seven Vietnamese children who, with their parents, had recently arrived in California (Gellermen, 1981). I shall now summarize the phenomena that were seen in these children during the last half of the second year.

RESULTS

The Appearance of Standards

Around 17 to 20 months of age, children display an obvious concern with a special class of events and actions whose attributes deviate from what adults regard as normative. Children now point with trepidation to small holes in clothing, tiny spots on furniture, dolls with chipped paint, missing bristles on a broom, or an almost invisible crack in a plastic toy and utter, with dysphoric tone, phrases like "Oh-oh." Hundreds of events, many of them subtle and instrumentally irrelevant, capture the child's attention and, on occasion, elicit a special facial reaction and verbal comment. Some one-word utterances have the qualities of a conceptual category. One of the 22-month-old children consistently called a "boo-boo" any place where an upholstered button was missing on a chair or sofa, a bowel movement, dirt on the floor, and a broken toy telephone. These events share no common physical quality. What they do share is that each is a variation on a normative experience which presumably has been associated with a communication from parents indicating that the event is disapproved.

In one of the cross-sectional studies, 14- and 19-month-old children were allowed to play for 20 minutes with a set of 22 toys. Ten toys were unflawed, without irregularities or tears—e.g. a fire engine, a car. Another set of 10 toys was purposefully flawed in some way. Examples included a boat with holes in the bottom, a doll with black streaks on the face, a broken telephone. Additionally, two of the toys were odd-shaped, meaningless wooden pieces that were unflawed. We inserted these two toys to test whether special concern with the flawed objects was due to the fact that their integrity was violated rather than to the fact that they were discrepant. No 14-month-old child behaved in any special way towards the flawed toys, while 57% of the older children showed unambiguous signs of concern with one or more of these objects. They would point to one of the flawed toys and vocalize, bring the toys to their mother, or say explicitly that something about the toy was unusual—"Fix it," "Broke," or "Yukky." No child behaved this way towards the meaningless forms.

Almost 50 years ago Charlotte Bühler (1935) also noted a sensitivity to parental standards during the second year. In her experiments one- to two-year-old children were forbidden to touch a toy by an adult. But when the adult left the room briefly, many touched the toy. When the adult returned, all of the 18-month-olds showed behavior that Bühler regarded as embarrassment or a frightened expression.

The language protocols from the six children we saw at home revealed that between 19 and 26 months the speech of every child contained reference to standards (*broken, boo-boo, dirty, wash hands, can't, hard do*). Similar data gathered by others (the sources are both English and German and include a 1928 diary by Stern and Stern) indicate that by 20 months most children are using words that refer to standards. The remarkable agreement in the time when children first use evaluative language implies the maturation of a new cognitive function (Bretherton et al., 1981). It is unlikely that all children decide by 24 months that a dirty blouse is a violation of a norm: they must first be exposed to some information which leads them to classify certain actions and associated outcomes in a special way. The most likely possibility is that certain events have provoked adult reactions which generated in the child a state of uncertainty. These reactions can be as subtle as an unexpected change in the timbre of the parent's voice or shape of her eyes, or as salient as a verbal reproof or spanking. The associations among the event (the norm violation), the unexpected parental reaction, and the subsequent state of uncertainty lead the child to award salience to the violation. Interviews with the Fijian parents revealed that the three most frequent behavioral categories regarded as "wrong" (*cakava cala*) were the destruction of property, acts potentially dangerous to the child's physical welfare, and aggression.

Because 18-month-olds can generate prototypic representations of events, detect deviations from those prototypes, and react to the detection, there is reason to believe that they are able to generate the idea of a proper or improper event, which they will eventually come to call "good" and "bad." One two-year-old became visibly upset because she held a small doll but a large toy bed and could not find a small toy bed, which she indicated was more appropriate for the doll. She had a representation of the proper object. What is required for the actualization of an evaluative frame are certain cognitive talents attained during the second year and experiences that permit children to associate some events with signs of adult displeasure.

I suggest that one critical function that emerges by the middle of the second year is the tendency to make inferences regarding the causes of an event. The child now expects events to have antecedents and automatically generates cognitive hypotheses as to their cause. Thus, when the child sees a crack in a toy he infers the flaw was caused by someone's action. Because that action is associated with displeasure, the child responds emotionally. The data from a linguistic inference task indicate that by the middle of the second year most children also are able to infer that events have names, and hence an unfamiliar word must name an unfamiliar object. The examiner first presents the child with a trio of known objects (a toy cat, car, and cup). After allowing the child to play with the toys for a bit, the examiner asks the child to hand her each of the objects on three separate questions. If the child is correct, the examiner then proceeds to the critical test trial. The examiner places two nameable objects (a doll and a dog) and one unfamiliar object that has no name (a wooden or styrofoam form) in front of the child. The examiner then says, "Give me the zoob." By 18 months the majority of children gave the unfamiliar object to the examiner. It is of interest that children learning sign language rather than oral speech first combine two signs in the middle of the second year. I suggest that the ability to combine two ideas is the essence of the inferential talent.

A second competence that matures in the second year is the ability to appreciate the psychological state of another. This competence permits empathy—what Hume called sympathy—and facilitates in a major way the control of aggression and excessive dominance toward another child, even without punishment for those acts. There is persuasive evidence for the two-year-old's ability to appreciate the perceptual and feeling states of another person. Novey (1975) visited children 18 and 27 months of age at home and invited them to play with either a pair of ski goggles that permitted vision or a pair that was opaque and gave a sense of blindness. A day later each child came to a laboratory setting and, after a period of play, watched the mother put on the opaque goggles. The 27-month-olds who had had previous experience with the opaque goggles behaved as if they had inferred that their mothers could not see. They tried to remove the goggles, asked the mother to remove them, and made fewer gestures toward her, in comparison with the children who had been exposed at home to the transparent goggles.

Longitudinal observations provided by mothers specially trained to record their children's reactions to the distress of others revealed a major change in behavior during the latter half of the second year. The two-year-old children behaved as if they were inferring the state of the victim, and accordingly, they issued appropriate responses. They hugged or kissed their victim, gave him a toy or food, and requested aid from an adult. Those behaviors were absent or infrequent to the same incentives during the early months of the second year (Cummings et al., 1981).

The combination of the ability to infer cause and to empathize with the states of another, combined with a preparedness to associate signs of disapproval with certain actions, permits the child to move into an evaluative frame. I view this preparedness as analogous to the suggestion that rats are prepared to associate gustatory stimuli with unpleasant visceral states, while birds are prepared to associate visual stimuli with the same internal states. This supposition is affirmed by interviews with the Fijian mothers who commented that children naturally become more responsible after their second birthday when they have acquired *vakayalo* (sense). As a result of this new competence, parents hold children more responsible for their actions. The recognition by the Fijians of a sudden appreciation of right and wrong is in accord with the belief of nineteenth century observers that young children are innately moral.

James Sully (1896) suggested that the child has an "inbred respect for what is customary and wears the appearance of a rule of life" and an "innate disposition to follow precedent and rule, which precedes education" (pp. 280-281). For "there is in the child from the first a rudiment of the true law abidingness . . . the day when the child first becomes capable of this putting himself into his mother's place and realizing, if only for an instant, the trouble he has brought on her, is an all-important one in his moral development" (pp. 289-290). Sully believed all children must, because they are human, realize that causing harm to another is immoral. Such knowledge can never be lost, regardless of any subsequent cruelty the child might experience. The child does not have to learn that hurting others is bad; it is an insight that accompanies growth.

In a popular text written at the turn of the century, two Americans, Tracy and Stimpfl (1909), asserted that the child is born with a disposition to be moral: "Moral ideas do not require to be created or implanted in the minds of children by their elders. Nothing is more certain than that the child is born potentially a moral being, possessing a moral nature which requires only to be evoked and developed by environmental conditions. . . . An empirical account of the derivation of the moral nature out of conditions in which no germs of it are to be found, fails utterly when tested by observed facts or by logical criticisms" (p. 179). After 1915, this theoretical view vanished from American texts in the wave of enthusiasm for social learning.

Because the concern with standards seems to be an inevitable event in the second year and one that appears long before linguistic or reproductive maturity, we might ask about the evolutionary advantage of this competence. Humans have the capacity for enduring resentment toward persons and a desire for personal property, together with the ability both to plan and to plot in order to attain these goals. Hence, it may have been necessary in human evolution to make sure that inhibitory functions would emerge early in development to curb these disruptive dispositions. An appreciation of proper and improper behavior facilitates the inhibition of aggression towards siblings, especially towards young infants. The importance of this inhibition is reflected in a rare event which occurred last November in Boston when a two-year-old boy killed his six-month-old younger sibling by stabbing him repeatedly with a kitchen knife. We are horrified by this event, in part because it is a freak phenomenon. But since all two-year-olds have the ability and occasional motivation to commit this action, why is it not more frequent? I suggest that one reason is that most children around the world have begun to establish standards on aggression by the second birthday.

Anxiety Over Potential Failure

Perhaps the most significant observation we made was the appearance of obvious signs of anxiety after the examiner modeled some acts in front of the child. After the child had played for about 15 minutes—in the laboratory or at home—the examiner and the mother joined the child on the floor and the examiner modeled three different acts with appropriate verbalizations while the child was watching. The acts became more complex as the child matured. For the children 22 months of age, the model made a doll talk on a telephone, made a doll cook some food in a pan and then had two dolls eat dinner, and made three animals take a walk and hide under a cloth in order to avoid getting wet. After she modeled the three acts, she simply said "Now it's your turn to play." She did not ask the child to imitate her actions. The child was then allowed to play for an additional 10 minutes. Distress was defined as the occurrence of any one of the following behaviors during the minute after the model completed her actions: fretting, crying, clinging to the mother, absence of any play with the toys during the entire minute, and protestations indicating the child did not want to play or wanted to go home. The most frequent reactions of distress were non-verbal and included clinging to the mother, inhibition of play, and crying. As shown in Fig. 1, the behavioral signs of distress appeared first around 15 months, grew with age, and reached a peak around the second birthday in all the samples. This display of distress is specific to this incentive and is independent of fearfulness to novelty. The Fijian one-year-olds, who had never seen a doll, showed extreme upset when the examiner showed them a doll. But fear of this stimulus waned during the second year, while signs of fear of the model increased in frequency, and at no age

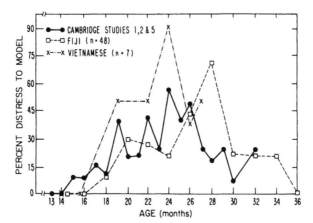

FIG. 1. Proportion of children showing distress to the model.

was there a correlation between fearful behavior toward the doll and distress following the model's behavior (Katz, 1981).

In order to eliminate alternative interpretations of this distress, we surmised that perhaps the child did not expect the adult to interrupt her play and, therefore, was upset by the unexpected interruption. But when we repeated the experiment with two other groups of children for whom the model scattered the toys and did not model behavior, no anxiety occurred. Thus the signs of anxiety seemed to be occasioned by the modeling of the actions. Additionally, if the model leaves the room right after acting, signs of distress are much less frequent (Jackowitz and Watson, 1980).

I believe this phenomenon reflects the emergence of at least two processes. First, the child experiences an obligation to implement the acts of the model, and second, has some awareness of her inability to do so, either because she forgot what the model did or because she recognizes she is unable to implement the acts. As a result, the child becomes uncertain and begins to cry or stop playing. If the child has no uncertainty over meeting the standard and believes she can be successful, she makes the attempt—a state nicely illustrative of Plato's axiom, "To know the good is to do the good."

The possibility of complete memory failure can be eliminated for, in many cases, seven or eight minutes after the distress, when the child had left the mother's side and begun to play again, she would display an exact or fragmented version of one of the model's prior actions and smile. There may have been a temporary forgetting of the model's behavior, but it was not permanent.

Because slightly fewer children showed distress when the mother rather than the less familiar examiner was the model, the familiarity of the social relationship between child and adult monitors the likelihood of uncertainty. Because the child had a less familiar relationship with the model, it is possible that she felt a stronger press to display the acts modeled by the examiner. Uncertainty in the social relationship could motivate the child to be concerned with the model's possible reactions toward her. If the child felt no obligation to imitate the model, she would not pass to the second stage of uncertainty over her inability to duplicate the acts she saw. These data reveal the exquisitely sensitive dependence of this behavior on subtle dimensions in the social relationship.

The suggestion that an inference of obligation is amplified during these months is supported by an investigation in which 16- and 23-month-old children watched a model display the same act, either with a toy as prop or without any prop at all. After the modeling the woman left the room, leaving the child with the toys and the mother. When the model had used toys, over 90% of both age groups imitated her. But when no prop was used, no 16-month-old implemented the act, while about 40% of the older children produced the imitation. The act modeled was clearly in the repertoire of the younger children, for they did act appropriately with the toy. But I suggest that with the adult model absent, the younger children did not experience an obligation to imitate what they had seen (Jackowitz and Watson, 1980).

Smiles of Mastery

A third phenomenon of this era is the occurrence of a smile after the child has attained a goal through effort—when she completes a tower, puts a final piece in a puzzle, or fits a dress on a doll. These are not social smiles, but private ones. The protocol for the seven Vietnamese children included the presentation of a puzzle and an invitation to the child to build a block tower on each visit to the home. Smiling upon mastery was rare at 17 months, increased after 19 months, and peaked at 25 months of age, when six of the seven children smiled privately upon completing one or both tasks. These private smiles that accompany mastery can be interpreted as signifying that the child had generated a goal for an external action sequence, persisted in attempts to gain that goal, and smiled upon attainment. The response is released when the child perceives that she has attained the cognitive representation of a previously generated goal following investment of effort. This assumption awards the child not only a disposition to generate goals, but the ability to know when that goal has been reached.

It seems useful, therefore, to posit one class of standards, called "normative," which contains representations of actions and events that have been linked with adult approval and disapproval. The familiar list of aggression, destruction, and cleanliness is prototypic. The second class, called "mastery standards," contains representations of goals to be attained through actions that have not necessarily been associated with adult displeasure or praise. I recognize that I am reinventing the distinction between the two components of the Freudian superego: the violations of a community's values and the representations that define the ego-ideal. I did not have that distinction in mind as I observed the children's behaviors; the data invited it.

There is a relation between the two classes of standards. Recognition of standards on aggression leads to inhibition of these behaviors. But recognition that one's behavior might not meet a private standard of mastery can lead to a reluctance to attempt problem solution or to deal with challenges that might be within the child's sphere of mastery. Hence timidity to challenge might be the price we pay for the socialization of disruptive acts. Some evolutionary biologists might argue about the relative advantages of withdrawal in a mastery situation compared with voluntary checks on aggression. But both properties may be packaged as a unit; the child cannot have one without the other.

Directives to Adults

A fourth phenomenon of this era is the emergence of behaviors that reflect the desire to influence the behavior of adults through requests or directives. The most frequent instances of this category include attempts to change the behavior of an adult or requests for help with a problem. Common examples include putting a toy telephone to the mother's ear and gesturing or vocalizing in a way to indicate that the child wants the mother to talk on the telephone, pointing to a place in the room where the child wants the mother to move, or giving the mother a doll and toy bottle and indicating, through gesture, that she wants the mother to feed the doll. The growth function for this behavior for the longitudinal sample of six American children studied at home is almost identical to the growth function for the seven Vietnamese children who displayed peak occurrence of this behavior at 21 months.

I suggest the child would not have begun to direct the behavior of an adult if she did not have an expectation that the request would be met. The enhancement of this class of response can be viewed as evidence that the child expects he can influence the behavior of others. It is true that eight-month-olds also point to desired objects and may whine, as if they are communicating that they want an object. But I believe that at this earlier age infants have no conscious conception that the cry or gesture will change the behavior of the adult. The response simply follows their seeing the desired object or their frustration at not having it. The pointing of the eight-month-old may resemble superficially the request for help with a puzzle seen in a 20-month-old. But the two responses are profoundly different with respect to the underlying cognitive competences. The monkey, the four-month-old baby, and the two-year-old can be operantly conditioned to make a motor response when it is followed by a reinforcement consisting of a change in visual stimulation. But this similarity does not mean that the accompanying cognitive processes are necessarily the same in all three organisms.

Self-descriptive Utterances

The speech of the six American children studied at home provided additional evidence for the growth of a function related to self-awareness. All of the utterances and associated contexts during the play session were recorded by one of the observers. Over 90% of the utterances were spontaneous remarks. As others have reported, when speech first emerges, the vast majority of one-word utterances name objects in the child's visual field. The next most frequent class of utterance during the first stage of speech is to communicate a desire for an object or event, or to point to an object and say its name with a tone of voice that signifies a frustrated need. I am concerned here with a type of utterance we called self-descriptive utterances. These were defined narrowly as utterances that occurred while the child was engaged in an action and referred to that action (*climb*, as the child was climbing up on a chair; *up*, as the child tried to get up on a box), and utterances containing the words *I*, *my*, *mine*, or the child's name with a predicate (my book, I sit, Mary eat). Once the child began to speak two- and three-word utterances, there was little difficulty in deciding whether a phrase was self-descriptive. The average reliability for coding this variable was 0.95. Self-descriptive utterances were absent at 17, 18, and 19 months, increased dramatically around the second birthday, and were sophisticated by 27 months, including phrases like "I do it myself," or "I can't do it." All the children showed similar growth functions for this class of utterance, with a major increase between 19 and 24 months. Lois Bloom and her colleagues (Bloom et al., 1975) have collected a similar set of protocols from four children over the course of repeated visits to their homes. When I coded her data for self-descriptive utterances, the proportion was remarkably similar to that found for our children: namely, about 35%. It is important to note that the proportion of self-descriptive utterances was relatively independent of the child's mean length of utterance. I believe that when the child becomes aware of his ability to gain goals through his actions, he feels pressed to comment upon his behavior. The child's actions have suddenly become a salient incentive for linguistic description, or at least more salient than the activities or qualities of other people. The child does not begin to talk about himself because he is able to utter predicates, but rather because the child is suddenly aware of a fresh experience. He is aware of what he is doing.

The Replacement of Self in Symbolic Play

Finally, there is a significant qualitative change in the child's symbolic play with toys during the months before the second birthday. During these months the child substitutes a toy for the self in pretend sequences. The child now puts a telephone to a doll's head rather than her own, a bottle to a toy animal's mouth rather than her own mouth. This transformation implies that the child is playing the role of director and distancing self from the simple sensory–motor play that is seen near the first birthday.

The studies implemented by Lewis and Brooks-Gunn (1979) are most relevant to this work. They administered a variety of procedures to children between 9 and 24 months of age in order to determine the time when those children showed signs of self-recognition. They concluded, "Between 18 and 21 months of age a large increase in the number of infants demonstrating self-recognition abilities is seen across a wide range of representative modes. . . . Clearly, self-recognition is well-established by 21 months of age" (p. 215). Their most dramatic evidence involves a procedure originally reported by Amsterdam (1972) in which infants are first allowed to look at themselves in a mirror. Their noses are then unobtrusively marked with a spot of rouge, and they are brought back to the mirror to observe their reflection. The behavior of interest is whether the child reaches for the place where the rouge has been put. Although no nine- or 12-month-olds touched their noses, this behavior increased dramatically from 15 to 24 months of age, and over 60% of the 21- and 24-month-olds touched their noses. It cannot be a coincidence that this is the time when distress to the model, directives to adults, and mastery smiles also show a sharp increase in frequency.

The appreciation of standards on proper behavior and awareness of one's competences to meet these standards imply that children should now show a major improvement in performance on tasks presented by adults. The data affirm that prediction.

Memory for Locations

The children in most of the studies showed a major improvement between 17 and 23 months in performance on a memory for locations task. The child was seated on the mother's lap, facing the experimenter and a stage. The child watched the examiner hide a prize (a raisin or a cheerio) under one of many receptacles. The receptacles were screened by an opaque screen for delays of one, five, or ten seconds. The screen was lifted and the examiner asked the child to find the prize. The child was first tested under one-second delays, using two, four, six, or eight receptacles of different colors, shapes, and sizes. After solving this problem the examiner proceeded to four, six, and eight containers, with the hardest problem being eight receptacles at a ten-second delay. Figure 2 shows the growth function for this performance. Children showed a major improvement in the months before the second birthday, the same time when other indexes of self-awareness and of standards were growing. By two years of age, almost all the children in all the samples solved the problem of eight different receptacles with a ten-second delay. Even though the task requirements and materials were probably less familiar to the Fijians than to the Americans, the Fijian children showed enhanced performance at the same time. I view this improvement as reflecting an enhancement in the motivation to meet a standard of competence, rather than a fundamental change in memory capacity.

This suggestion is supported by the fact that many three-year-old American children, especially those being reared in families encouraging

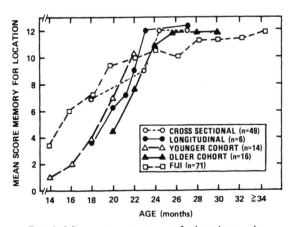

FIG. 2. Mean score on memory for locations task.

autonomy, perform less well than two-year-olds. I believe this is because the increasing enhancement of self that occurs during the third year provokes the older child to resist accommodation—or conformity—to all adult requests. After the third birthday the child is made uncertain by contemplation of violation of adult standards. He will occasionally violate them in order to resolve and control the disquiet. Because modern Western parents do not want a fearful or timid 10-year-old, they tolerate these violations, which we have come to call the disobedience of the "terrible twos."

Drawing a Face

In another procedure the child first watched the examiner draw a schematic face consisting of a circle containing two dots for eyes, a vertical line for the nose, and curved line for the mouth. The child was then given a crayon and paper and asked to draw the face, while the examiner's drawing remained in view. The child's first attempt to copy the face was a scribbling of lines. In the next stage the child approximated a crude circle, but without any internal elements. In the final stage the child included some elements in the circles. The tendency to place elements in the circle grew around the second birthday. The drawing of a circle is probably determined both by the child's familiarity with materials and improved motor coordination, but the ability to place a few marks inside a circle cannot be due to enhanced motor coordination, for no unusual skill is required to scratch a few lines inside the circular frame. I suggest that the placing of marks inside the circle, like memory for locations, indicates that the children were reflecting more seriously on the standard posed by the examiner and had an expectation of meeting that standard. Hence they made the attempt.

DISCUSSION

I should now like to impose some interpretive frames on the evidence and use these data to address some broader philosophical issues. The evidence suggests that the central psychological victories of the last half of the second year include the appreciation of standards on proper behavior and the emergence of awareness of one's actions, intentions, states, and competences. I choose the phrase *self-awareness* to name the second set of related psychological functions, but not as an explanatory construct. Many readers may prefer a different name. My use of the term *self-awareness* is motivated by the behaviors quantified during the last half of the second year: namely, mastery smiles, directives to adults, distress to the model, and self-descriptive utterances. I do not declare that the eight-month-old is not aware that she is hungry. This statement should not be taken as announcing a sudden timidity over my conclusions. Quite the contrary. The use of the construct *intelligence* to summarize a set of responses to the Wechsler Intelligence Scale for Children does not have the same meaning as the intelligence that describes a six-year-old's correct solutions to a series of conservation problems. Similarly, the use of *anxiety* to explain or describe the increase in frequency of distress to unexpected events across the period from 7 to 15 months of age is not the same anxiety inferred from the increase in phobias among four-year-olds. In commenting on the Heisenberg uncertainty principle, Bridgman (1958) noted "It is well recognized that there is no sharp dividing line between the instrument of knowledge and the object of knowledge, and that for different purposes the line may be drawn at different places" (p. 62). If the psychologist's procedures are substituted for "instruments of knowledge," then what may appear as timidity becomes a principle of understanding.

Words used as constructs have meaning only with reference to a specific set of data. For example, Weiskrantz (1977) has shown that the truth value of statements describing the cross-modality matching ability of monkeys (haptic to visual) depends on the procedures used by the investigator. The monkeys fail on some procedures; they succeed on others.

This is not an idle issue in the social sciences. There is far greater consensus among physicists and chemists than among psychologists over the methods appropriate to particular descriptions or theoretical statements. When a chemist writes about the acidity or temperature of a solution, his colleagues know and agree on the selection of the evidential source of that statement and appreciate the relation between the observation and the construct. For controversial classifications like "particle," the physicist is careful to tell his colleagues whether his observations came from a Wilson cloud chamber or a linear accelerator, for the meaning of *particle* is not identical in these two procedures.

Psychologists, however, work with far less agreement than physical scientists and, unfortunately, with less concern over the degree of consensus regarding the relation of a classification construct to its source. Psychologists argue, for example, about the effect of surrogate care on the infant's attachment to its caretaker. One reason for the controversy is an indifference to the fact that some investigators use behavior generated in the Ainsworth Strange Situation as the measure of attachment;

others use clinging to the mother in the home; and still others use separation anxiety. Since these procedures do not produce theoretically equivalent behavior, statements about an infant's attachment do not have the same meaning. Similar criticisms hold for conclusions about memory, imitation, motivation, affect, and a host of other psychological terms.

Other observers have used different names for the psychological changes that characterize this era of growth. Tiedemann (1787) remarked that the child develops *Eigenliebe* (love of self) during the same period; Preyer (1888) suggested that *Ichheit* (selfhood) emerges during the second year. But the Utku of Hudson Bay believe the child develops *ihuma* (reason), and the Fijians say the child has now acquired *vakayalo* (sense).

Important premises are hidden in each of these phrases. Although Tiedemann and Preyer assumed that the behavioral changes indexed a new appreciation of individuality, the Utku and the Fijians, like most non-Western societies, emphasized the child's ability to appreciate the difference between right and wrong (Briggs, 1970). It is understandable, after the fact, that urban Europeans would wonder about the origins of the narcissistic, autonomous, and actualizing ego, while small, isolated, hunting or agricultural communities would be more concerned with the child's adherence to social norms. The name chosen for a complex phenomenon has significant connotations for empirical work. If the complex event that geneticists call "mutation" had been named "replacement," different experiments might have been performed. Self and self-awareness are very popular ideas in the West: hence the contemporary scholar's mind leaps to these words quickly. If these same data had been discovered by a seventeenth-century Chinese observer, he would doubtless have used a different term.

Changes in the quality of the child's play during the second year suggest a slightly different and more speculative way of describing the victories of this era. One of the most striking changes is the increased duration of a play epoch. Brenner and Mueller (unpublished manuscript) have reported a major increase in the duration of social interaction sequences among boys observed longitudinally during the second year. I believe that a central change of this interval is the ability to sustain ideas and action plans. The psychological stage on which schemata interact and guide action does not collapse every half-minute or so. As a result, the child does not forget the goals he is pursuing, asks his mother for help if he is unsuccessful, and smiles upon attaining a self-generated goal. Perhaps what I have been calling *self-awareness* is better categorized as the "capacity to hold cognitive representations on the stage of active memory." Maturing central nervous system structures and functions permit schemata to remain in consciousness for a longer period of time. This argument is appealing, because available knowledge about the relation between brain function and psychological phenomena implies that damage to specific frontal and temporal areas of the brain is often accompanied by a loss of ability to retrieve past memories or to hold ideas on the stage that is called "active memory." Retrieval, maintenance, and operation upon information seem to be yoked to central nervous system functioning in a fundamental way.

The suggestion that the enhancement of the behaviors we have considered is a direct consequence of brain growth finds persuasive support in data on histological changes in the young cerebral cortex. The length and degree of branching of dendrites in the human cerebral cortex do not approach adult magnitudes until two years of age. And Rabinowicz (1979) has concluded that neuronal density (the number of neurons per unit volume) decreases very rapidly until birth: "From birth to between three and six months the decrease is slower and it ceases at about 15 months . . . one has to deduce that a very important moment in cortical maturation appears to be the period between 15 and 24 months, a period when almost all the layers reach, for the first time, a similar state of maturation" (p. 122).

I do not think it a coincidence that this period corresponds to the interval when the child displays the behaviors that are regarded as indicative of self-awareness. If the changes I have described are inevitable, psychological consequences of maturational events in the central nervous system, as long as the child lives in a world of objects and people, both current and traditional descriptions of the emergence of a sense of self may be misleading. Theorists in the psychoanalytic tradition, like Margaret Mahler (1968), have assumed that initially self was merged with another person and the infant gradually differentiated itself from the parent. But perhaps there is no self prior to the second year, as there is no frog in the tadpole and no morphemes hidden in the babbling of a three-month-old.

The most popular view, supported by theorists with diverse agendas, insists that a sense of self develops gradually, as a direct consequence of action. Preyer (1888) was reluctant to attribute the "I"-function only to endogenous changes in the central nervous system and, in agreement with the associational beliefs of his period, declared that it was through the child's actions and sense experiences that the "I"-feeling emerged.

Guillaume (1971) suggested that the first phase of self was dependent upon imitation of others. The pragmatist George Herbert Mead (1934) made social interaction a mandatory requirement for the first stage of self, and wrote that the self "arises in the process of social experience and activity. . . . It is impossible to conceive of a self arising outside of social experience" (pp. 135, 140).

Charles Cooley (1902) was closer to nineteenth-century suppositions in awarding more influence to the perceptual and affective components of the self than to the action sector. Nonetheless, he too insisted that acts informing the young child of her effectiveness are prerequisites for the feeling of self, which "appears to be associated chiefly with ideas of the exercise of power and of being a cause" (p. 177). Piaget (1976) wrote on the relevance of interaction: "The subject only learns to know himself when acting on the object and the latter can become known only as the result of progress of the actions carried out on it" (p. 353).

Lewis and Brooks-Gunn (1979) also argued that the child's awareness of self "has as its source the interaction of the young organism with others—both people and objects . . . it is from action that knowledge develops" (p. 241), in a connected, stage-like sequence. Although these psychologists did not explicitly deny that the maturation of a new competence lies at the root of self-recognition, they awarded to accumulated interactions with objects and people the major bases for the appearance of self-awareness and self-recognition.

The British psychologist Crook (1980) is unusual among modern theorists in his emphasis on cognitive maturation as an element in the emergence of consciousness: "The child's emerging sense of self is dependent upon the growth of its cognitive abilities in categorization, its experiences of contingency and agency in interaction with care-givers, and its experience of the emotional quality of its own conscious states" (p. 254).

I, too, believe that a child isolated from all people and objects will not develop self-awareness. But I am less certain that these processes and their attendant structures are necessarily created out of specific forms of feedback from imitation of others, play with parents, and the directing of adults. It is possible that the American children in Cambridge, the Fijians, and the Vietnamese refugees all displayed signs of apprehension to the modeling of acts during the last half of the second year because their patterns of social experience were similar. However, the remarkable temporal concordance for the appearance of distress to the model, across all samples, exceeded that for the onset of speech, which most scientists acknowledge depends in part on the maturation of new capacities. Perhaps no special class of social interaction is necessary for these competences to develop. Perhaps all that is required for the capacities called "self-awareness" to appear is any information resulting from the child's actions and feelings. The neurons of the visual cortex require patterned stimulation in order to mature and permit the psychological competence of discrimination. But almost any form of patterned stimulation will do. Similarly, certain species of birds living in isolated cages will sing their characteristic song at maturity if they only hear a tape-recorded version of it at the proper time; interaction with other birds is irrelevant.

Rhesus monkeys raised only with an inanimate object and isolated from all contingent interaction with any living creature showed maximal signs of fear when put in a novel environment at four months. This is the same age as monkeys who had been raised with dogs, even though the magnitude of the reaction was muted in the completely isolated monkeys. It appears that the fear reaction—as evidenced by higher heart rate and distress calls—was an inevitable consequence of the maturation of the central nervous system in these isolated animals (Mason, 1978).

Similarly, it is of interest that one species of Macaque—called crab eaters—displayed normal patterns of social behavior despite the fact that they spent the first six months of life in complete isolation. The investigators wrote ". . . extended social experience is not necessary for the development of species' typical social behavior in crab eating Macaques. . . . Whether early social experience is or is not necessary seems to depend on genotypic differences—a sorry state of affairs for the generality of social development theories based on environmental factors" (Sackett et al., 1981, p. 316).

By contrast, rhesus and pigtail monkeys raised in isolation showed more serious disturbances in social behavior. Obviously, social interaction contains a rich and complex source of information and probably hastens the development of these processes. But it is neither theoretically obvious nor empirically demonstrable that a child who has few material encounters with people will fail to develop the behaviors reflective of self-awareness, albeit at a slower rate. It is useful to take a strong sceptical stand, if only to stimulate relevant research.

The speculation that self-awareness is a consequence of a cumulative and rather lengthy history of material experiences with objects and people probably owes some of its popularity to the fact that most Western scholars have been reluctant to posit discrete endogenous mechanisms, relatively independent of specific external events, which might be responsible for the emergence of new behaviors. During the last decade of the nineteenth century and the first decade of the twentieth, biologists were generally opposed to the idea that spontaneous mutation in genes, rather than the cumulative effects of natural selection, was the major force in evolution. After the geneticists gained power around World

War I, natural selection was given decreased potency. It was not until the 1930s that the modern synthesis of discrete endogenous genetic forces and natural selection became acceptable doctrine.

Similarly, many physiologists during most of this century have resisted the idea that the central nervous system did not require feedback from sense organs in order to generate coherent sequences of rhythmic movement during repetitive behavior, locomotion being the classic example. Most physiologists wanted to have sensory processes control basic movement patterns. But recent experimental evidence has led Delcomyn (1980) to argue persuasively that "Isolation of the nervous system from all possible sources of sensory feedback does not abolish the normal pattern of rhythmic bursts in motoneurons. . . . Timing of the repetitive movements that constitute any rhythmic behavior is regulated by intrinsic properties of the central nervous system rather than by sensory feedback from moving parts of the body" (p. 493).

Both physiologists and psychologists have wanted to believe that external events, potentially quantifiable, are the primary causes of action, because this premise is more in accord with an epistemology of mechanism and a philosophy of logical positivism than with a presupposition that awards potency to invisible entities that seem to have direction and structure from the beginning. The latter view leaves the investigator frustrated in his search for the chain of manipulable causes for the observed event.

Additionally, these data speak to the premise of gradual growth, for there is a deep prejudice against postulating significant entities that can arise with a short history. Western scientists prefer to impose gradualism on all instances of change. Thomas Henry Huxley warned Darwin that his insistence on gradual evolution represented "an unnecessary difficulty" in the theory, and both Gould and Stanley (Eldredge and Gould, 1972; Stanley, 1981) have argued that, on occasion, speciation can be rapid—a phenomenon called "punctuated equilibria." It has been suggested that the appearance of most of the extraordinary variety of mammalian species now present on earth, derived from a small rodent-like animal, occurred in a relatively brief span of about 12 million years—only 20% of the interval from the extinction of the dinosaurs 60 million years ago to the present.

Increasingly sophisticated studies of morphological embryogenesis are verifying Weiss' (1968) suggestion that the differentiation of cells "produces a definite number of discrete, distinct, discontinuous and more or less sharply delimited cell types which are not connected by intergradations" (p. 212). Biologists now describe aspects of organ development in terms that explicitly assume abruptness of change. Newman and

Frisch (1979) suggested that in the early formation of the chick limb there appear to be sudden structural changes in the conditions surrounding developing cartilage cells. If the morphological growth of the embryo provides a useful model for early psychological growth, then a relatively sudden change in central nervous system function may be more important for selected psychological competences like self-awareness than the amount of time the child has spent in a particular class of interaction. New developmental forms can occur without long periods of transition. D'Arcy Wentworth Thompson has noted, "We cannot transform an invertebrate into a vertebrate nor a coelenterate into a worm by any single and legitimate deformation. . . . Nature proceeds from one type to another. . . . To seek for stepping-stones across the gaps between is to seek in vain forever" (in Gould, 1980, p. 193).

I believe that the growth of the functions I have called self-consciousness is composed of the maturation of at least five competences: recognition of the past, retrieval of prior schemata, inference, awareness of one's potentiality for action, and, finally, awareness of self as an entity with symbolic attributes. The degree of connectedness among these five functions is obscure. Although the first four are all presumed by awareness of the self as an entity, it need not emerge from them. That is, awareness of the self as an object with attributes is not an inevitable process: some new processes must be inserted into the developmental sequence if it is to appear. Once again we encounter the ancient enigma in historical sequence. What propositions must we invent to describe how novel properties use and subsume earlier ones, but are not produced by them? The biologist who wishes to explain morphological changes in phylogeny faces the same problem. The convolutions of the cerebral cortex depend on the prior existence of a forebrain. But without the mutations that were a part of evolution, no convolutions would have occurred. Unique endogenous changes are required if the novel structure is to appear. Thus recognition, retrieval, inference, and self-awareness are necessary for awareness of the self as an entity with attributes, but they are not sufficient. The half year that begins with the first smile following completion of a puzzle and ends with the embarrassed statement, "I can't do that," contains one of the most significant sets of competences to appear in our species.

SUMMARY

Longitudinal and cross-sectional investigations of children from three different cultural settings reveal the emergence of behaviors during the last half of the second year that imply the first appreciation of standards on prohibited actions, recognition of the ability to gain goals, and awareness of the self's feeling states. It was suggested that these competences were inevitable consequences of maturational changes in the central nervous system as long as children were growing in a world of objects and people. The foundations for a moral evaluation of aggression and self-consciousness appear to be universal milestones of the second year of life.

Acknowledgements—The research was supported by a grant from the Foundation for Child Development. A more detailed exposition can be found in my book, *The Second Year* (1981). I thank M. Katz and R. Gellerman for permitting me to summarize the results of their doctoral research.

REFERENCES

Amsterdam, B. K. (1972). Mirror self image reactions before age two. *Developmental Psychology*, 5:297-305.

Bloom, L., Lightbown, P. and Hood, L. (1975). Structure and variation in child language. *Monographs of the Society for Research in Child Development*, 40: 1.

Bretherton, I., McNew, S. and Beeghly-Smith, M. (1981). Early person knowledge as expressed in gestural and verbal communications. In *Infant Social Cognition*, M. E. Lamb and L. R. Sherrod, eds., pp. 333-377. Hillsdale, NJ: Erlbaum.

Bridgman, P. W. (1958). Determinism in modern science. In *Determinism and Freedom in the Age of Modern Science*, S. Hook, ed., pp. 43-63. New York: New York University Press.

Briggs, J. L. (1970). *Never in Anger*. Cambridge, MA: Harvard University Press.

Buhler, C. (1975). *The First Year of Life*. New York: Arno (New York: John Day, 1930).

Cooley, C. H. (1902). *Human Nature and the Social Order*. New York: Charles Scribners.

Crook, J. H. (1980). *The Evolution of Human Consciousness*. Oxford: Clarendon Press.

Cummings, E. M., Zahn-Waxler, C. and Radke-Yarrow, M. (1981). Young children's responses to expressions of anger and affection by others in the family. *Child Development*, 52: 1274-1282.

Delcomyn, F. (1980). Neural bases of rhythmic behavior in animals. *Science*, 210:492-498.

Eldredge, N. and Gould, S. J. (1972). Punctuated equilibria. In *Models in Paleobiology*, T. J. N. Schopf, ed., pp. 82–115. San Francisco: Freeman.

Gellerman, R. L. (1981). Psychological Development of the Vietnamese Child in the Second Year of Life. Doctoral dissertation, Harvard University.

Gould, S. J. (1980). *The Panda's Thumb*. New York: W. W. Norton.

Guillaume, P. (1971). *Imitation in Children*. Translated by E. D. Halperin. Chicago: University of Chicago Press (Press Universitaires de France, Paris, 1926).

Jackowitz, E. R. and Watson, M. W. (1980). Development of object transformations in early pretend play. *Developmental Psychology*, 16:543–549.

Kagan, J. (1971). *Change and Continuity in Infancy*. New York: John Wiley.

Kagan, J. (1981). *The Second Year*. Cambridge, MA: Harvard University Press.

Kagan, J. and Moss, H. A. (1962). *Birth to Maturity*. New York: John Wiley.

Kagan, J., Kearsley, R. B. and Zelazo, P. R. (1978). *Infancy: Its Place in Human Development*. Cambridge, MA: Harvard University Press.

Katz, M. M. W. (1981). Gaining Sense at Age Two in the Outer Fiji Islands. Doctoral dissertation, Harvard Graduate School of Education.

Lewis, M. and Brooks-Gunn, J. (1979). *Social Cognition and the Acquisition of Self*. New York: Plenum.

Mahler, M. S. (1968). *Human Symbiosis and the Vicissitudes of Individuation*, Vol. 1. *Infantile Psychosis*. New York: International Universities press.

Mason, W. A. (1978). Social experience in primate cognitive development. In *The Development of Behavior*, G. H Burghardt and M. Bekoff, eds. pp. 233–251. New York: Garland.

Mead, G. H. (1934). *Mind, Self, and Society*. Chicago: University of Chicago Press.

Newman, S. A. and Frisch, H. L. (1979). Dynamics of skeletal pattern formation in developing chick limb. *Science*, 205:662–668.

Novey, M. S. (1975). The Development of Knowledge of Others' Ability to See. Doctoral dissertation, Harvard University.

Piaget, J. (1976). *The Grasp of Consciousness*. Cambridge, MA: Harvard University Press.

Preyer, W. (1888). *The Mind of the Child*, Part 1. *The Senses and the Will*. New York: Appleton.

Rabinowicz, T. (1979). The differentiate maturation of the human cerebral cortex. In *Human Growth*, Vol. 3, F. Faulkner and J. M. Tanner, eds., pp. 97–123. New York: Plenum.

Sackett, G. P., Ruppenthal, G. C., Rahrenbruch, C. E., Holm, R. A. and Greenough, W. T. (1981). Social isolation rearing effects in monkeys vary with genotype. *Developmental Psychology*,. 17: 313–318.

Stanley, S. M. (1981). *The New Evolutionary Timetable*. New York: Basic Books.

Stern, C. and Stern, W. (1928). *Die Kindersprache: Eine Psychologische und Sprachtheoritische Untersuchwag*. 4th Edn. Leipzig: Barth.

Sully, J. (1896). *Studies of Childhood*. New York: Appleton.

Tiedemann, D. (1787). *Beobachtungen uber die Entwicklung der Seelenfahigkeiten*. Altenburg: Oskar Bonde.

Tracy, F. and Stimpfl, J. (1909). *The Psychology of Childhood*. 7th Edn. Boston: D. C. Heath.

Weiskrantz, L. (1977). Trying to bridge some neuropsychological gaps between monkey and man. *British Journal of Psychology*. 68: 431–445.

Weiss, P. A. (1968). *Dynamics of Development*. New York: Academic Press.

2

Attachment and Loss: Retrospect and Prospect

John Bowlby

Honorary Consultant Psychiatrist, Tavistock Clinic, London

An historical sketch of the manner in which evidence has accumulated showing the ill effects of separation, loss, and maternal deprivation during the early years, and of how, in the light of this evidence, a new conceptual framework, often referred to as attachment theory, has been formulated for understanding personality development and psychopathology.

When the American Orthopsychiatric Association honored me by conferring on me the Fourth Blanche F. Ittleson Memorial Award, I gave a brief, informal account of the way my ideas had developed over the years. In doing so I was especially glad to have an opportunity to express the deep gratitude I feel for the generous support given to me and to my research group by a number of American foundations, and to express also my deep indebtedness to the colleagues with whom I have worked and without whose help I could have done very little. In this article the editor has suggested I attempt something different and very much harder, namely, to give an account of what we know today in the field I have been exploring, how we arrived at the knowledge, and the directions that further research might take. Since I am in no position to

Reprinted with permission from the *American Journal of Orthopsychiatry*, 1982, Vol. 52, No. 4, 664–678. Copyright 1982 by the American Orthopsychiatric Association, Inc.

Based on the Fourth Annual Blanche F. Ittleson Memorial Lecture, presented at the Presidential Session of the American Orthopsychiatric Association's 1981 annual meeting, in New York.

be an objective historian in a field that is only now ceasing to be controversial, my aim must be more modest. All I can attempt is to describe the story as I recall it and a few of the empirical studies and theoretical ideas that have been influential in shaping it. My personal biases will be everywhere evident.*

EARLY WORK

During the 1930s and '40s a number of clinicians on both sides of the Atlantic, mostly working independently of each other, were making observations of the ill effects on personality development of prolonged institutional care or frequent changes of mother-figure during the early years of life. Influential publications followed, including, in alphabetical order, publications by Bender,[8,9] Bowlby,[10,11] Burlingham and Freud,[25,26] Goldfarb,[35-38] Levy,[52] and Spitz.[71,72] Since each of the authors was a qualified analyst (except for Goldfarb, who trained later), it is no surprise that the findings created little stir outside analytical circles.

Late in 1949, an imaginative young British psychiatrist, analytically oriented and recently appointed to be Chief of the Mental Health Section of the World Health Organization, stepped in. Requested to contribute to a United Nations study of the needs of homeless children, Ronald Hargreaves** decided to appoint a short-term consultant to report on the mental health aspects of the problem and, knowing of my interest in the field, invited me to undertake the task. For me this was a golden opportunity. After five years as an army psychiatrist, I had returned to child psychiatry determined to explore further the problems I had begun working on before the war; and I had already appointed as my first research assistant James Robertson, a newly qualified psychiatric social worker who had worked with Anna Freud in the Hampstead Nurseries during the war. The six months I spent with the World Health Organization in 1950 gave me the chance not only to read the literature and to discuss it with the authors but also to meet many others in Europe and the United States with experience in the field. Soon after the end of my contract I submitted my report,[12] in which I reviewed the far from negligible evidence then available regarding the adverse influences on personality development of inadequate maternal care during early child-

---

*The origins of my interests, and why I selected separation of young child from mother-figure as a point of entry for systematic research into the broader field of the influence of family experience on personality development, are described in two recent publications.[18,20]

**Hargreaves's premature death in 1962, when professor of psychiatry at Leeds, was a grievous loss to preventive psychiatry.

hood, called attention to the acute distress of young children who find themselves separated from those they know and love, and made recommendations of how best to avoid, or at least mitigate, the short-term and the long-term ill effects.

Influential though the written word may often be, it has nothing like the emotional impact of a movie. Throughout the 1950s, Spitz's early film, *Grief: A Peril in Infancy*,[73] soon followed by Robertson's *A Two-Year-Old Goes to Hospital*,[64] together had an enormous influence. Not only did they draw the attention of professional workers to the immediate distress and anxiety of young children in an institutional setting, but they proved powerful instruments for promoting changes in practice. In this field, Robertson was to play a leading part.[65,66]

Although by the end of the 1950s a great many of those working in child psychiatry and psychology and in social work, and some also of those in pediatrics and nursing, had accepted the research findings and were implementing change, the sharp controversy aroused by the early publications and films continued. Psychiatrists trained in traditional psychiatry and psychologists who adopted a learning theory approach never ceased to point to the deficiencies of the evidence and to the lack of an adequate explanation of how the types of experience implicated could have the effects on personality development that were claimed. Many psychoanalysts, in addition, especially those whose theory focused on the role of fantasy in psychopathology to the relative exclusion of the influence of real life events, remained unconvinced and sometimes very critical. Meanwhile, research continued. For example, at Yale, Provence and Lipton[61] were making a systematic study of institutionalized infants, in which they compared their development with that of infants living in a family. At the Tavistock members of my small research group were active collecting further data on the short-term effects on a young child of being in the care of strange people in a strange place for weeks and sometimes months at a time,[41,42] whilst I addressed myself to the theoretical problems posed by our data.

The field was continually changing. One important influence was the publication in 1962 by the World Health Organization of a collection of articles in which the manifold effects of the various types of experience covered by the term "deprivation of maternal care" were reassessed. Of the six articles, by far the most comprehensive was that by my colleague Ainsworth.[1] In it she not only reviewed the extensive and diverse evidence and considered the many issues that had given rise to controversy but also identified a large number of problems requiring further research.

A second important influence was the publication, beginning during the late '50s, of Harlow's studies of the effects of maternal deprivation on rhesus monkeys; once again film played a big part. Harlow's work in the United States had been stimulated by Spitz's reports. In the United Kingdom complementary studies by Hinde had been stimulated by our work at the Tavistock. For the next decade a stream of experimental results from those two scientists,[39,44] coming on top of the Ainsworth review, undermined the opposition. Thereafter, little more was heard of the inherent implausibility of our hypotheses, and criticism became more constructive.

Much, of course, remained uncertain. Even if the reality of short-term distress and behavioral disturbance is granted, what evidence is there, it was asked, that the ill effects can persist? What features of the experience, or combination of features, are responsible for the distress? And, should it prove true that in some cases ill effects do persist, how is that to be accounted for? How does it happen that some children seem to come through very unfavorable experiences relatively unharmed? How important is it that a child should be cared for most of the time by one principal caregiver? In less developed societies, it was claimed (wrongly, as it turns out), multiple mothering is not uncommon. In addition to all these legitimate questions, moreover, there were misunderstandings. Some supposed that advocates of the view that a child should be cared for most of the time by a principal mother-figure held that that had to be the child's natural mother—the so-called blood-tie theory. Others supposed that, in advocating that a child should "experience a warm intimate and continuous relationship with his mother (or permanent mother-substitute)," proponents were prescribing a regime in which a mother had to care for her child 24 hours a day, day in and day out, with no respite. In a field in which strong feelings are aroused and almost everyone has some sort of vested interest, clear unbiased thinking is not always easy.

A NEW LOOK AT THEORY

The monograph, *Maternal Care and Mental Health*,[12] is in two parts. The first reviews the evidence regarding the adverse effects of maternal deprivation, the second discusses means for preventing it. What was missing, as several reviewers pointed out, was my explanation of how experiences subsumed under the broad heading of maternal deprivation could have the effects on personality development of the kinds claimed. The reason for this omission was simple: the data were not accommodated by any theory then current and in the brief time of my employment by WHO there was no possibility of developing a new one.

The Child's Tie to the Mother

At that time it was widely held that the reason a child develops a close tie to his mother is that she feeds him. Two kinds of drive are postulated, primary and secondary. Food is thought of as primary; the personal relationship, referred to as "dependency," as secondary. This theory did not seem to me to fit the facts. For example, were it true, an infant of a year or two should take readily to whomever feeds him and this clearly was not the case. An alternative theory, stemming from the Hungarian school of psychoanalysis, postulated a primitive object relation from the beginning. In its best known version, however, the one advocated by Melanie Klein, mother's breast is postulated as the first object, and the greatest emphasis is placed on food and orality and on the infantile nature of "dependency." None of these features matched my experience of children. But if the current dependency theories were inadequate, what was the alternative?

During the summer of 1951 a friend mentioned to me the work of Lorenz on the following responses of ducklings and goslings.[53] Reading about this and related work on instinctive behavior revealed a new world, one in which scientists of high caliber were investigating in nonhuman species many of the problems with which we were grappling in the human, in particular the relatively enduring relationships that develop in many species, first between young and parents and later between mated pairs, and some of the ways in which these developments can go awry. Could this work, I asked myself, cast light on a problem central to psychoanalysis, that of "instinct" in humans?

Next followed a long phase during which I set about trying to master basic principles and to apply them to our problems, starting with the nature of the child's tie to his mother. Here Lorenz's work was of special interest. It showed that in some animal species a strong bond to an individual mother-figure could develop without the intermediary of food: for these young birds *are not fed by parents* but feed themselves by catching insects. Here then was an alternative model to the traditional one, and one that had a number of features that seemed possibly to fit the human case. Thereafter, as my grasp of ethological principles increased and I applied them to one clinical problem after another, I became increasingly confident that this was a promising approach. Thus, having adopted this novel point of view, I decided to "follow it up through the material as long as the application of it seems to yield results" (to borrow a phrase of Freud's).

From 1957, when *The Nature of the Child's Tie to His Mother*[13] was first presented, through 1969, when *Attachment*[16] appeared, until 1980, with the publication of *Loss*,[19] I concentrated on this task. The resulting conceptual framework* is designed to accommodate all those phenomena to which Freud called attention—for example, love relations, separation anxiety, mourning, defense, anger, guilt, depression, trauma, emotional detachment, sensitive periods in early life—and so to offer an alternative to the traditional metapsychology of psychoanalysis and to add yet another to the many variants of the clinical theory now extant. How successful these ideas will prove only time will tell.

As Kuhn has emphasized, any novel conceptual framework is difficult to grasp, especially so for those long familiar with a previous one. Of the many difficulties met with in understanding the framework advocated, I describe only a few. One is that, instead of starting with a clinical syndrome of later years and trying to trace its origins retrospectively, I have started with a class of childhood traumata and tried to trace their sequelae prospectively. A second is that, instead of starting with the private thoughts and feelings of a patient, as expressed in free associations or play, and trying to build a theory of personality development from those data, I have started with observations of the behavior of children in certain sorts of defined situations, including records of the feelings and thoughts they express, and have tried to build a theory of personality development from there. Other difficulties arise from my use of concepts such as control system (instead of psychic energy) and developmental pathway (instead of libidinal phase) which, although now firmly established as key concepts in all the biological sciences, are still foreign to the thinking of a great many psychologists and clinicians.

Having discarded the secondary drive, dependency theory of the child's tie to his mother, and also the Kleinian alternative, a first task was to formulate a replacement. This led to the concept of attachment behavior as a special class of behavior with its own dynamics distinct from the behavior and dynamics of either feeding or sex, the two sources of human motivation long regarded as the most fundamental. Strong support for this step soon came from Harlow's finding that, in another primate species—rhesus macaques—infants show a marked preference for a soft dummy "mother," despite its providing no food, to a hard one that does provide food.[40]

Attachment behavior is any form of behavior that results in a person attaining or maintaining proximity to some other clearly identified individual who is conceived as better able to cope with the world. It is most obvious whenever the person is frightened, fatigued, or sick, and is

---

*This is the term Kuhn recently used[51] to replace "paradigm," the term he used in his earlier work.[50]

assuaged by comforting and caregiving. At other times the behavior is less in evidence. Nevertheless, the knowledge that an attachment figure is available and responsive provides a strong and pervasive feeling of security, and so encourages the person to value and continue the relationship. Whilst attachment behavior is at its most obvious in early childhood, it can be observed throughout the life cycle, especially in emergencies. Since it is seen in virtually all human beings (though in varying patterns), it is regarded as an integral part of human nature and one we share (to a varying extent) with members of other species. The biological function attributed to it is that of protection. To remain within easy access of a familiar individual known to be ready and willing to come to our aid in an emergency is clearly a good insurance policy, whatever our age.

By conceptualizing attachment in this way, as a fundamental form of behavior with its own internal motivation distinct from feeding and sex, and of no less importance for survival, the behavior and motivation are accorded a theoretical status never before given them—though parents and clinicians alike have long been intuitively aware of their importance. Hitherto the concepts of "dependency" and "dependency need" have been used to refer to them, but these terms have serious disadvantages. In the first place, dependency has a pejorative flavor; in the second, it does not imply an emotionally charged relationship to one or a very few clearly preferred individuals; and, in the third, no valuable biological function has ever been attributed to it.

It is now 25 years since the notion of attachment was first advanced as a useful way of conceptualizing a form of behavior of central importance not only to clinicians and to developmental psychologists but to every parent as well. During that time attachment theory has been greatly clarified and amplified. The most notable contributors have been Hinde, who, in addition to his own publications,[43] has constantly guided my own thinking, and Ainsworth who, starting in the late '50s, has pioneered empirical studies of attachment behavior both in Africa[2,3] and in the U.S.,[6,7] and has also helped greatly to develop theory.[4,5] Her work, together with that of her students and others influenced by her,[22,55,74,75] has led attachment theory to be widely regarded as probably the best supported theory of socioemotional development yet available.[59,62,69]

Because my starting point in developing theory was observations of behavior, some clinicians[23]* have assumed that the theory amounts to

---

*Judging by publications cited, Brody's criticisms[23] seem to have been made without having studied the third volume of *Attachment and Loss*,[19] in which the structural properties of the theory are most fully described. Likewise, the rather similar criticisms by Kernberg[43] appear to have been made without his having studied the second[17] or third[19] volumes.

no more than a version of behaviorism. This perception is due in large part to the unfamiliarity of the conceptual framework proposed and in part to my own failure in early formulations to make clear the distinction to be drawn between an attachment and attachment behavior. To say of a child (or older person) that he is attached to, or has an attachment to, someone means that he is strongly disposed to seek proximity to and contact with that individual and to do so especially in certain specified conditions. The disposition to behave in this way is an attribute of the attached person, a persisting attribute that changes only slowly over time and that is unaffected by the situation of the moment. Attachment behavior, by contrast, refers to any of the various forms of behavior that the person engages in from time to time to obtain or maintain a desired proximity.

There is abundant evidence that almost every child habitually prefers one person, usually the mother-figure, to turn to when in distress but, in her absence, will make do with someone else, preferably someone well known to the child. On these occasions most children show a clear hierarchy of preference so that, in extremity and with no one else available, even a kindly stranger may be approached. Thus, whilst attachment behavior may in differing circumstances be shown to a variety of individuals, an enduring attachment, or attachment bond, is confined to very few. A child who fails to show such clear discrimination is likely to be severely disturbed.

The theory of attachment is an attempt to explain both attachment behavior, with its episodic appearance and disappearance, and also the enduring attachments that children and other individuals make to particular others. In this theory the key concept is that of behavioral system. This is conceived on the analogy of a physiological system organized homeostatically to ensure that a certain physiological measure, such as body temperature or blood pressure, is held between appropriate limits. In proposing the concept of a behavioral system to account for the way a child or older person maintains his relation to his attachment figure between certain limits of distance or accessibility, no more is done than to use these well-understood principles to account for a different form of homeostasis, namely one in which the set-limits concern the organism's relation to clearly identified persons in, or other features of, the environment and in which the limits are maintained by behavioral instead of physiological means.

In thus postulating the existence of an internal psychological organization with a number of highly specific features, which include representational models of the self and of attachment figure(s), the theory proposed can be seen as having all the same basic properties as those that characterize other forms of structural theory, of which the variants of psychoanalysis are some of the best known, and that differentiate them so sharply from behaviorism in its many forms. Historically, attachment theory was developed as a variant of object relations theory.

The reason that I have given so much space in this account to the concept and theory of attachment is that, once those principles are grasped, there is little difficulty in understanding how the many other phenomena of central concern to clinicians are explained within the framework proposed.

Separation Anxiety

For example, a new light is thrown on the problem of separation anxiety, namely anxiety about losing, or becoming separated from, someone loved. Why "mere separation" should cause anxiety has been a mystery. Freud wrestled with the problem and advanced a number of hypotheses.[32,76] Every other leading analyst has done the same. With no means of evaluating them, many divergent schools of thought have proliferated.

The problem lies, I believe, in an unexamined assumption, made not only by psychoanalysts but by more traditional psychiatrists as well, that fear is aroused in a mentally healthy person only in situations that everyone would perceive as intrinsically painful or dangerous, or that are perceived so by a person only because of his having become conditioned to them. Since fear of separation and loss does not fit this formula, analysts have concluded that what is feared is really some other situation; and a great variety of hypotheses have been advanced.

The difficulties disappear, however, when an ethological approach is adopted. For it then becomes evident that man, like other animals, responds with fear to certain situations, not because they carry a *high* risk of pain or danger, but because they signal an *increase* of risk. Thus, just as animals of many species, including man, are disposed to respond with fear to sudden movement or a marked change in level of sound or light because to do so has survival value, so are many species, including man, disposed to respond to separation from a potentially caregiving figure and for the same reasons.

When separation anxiety is seen in this light, as a basic human disposition, it is only a small step to understanding why threats to abandon a child, often used as a means of control, are so very terrifying. Such threats, as well as threats of suicide by a parent, are, we now know, common causes of intensified separation anxiety. Their extraordinary neglect in traditional clinical theory is due, I suspect, not only to an inadequate theory of separation anxiety but to a failure to give proper weight to the powerful effects, at all ages, of real life events.

Not only do threats of abandonment create intense anxiety, they also arouse anger, often also of intense degree, especially in older children and adolescents. This anger, the function of which is to dissuade the attachment figure from carrying out the threat, can easily become dysfunctional. It is in this light, I believe, that we can understand such absurdly paradoxical behavior as the adolescent, reported by Burnham,[27] who, having murdered his mother, exclaimed, "I couldn't stand to have her leave me."

Other pathogenic family situations are readily understood in terms of attachment theory. One fairly common example is that of the child who has such a close relationship with his mother than he has difficulty in developing a social life outside the family, a relationship sometimes described as symbiotic. In a majority of such cases the cause of the trouble can be traced to the mother who, having grown up anxiously attached as a result of a difficult childhood, is now seeking to make her own child her attachment figure. Far from the child being overindulged, as is sometimes asserted, he is being burdened with having to care for his own mother. Thus, in these cases, the normal relationship of attached child to caregiving parent is found to be inverted.

Mourning

Whilst separation anxiety is the usual response to a threat or some other risk of loss, mourning is the usual response to a loss after it has occurred. During the early years of psychoanalysis a number of analysts identified losses, occurring during childhood or in later life, as playing a causal role in emotional disturbance, especially in depressive disorders; by 1950 a number of theories about the nature of mourning, and other responses to loss, had been advanced. Moreover, much sharp controversy had already been engendered. This controversy, which began during the 1930s, arose from the divergent theories about infant development that had been elaborated in Vienna and London. Representative examples of the different points of view about mourning are those expressed by Deutsch[29] and by Klein.[46] Whereas Deutsch held that, due to inadequate psychic development, children are unable to mourn, Klein held that they not only can mourn but do. In keeping with her strong emphasis on feeding, however, she held that the object mourned was the lost breast; in addition, she attributed a complex fantasy-life to the infant. Opposite though these theoretical positions are, both were constructed using the same methodology, namely by inferences about earlier phases of psychological development based on observations made during the analysis of older, and emotionally disturbed, subjects. Neither theory has been checked by direct observation of how ordinary children of different ages respond to a loss.

Approaching the problem prospectively, I was led to different conclusions. During the early 1950s Robertson and I had generalized the sequence of responses seen in young children during temporary separation from mother as those of protest, despair, and detachment.[67] A few years later, when reading a study by Marris[56] of how widows respond to loss of husband, I was struck by the similarity of the responses he described to those of young children. This led me to a systematic study of the literature on mourning, especially the mourning of healthy adults. The sequence of responses that commonly occur, it became clear, was very different from what clinical theorists had been assuming. Not only does mourning in mentally healthy adults last far longer than the six months often suggested in those days, but several component responses widely regarded as pathological were found to be common in healthy mourning. These include anger, directed at third parties, the self, and sometimes at the person lost; disbelief that the loss has occurred (misleadingly termed denial); and a tendency, often though not always unconscious, to search for the lost person in the hope of reunion. The clearer the picture of mourning responses in adults became, the clearer became their similarities to the responses observed in childhood. This conclusion, when first advanced,[14,15] was much criticized; but it has now been amply supported by a number of subsequent studies.[33,48,58,63]

Once an accurate picture of healthy mourning has been obtained it becomes possible to identify features that are truly indicative of pathology. It becomes possible also to discern many of the conditions that promote healthy mourning and those that lead in a pathological direction. The belief that children are unable to mourn can then be seen to derive from generalizations that had been made from the analyses of children whose mourning had followed an atypical course. In many cases this had been due either to the child never having been given adequate information about what had happened or else to there having been no one to sympathize with him and help him gradually come to terms with his loss, his yearning for his lost parent, his anger and his sorrow.

Defensive Processes

The next step in this reformulation of theory was to consider how defensive processes could best be conceptualized, a crucial step since defensive processes have always been at the heart of psychoanalytic theory. Although as a clinician I have inevitably been concerned with the whole range of defenses, as a research worker I have directed my attention especially to the way a young child behaves toward his mother after a spell in a hospital or residential nursery unvisited. In such circumstances it is common for a child to begin by treating his mother almost as though she were a stranger; then, after an interval, usually of hours or days, the child becomes intensely clinging, anxious lest he lose her again, and angry with her should he think he may. In some way all his feeling for his mother and all the behavior toward her we take for granted (keeping within range of her and, most notably, turning to her when frightened or hurt) have suddenly vanished—only to reappear again after an interval. That was the condition Robertson and I termed detachment, and that we believed was a result of some defensive process operating within the child.

Whereas Freud in his scientific theorizing felt confined to a conceptual model that explained all phenomena, whether physical or biological, in terms of the disposition of energy, today we have available conceptual models of much greater variety. Many draw on such interrelated concepts as organization, pattern, and information, while the purposeful activities of biological organisms can be conceived in terms of control systems structured in certain ways. With supplies of physical energy available to them, these systems become active on receipt of certain sorts of signals and inactive on receipt of signals of other sorts. Thus the world of science in which we live is radically different from the world Freud lived in at the turn of the century, and the concepts available to us immeasurably better suited to our problems than were the very restricted ones available in his day.

Returning now to the strange detached behavior a young child shows after being away for a time with strange people in a strange place, what is so peculiar about it is, of course, the absence of attachment behavior in circumstances in which we would confidently expect to see it. Even when he has hurt himself severely such a child shows no sign of seeking comfort. Thus, signals that would ordinarily activate attachment behavior are failing to do so. This suggests that, in some way and for some reason, these signals are failing to reach the behavioral system responsible for attachment behavior, that they are being blocked off and the behavioral system itself thereby immobilized. What this means is that a system controlling such crucial behavior as attachment can in certain circumstances be rendered either temporarily or permanently incapable of being activated, and the whole range of feeling and desire that normally accompanies it can thus be rendered incapable of being aroused.

In considering how this deactivation might be effected, I turn to the work of the cognitive psychologists[30,31,57] who, during the past 20 years, have revolutionized our understanding of how we perceive the world and how we construe the situations we are in. Amongst much else that is clinically congenial, this revolution in cognitive theory not only gives unconscious mental processes the central place in mental life that analysts have always claimed for them, but presents a picture of the mental apparatus as well able to shut off information of certain specified types and of doing so selectively without the person being aware of what is happening.

In the emotionally detached children described earlier—and also, I believe, in adults who have developed the kind of personality that Winnicott[77] described as "false self" and Kohut[49] as "narcissistic"—the information being blocked off is of a very special type. Far from its being the routine exclusion of irrelevant and potentially distracting information that we engage in all the time and that is readily reversible, what is being excluded in these pathological conditions are the signals, arising from both inside and outside the person, that would activate their attachment behavior and that would enable them both to love and to experience being loved. In other words, the mental structures responsible for routine selective exclusion are being employed (one might say exploited) for a special and potentially pathological purpose. This form of exclusion I refer to, for obvious reasons, as defensive exclusion, which is, of course, only another way of describing repression. And, just as Freud regarded repression as the key process in every form of defense, so I see the role of defensive exclusion.* A fuller account of this, an information processing approach to the problem of defense, in which defenses are classified into defensive processes, defensive beliefs, and defensive activities, is given in an early chapter of *Loss*.[19]

An Alternative Framework

During the period in which the conceptual framework described here was developed, Margaret Mahler has been concerned with many of the same clinical problems and some of the same features of children's be-

---

*As Spiegel[70] has pointed out, my term "defensive exclusion" carries a meaning very similar to Sullivan's term "selective inattention."

havior; she also has been developing a revised conceptual framework to account for them, set out fully in *The Psychological Birth of the Human Infant.*[54] To compare alternative frameworks is never easy, as Kuhn[50] emphasized, and no attempt is made to do so here. Elsewhere[21] I have described what I believe to be some of the strengths of the framework I favor, including its close relatedness to empirical data, both clinical and developmental, and its compatibility with current ideas in evolutionary biology and neurophysiology; the shortcomings of Mahler's framework have been trenchantly criticized by Peterfreund[60] and Klein.[47] In brief, Mahler's theories of normal development, including her postulated normal phases of autism and symbiosis, are shown to rest not on observation but on preconceptions based on traditional psychoanalytic theory and, in doing so, to ignore almost entirely the remarkable body of new information about early infancy that has been built up from careful empirical studies over the past two decades. Although some of the clinical implications of Mahler's theory are not very different from those of attachment theory, and her concept of return to base to "refuel" is similar to that of use of attachment figure as secure base from which to explore, the key concepts with which the two frameworks are built are very different.

RESEARCH

Nothing has been so rewarding as the immense amount of careful research to which the early work on maternal deprivation has given rise. The literature is now enormous and far beyond the compass of an account of this sort to summarize. Fortunately, moreover, it is unnecessary since a new, comprehensive, and critical review of the field has recently been published by Rutter,[68] who concluded by referring to the "continuing accumulation of evidence showing the importance of deprivation and disadvantage on children's psychological development" and expressing the view that the original arguments "have been amply confirmed." A principal finding of recent work is the extent to which two or more adverse experiences interact so that the risk of a psychological disturbance following is multiplied, often many times over. An example of this interactive effect of adverse experiences is seen in the findings of Brown and Harris,[24] derived from their studies of depressive disorders in women.

Not only is there this strongly interactive effect of adverse experiences, there is also an increased likelihood for someone who has had one adverse experience to have another. For example,

... people brought up in unhappy or disrupted homes are more likely to have illegitimate children, to become teenage mothers, to make unhappy marriages, and to divorce.[68]

Thus, adverse childhood experiences have effects of at least two kinds. First, they make the individual more vulnerable to later adverse experiences. Secondly, they make it more likely that he or she will meet with further such experiences. Whereas the earlier adverse experiences are likely to be wholly independent of the agency of the individual concerned, the later ones are likely to be the consequences of his or her own actions, actions that spring from those disturbances of personality to which the earlier experiences have given rise.

Of the many types of psychological disturbance that are traceable, at least in part, to one or another pattern of maternal deprivation, the effects on parental behavior and thereby on the next generation are potentially the most serious. Thus a mother who, due to adverse experiences during childhood, grows up to be anxiously attached is prone to seek care from her own child and thereby lead the child to become anxious, guilty, and perhaps phobic.[17] A mother who as a child suffered neglect and frequent severe threats of being abandoned or beaten is more prone than others to abuse her child physically,[28] resulting in the adverse effects on the child's developing personality recorded by, amongst others, George and Main.[34] Systematic research into the effects of childhood experiences on the way mothers and fathers treat their children has only just begun and seems likely to be one of the most fruitful of all fields for further research. Other research leads are described in a recent symposium edited by Parkes and Stevenson-Hinde.[59]

CONCLUSION

My reason for giving so much space in this account to the development of theory is not only because it has occupied so much of my time but because, as Kurt Lewin remarked long ago, "There is nothing so practical as a good theory," and, of course, nothing so handicapping as a poor one. Without good theory as a guide, research is likely to be difficult to plan and to be unproductive, and findings are difficult to interpret. Without a reasonably valid theory of psychopathology, therapeutic techniques tend to be blunt and of uncertain benefit. Without a reasonably valid theory of etiology, systematic and agreed measures of prevention will never be supported. My hope is that, in the long term, the greatest value of the theory proposed may prove to be the light it throws on the conditions most likely to promote healthy personality development. Only when those conditions are clear beyond doubt will parents know what is best for their children and will communities be willing to help them provide it.

REFERENCES

1. Ainsworth, M. (1962). The effects of maternal deprivation: A review of findings and controversy in the context of research strategy. In *Deprivation of Maternal Care: A Reassessment of Its Effects*, Public Health Papers No. 14. World Health Organization, Geneva.
2. Ainsworth, M. (1963). The development of infant-mother interaction among the Ganda. In *Determinants of Infant Behavior*, Vol. 2, B. Foss, ed. New York: John Wiley.
3. Ainsworth, M. (1967). *Infancy in Uganda: Infant Care and the Growth of Attachment*. Baltimore: Johns Hopkins Press.
4. Ainsworth, M. (1969). Object relations, dependency and attachment: A theoretical review of the infant-mother relationship. *Child Development*, 40:969–1025.
5. Ainsworth, M. (1982). Attachment: Retrospect and prospect. In *The Place of Attachment in Human Behavior*, C. Parkes and J. Stevenson-Hinde, eds. New York: Basic Books.
6. Ainsworth, M. et al. (1978). *Patterns of Attachment: Assessed in the Strange Situation and at Home*. Hillsdale, NJ: Erlbaum Associates.
7. Ainsworth, M. and Wittig, B. (1969). Attachment and exploratory behavior in one-year-olds in a strange situation. In *Determinants of Infant Behavior*, Vol. 4, B. Foss, ed. New York: Barnes & Noble.
8. Bender, L. (1947). Psychopathic behavior disorders in children. In *Handbook of Correctional Psychology*, R. Lindner and R. Seliger, eds. New York: Philosophical Library.
9. Bender, L. and Yarnell, H. (1941). An observation nursery. *American Journal of Psychiatry*, 97:1158–1174.
10. Bowlby, J. (1940). The influence of early environment of the development of neurosis and neurotic character. *International Journal of Psychoanalysis*, 21:154–178.
11. Bowlby, J. (1944). Forty-four juvenile thieves: Their characters and home life. *International Journal of Psychoanalysis*, 25:19–52, 107–127.
12. Bowlby, J. (1951). *Maternal Care and Mental Health*. New York: Columbia University Press.
13. Bowlby, J. (1958). The nature of the child's tie to his mother. *International Journal of Psychoanalysis*, 39:350–373.
14. Bowlby, J. (1960). Grief and mourning in infancy and early childhood. *Psychoanalytic Study of the Child*, 15:9–52.
15. Bowlby, J. (1961). Processes of mourning. *International Journal of Psychoanalysis*, 42:317–340.
16. Bowlby, J. (1969). *Attachment and Loss Vol. 1: Attachment*. New York: Basic Books.
17. Bowlby, J. (1973). *Attachment and Loss Vol. 2: Separation—Anxiety and Anger*. New York: Basic Books.
18. Bowlby, J. (1979). Psychoanalysis as art and science. *International Review of Psychoanalysis*, 6:3–14.
19. Bowlby, J. (1980). *Attachment and Loss Vol. 3: Loss—Sadness and Depression*. New York: Basic Books.

20. Bowlby, J. (1981). Perspective: A contribution. *Bulletin of the Royal College of Psychiatry*, 5:2–4.
21. Bowlby, J. (1981). Psychoanalysis as a natural science. *International Review of Psychoanalysis*, 8:243–256.
22. Bretherton, I. (1980). Young children in stressful situations: The supporting role of attachment figures and unfamiliar caregivers. In *Uprooting and Development*, G. Coelho and P. Ahmed, eds. New York: Plenum Press.
23. Brody, S. (1981). The concepts of attachment and bonding. *Journal of American Psychoanalytic Association*, 29:815–829.
24. Brown, G. and Harris, T. (1978). *The Social Origins of Depression*. London: Tavistock.
25. Burlingham, D. and Freud, A. (1942). *Young Children in War-Time London*. London: Allen and Unwin.
26. Burlingham, D. and Freud, A. (1944). *Infants Without Families*. London: Allen and Unwin.
27. Burnham, D. (1965). Separation anxiety. *Archives of General Psychiatry*, 13:346–358.
28. De Lozier, P. (1982). Attachment theory and child abuse. In *The Place of Attachment in Human Behavior*, C. Parkes and J. Stevenson-Hinde, eds. New York: Basic Books.
29. Deutsch, H. (1937). Absence of grief. *Psychoanalytic Quarterly*, 6:12–22.
30. Dixon N. (1971). *Subliminal Perception: The Nature of a Controversy*. London: McGraw-Hill.
31. Dixon, N. (1981). *Preconscious Processing*. New York: John Wiley.
32. Freud, S. (1926). Inhibitions, symptoms and anxiety. In *Standard Edition*, Vol. 20. London: Hogarth Press.
33. Furman, E. (1974). *A Child's Parent Dies*. New Haven: Yale University Press.
34. George C. and Main M. (1979). Social interactions of young abused children: Approach, avoidance and aggression. *Child Development*, 50:306–318.
35. Goldfarb, W. (1943). Infant rearing and problem behavior. *American Journal of Orthopsychiatry*, 13:249–265.
36. Goldfarb, W. (1943). The effect of early institutional care on adolescent personality. *Child Development*, 14:213–223.
37. Goldfarb W. (1943). The effects of early institutional care on adolescent personality. *Journal of Experimental Education*, 12:106.
38. Goldfarb, W. (1955). Emotional and intellectual consequences of psychologic deprivation in infancy: A revaluation. In *Psychopathology of Childhood*, P. Hoch and J. Zubin, eds. New York: Grune & Stratton.
39. Harlow H. and Harlow, M. (1965). The affectional systems. In *Behavior of Nonhuman Primates*, Vol. 2. A. Schrier, H. Harlow and F. Stollnitz, eds. New York: Academic Press.
40. Harlow, H. and Zimmermann, R. (1959). Affectional responses in the infant monkey. *Science*, 130:421.
41. Heinicke, C. (1956). Some effects of separating two-year-old children from their parents: A comparative study. *Human Relations*, 9:105–176.
42. Heinicke, C. and Westheimer, I. (1966). *Brief Separations*. New York: International Universities Press.
43. Hinde, R. (1974). *Biological Bases of Human Social Behavior*. New York: McGraw-Hill.
44. Hinde, R. and Spencer-Booth, Y. (1971). Effects of brief separation from mother on rhesus monkeys. *Science*, 173:111–118.
45. Kernberg, O. (1980). *Internal World and External Reality: Object Relations Theory Applied*. New York: Aronson.

46. Klein, M. (1940). Mourning and its relation to manic-depressive states. In *Love, Guilt and Reparation and Other Papers, 1921–1946*. Boston: Seymour Lawrence/Delacorte.
47. Klein, M. (1981). On Mahler's autistic and symbiotic phases: An exposition and evaluation. *Psychoanalytic Contemporary Thought*, 4:69–105.
48. Kliman, G. (1965). *Psychological Emergencies of Childhood*. New York: Grune & Stratton.
49. Kohut, H. (1977). *The Restoration of the Self*. New York: International Universities Press.
50. Kuhn, T. (1962). *The Structure of Scientific Revolutions*. Chicago: University of Chicago Press.
51. Kuhn, T. (1974). Second thoughts on paradigms. In *The Structure of Scientific Theory*, F. Suppe, ed. Urbana, IL: University of Illinois Press.
52. Levy, D. (1937). Primary affect hunger. *American Journal of Psychiatry*, 94:643–652.
53. Lorenz, K. (1935). Der Kumpan in der Umwelt des Vogels. *J. Orn. Berl.* 83. (In *Instinctive Behavior*, C. Schiller ed. 1957. New York: International Universities Press.)
54. Mahler, M., Pine, F. and Bergman, A. (1975). *The Psychological Birth of the Human Infant*. New York: Basic Books.
55. Main, M. (1977). Analysis of a peculiar form of reunion behavior in some day-care children: Its history and sequelae in children who are home-reared. In *Social Development in Childhood: Day-Care Programs and Research*, R. Webb, ed. Baltimore: Johns Hopkins University Press.
56. Marris, P. (1958). *Widows and Their Families*. London: Routledge & Kegan Paul.
57. Norman, D. (1976). *Memory and Attention: Introduction to Human Information Processing* (2nd Ed.). New York: John Wiley.
58. Parkes, C. (1972). *Bereavement: Studies of Grief in Adult Life*. New York: International Universities Press.
59. Parkes, C. and Stevenson-Hinde, J. (Eds.) (1982). *The Place of Attachment in Human Behavior*. New York: Basic Books.
60. Peterfreund, E. (1978). Some critical comments on psychoanalytic conceptualizations of infancy. *International Journal of Psychoanalysis*, 59:427–441.
61. Provence, S. and Lipton, R. (1962). *Infants in Institutions*. New York: International Universities Press.
62. Rajecki, D., Lamb, M. and Obmascher, P. (1978). Towards a general theory of infantile attachment: A comparative review of aspects of the social bond. *Behav. Brain Sci.*, 3:417–464.
63. Raphael, B. (1982). The young child and the death of a parent. In *The Place of Attachment in Human Behavior*. C. Parkes and J. Stevenson-Hinde, eds. New York: Basic Books.
64. Robertson, J. (1952). *A Two-Year-Old Goes to Hospital*. New York: New York University Film Library (Film).
65. Robertson, J. (1958). *Going to Hospital with Mother*. New York: New York University Film Library (Film).
66. Robertson, J. (1970). *Young Children in Hospital* (2nd Ed.). London: Tavistock.
67. Robertson, J. and Bowlby, J. (1952). Responses of young children to separation from their mothers. *Courrier Centre Internationale Enfance*, 2:131–142.
68. Rutter, M. (1979). Maternal deprivation, 1972–1978: New findings, new concepts, new approaches. *Child Development*, 50:283–305.
69. Rutter, M. (Ed.) (1980). *Scientific Foundations of Developmental Psychiatry*. London: Heinemann Medical Books.
70. Spiegel, R. (1981). Review of Loss: Sadness and Depression by John Bowlby. *American Journal of Psychotherapy*, 35:598–600.

71. Spitz, R. (1945). Hospitalism: An enquiry into the genesis of psychiatric conditions in early childhood. *Psychoanalytic Study of the Child,* 1:53.
72. Spitz, R. (1946). Anaclitic depression. *Psychoanalytic Study of the Child,* 2:313–342.
73. Spitz, R. (1947). *Grief: A Peril in Infancy.* New York: New York University Film Library (Film).
74. Sroufe, A. (1982). Infant-caregiver attachment and patterns of adaptation in pre-school: The roots of maladaptation and competence. In *Minnesota Symposium in Child Psychology,* M. Perlmutter, ed. Minneapolis: University of Minnesota Press.
75. Sroufe, A. and Waters, E. (1977). Attachment as an organizational construct. *Child Development,* 48:1184–1199.
76. Strachey, J. (1959). Editor's introduction. In *Inhibitions, Symptoms and Anxiety, Standard Edition of the Works of Sigmund Freud,* Vol. 20. London: Hogarth Press.
77. Winnicott, D. (1960). Ego distortion in terms of true and false self. In *The Maturational Process and the Facilitating Environment,* D. Winnicott. New York: International Universities Press.

3

Infant Bonding: Mystique and Reality

Stella Chess and Alexander Thomas

Department of Psychiatry, New York University Medical Center

Current formulations of the crucial significance of the mother-infant relationship in the neonatal period and the first year of life for the child's psychological development have important theoretical and practical implications. This review examines these formulations in their historical context and concludes that they are not supported by the research literature. An alternative approach is suggested.

In middle-class American society the mother-infant relationship is invested with a special mystique both in the mass media and the professional literature. In the marketplace, the image of the blissful, nurturant mother with a happy contented baby is used as a symbol of all that is desirable and good; by juxtaposition, these qualities are presumably transferred to the advertised product, whether it be soap or automobiles.

In the mental health field, the concept of the decisive importance of the mother for the infant's development took hold gradually, starting in the 1920s with Freud and Watson's emphasis on the paramount importance of the first years of life.[17,45] Subsequent studies in the 1930s and 1940s on the effects of disturbed maternal functioning, such as maternal overprotection or rejection, buttressed this thesis, and were climaxed by Bowlby's 1951 report on maternal deprivation, with his conclusion that

Reprinted with permission from the *American Journal of Orthopsychiatry*, 1982, Vol. 52, No. 2, 213–222. Copyright 1982 by the American Orthopsychiatric Association, Inc.

> . . . mother love in infancy and childhood is as important for
> mental health as are vitamins and proteins for physical
> health.[4]

These reports did have a salutary influence in highlighting the psychological needs of the young child, and in emphasizing the importance
of a humane nurturant environment for the infant's healthy development. But such considerations are different from the professional ideology that crystallized by the 1950s, in which the causation of all
psychopathology, from simple behavior problems to juvenile delinquency to schizophrenia itself, was laid at the doorstep of the mother.
The guilt and anxiety created in mothers whose children had even minor
behavior deviations were enormous. The pressure on mothers in those
days was vividly described in 1954 by Bruch,[8] one of the few psychiatrists
who viewed this development with alarm:

> Modern parent education is characterized by the experts
> pointing out in great detail all the mistakes parents have made
> and can possibly make, and substituting "scientific knowledge"
> for the tradition of the "good old days." An unrelieved picture
> of model parental behavior, a contrived image of artificial
> perfection of happiness, is held up before parents who try
> valiantly to reach the ever receding ideal of "good parent
> hood" like dogs after a mechanical rabbit. . . . The new teach
> ing implies that parents are all-responsible and must assume
> the role of preventive Fate for their children.

We ourselves were motivated to initiate our longitudinal studies of temperament by the same concerns as Bruch's, by our own inability as clinicians to make linear one-to-one correlations between parental attitudes
and practices and the child's psychological development, by the considerable skepticism in the research literature of the validity of the "blame
the mother" ideology[24,32] and the indications that the child's own behavioral individuality, or temperament, was an active influence from birth
onward in the parent-child interactional process.[11,40]

CONCEPTUAL REVISIONS IN THE 1960S AND '70S

In succeeding years, into the mid-1970s, this professional ideology
which held the parents, primarily the mother, all-responsible for their
child's developmental course came to be increasingly challenged. Our

own findings on the importance of the child's own characteristics, which are independent of parental attitudes and practices, played a part. This thesis was buttressed by an influential article by Bell[3] with a similar emphasis. Studies of physically handicapped children, such as the deaf or blind, demonstrated the plasticity of the brain and the capacity of the infant for effective coping and mastery in the face of a highly stressful environment.[9] Clinical and research studies confirmed the evidence that the infant's development was not related in any linear fashion to parental characteristics.[2,38] The formulation of maternal deprivation and its pathological consequences came in for critical review.[35] The concept of imprinting and critical periods derived from animal behavior studies, which had been freely used as support for the assertion that the mother's attitudes and behavior could have a decisive and permanent effect on the human infant, was scrutinized in several systematic reviews, with the conclusion that the terms be abandoned.[13,48] Most important, perhaps, have been the data that have come from the major longitudinal studies, including our own—the type of study that is uniquely suited to examine the issue of the consequences of parental attitudes and behavior in infancy for the child's subsequent development. With impressive unanimity, these studies reported that the child's experiences in the first few years of life, including the mother-child relationship, were unreliable predictors of later behavior.[22,27,31,40,42] Strong confirmation also came from the comprehensive reviews of the literature on early development by Sameroff[37] and by the Clarkes.[12]

Thus, by the mid-1970s it could be said that a new consensus had been established by research psychiatrists and developmental psychologists. The mother was certainly an important influence on the child's development, and in some cases even a highly significant one. But other factors were also important—the father, sibs, the pattern of family organization and function, the school, peer groups, the larger social environment, and the child's own characteristics. Development proceeded by the sequences of interaction among all these influences at succeeding age-periods, and no one factor or age-period could be considered all-important and decisive by itself. Attempts to reassert earlier concepts, such as the proposition that the parents determine the child's future cognitive abilities by what they do in the first three years,[47] received little support.

This consensus had a most salutary impact on the "blame the mother" ideology, which had previously been so pervasive among mental health professions. Child-care experts from various disciplines could reassure mothers that a child's problems could stem from many causes. Also, mistakes in parental handling or judgment were not irrevocable and their correction could reverse an unhealthy trend in the child's development. Parents did not have "to try valiantly to reach the ever receding ideal of 'good parenthood' like dogs after a mechanical rabbit."[8] Unnecessary and destructive maternal guilt was relieved, with positive effects for both mother and child.

INFANT BONDING: THE PRESENT SCENE

The past few years, however, have witnessed the disruption of this consensus. New formulations have appeared in the developmental research field reasserting the thesis that the early relationship with the mother is of decisive importance for the child's psychological future. The earlier formulations placed the "critical period" through the first five years of life; the new statements place it in the first year, even the first hour after birth. Already, we are witnessing a resurgence of anxiety and guilt in educated young mothers over this new "scientific knowledge." What are these new formulations? What are their implications? And how valid are the findings on which they are based?

BONDING IN THE FIRST YEAR

Two separate but closely related formulations of infant bonding are made, one concerning the neonatal period, the other with regard to the later months of the first year.

For the neonatal period the most emphatic and influential formulation is that of Klaus and Kennell in the volume *Maternal-Infant Bonding*, published in 1976.[25] Their thesis is clearly stated:

> This original mother-infant bond is the wellspring for all the infant's subsequent attachments and is the formative relationship in the course of which the child develops a sense of himself. Throughout his lifetime the strength and character of this attachment will influence the quality of all future bonds to other individuals. (pp. 1–2)

And furthermore:

> This is one of our principles of attachment—that early events have long-lasting effects. Anxieties a mother has about her baby in the first few days after birth, even about a problem

that is easily resolved, may affect her relationship with the child long afterward. (p. 52)

The "critical period" concept is reintroduced:

> ... we strongly believe that an essential principle of attachment is that there is a *sensitive period* in the first minutes and hours after an infant's birth which is optimal for the parent-infant attachment. (pp. 65–66)

If the child is separated from the mother during these first hours after birth, so the thesis goes, optimal development will not occur.

Formulations of the mother-infant relationship in the latter half of the first year of life have relied heavily on the fact that most infants begin to show at that time negative reactions to strangers, especially if associated with separation from the mother. This response has been rated in a standard procedure by Ainsworth,[1] which has been widely used. In this Ainsworth Strange Situation, the infant's reactions are recorded in detail when the mother leaves the child, once alone and once with a stranger, and then returns a few minutes later. Those children who show mild distress at the mother's leaving, approach the mother on her return, and are quickly soothed are categorized as having a secure attachment or bond to the mother. Those infants who do not show distress at the mother's leaving and actively turn away at reunion or who are difficult to comfort and resistant to contact on the mother's return are considered anxiously attached.[1] The "securely attached" infant is presumed to be the one whose mother is appropriately sensitive and responsive to the infant's signals.

Sroufe and his co-workers[29,43] have reported that the Ainsworth measure of attachment correlates significantly with the quality of play and problem-solving behavior at age 2, and to interpersonal competence with peers at 3½ years of age. The authors consider that a "secure" attachment, in the Ainsworth sense,

> ... is an important aspect of infant emotional development, the secure base serving as a context within which the infant develops its first reciprocal relationship with another individual, its rudimentary senses of self, and its first sense of the emotional availability and sensitivity of others.[29] (p. 554)

Thus, in this formulation, the infant's attachment to the mother, as measured in one specific experimental situation, becomes a decisive influence for the course of emotional and task-competence development. And it is the mother who shapes the nature of this attachment. Ominous consequences are predicted if "bonding" is "inadequate" in the first year of life. As one influential mental health professional put it:

> Love of a partner and sensual pleasure experienced with that partner begin in infancy, and progress to a culminating experience, "falling in love," the finding of a permanent partner, the achievement of sexual fulfillment. In every act of love in mature life, there is a prologue which originated in the first year of life.[16] (pp. 31–32)

IMPLICATIONS OF INFANT BONDING CONCEPTS

Klaus and Kennell's writings have had important positive consequences. Newborn nurseries, especially for the premature and sick infant, had been private, sterile, and impersonal preserves from which parents had been barred on the excuse of protecting the fragile infants from infection. Klaus and Kennell, with their insistence that this concern was of minor importance, that the establishment of a human sensuous contact between mother and newborn infant took precedence and that this contact might even reduce the incidence of infections, pioneered in the reopening of nurseries to parents and their families. With our current knowledge of the capacities of the neonate for entering into reciprocal active human relationships with the primary caretakers, this is both humane and developmentally desirable.[18,41] The mother of the older infant is also reassured that her influence depends on objective behavior, on the responsiveness to overt stimuli and messages coming from the baby, rather than a mystical, unconscious, uncontrollable "mother love."

But what price is being paid for these gains? And is this price necessary? What about the mothers who are unavoidably unable to have this immediate skin-to-skin contact with their newborns, either because of illness in the baby or mother, or because of inflexible hospital routines? Are these babies doomed to less than "optimal development"? Klaus and Kennell themselves, as sensitive clinicians, are concerned with these questions, but, within the framework of their conceptual commitments, find this an insoluble dilemma.[23] They can reassure mothers separated from their infants in the neonatal period that all is not lost, but their categorical insistence on the vital importance of close mother-infant contact in the first hours after birth[25] makes such reassurances of dubious value.

And what about the many young children who will exhibit patterns of deviant development, whether transient or of long duration? Are their mothers now to conclude this was their fault, that they were insensitive to the baby's signals, that they failed to fulfill their maternal responsibilities? These are not speculative questions. Already mothers separated from their newborns who are in premature or intensive care units are showing anxiety and guilt reactions. And mental health authorities are laying down the line for the good mother. As one influential article[19] put it, the "adaptive caretaker" in the infant's first three months of life should be

> . . . invested, dedicated, protective, comforting, predictable, engaging and interesting.

How many mothers struggling to cope with the innumerable demands, responsibilities, and frustrations of managing their households, and perhaps having to work on the outside in addition, can expect to meet such standards, which seem more appropriate to the world of television advertisements than to the world in which most mothers live.

What are the facts? Is "infant bonding" so unique and crucial to subsequent development? What is the thrust of research findings in this area?

CRITIQUE OF NEONATAL INFANT BONDING CONCEPTS

The concept of the crucial importance of immediate postnatal mother-infant contact for later development has two implications. Firstly, the mother's (or other primary caretaker's) relationship to the child has some special and even unique quality. Secondly, there is a "critical period" for the initiation of this relationship, the immediate postnatal period, and, if this is missed, adequate compensation subsequently is not possible. Rutter, in a recent revision[36] of his 1972 classic review of maternal deprivation,[35] has carefully examined the evidence for a special quality to the mother-infant relationship. His conclusion is definitive:

> The . . . proposition is that the first or main attachment differs *in kind* from all other subsidiary ones. Most research findings suggest that this is not the case. . . . Bowlby's argument is that the child's relationship with mother differs from other relationships specifically with respect to its *attachment* qualities, and the evidence indicates that this is not so. (pp. 141–142)

As to the "critical period" concept, the validity of this formulation for human development has come into serious question.[12,48] From the vantage point of developmental theory, a critical-period hypothesis also stands in opposition to the basic interactionist formulation, in which psychological development is seen as a sequential dynamic process of continuous and mutual interaction between organism and environment.[37,41]

Klaus and Kennell[25] reported a number of studies to support their view of the special importance of neonatal mother-child contact. Some are animal studies, with applicability to the human situation that is highly debatable. Almost all the others are reports of short-term effect, which do not deal with the possibility of a "greenhouse effect." In other words, greater neonatal contact may have a forcing effect on one or another aspect of development, but in the long-run the others catch up. This phenomenon is illustrated by our study of the frequency of social interactions of children with their peers in nursery school.[33] At four years old, those children with a previous year of nursery school attendance showed a significantly higher frequency of such interactions than did the children with no previous school experience. By age five, the first group had leveled off, the second group had reached the first group's level, and those starting school for the first time at age five were at the same level as were the two other groups.

Klaus and Kennell did report that a group of mothers with extended neonatal contact with their babies showed more active linguistic behavior toward their children at two years than did a control group. At five years, the children also had significantly higher IQs than the control group. The sample size, however, was small (9 versus 10) and there are insufficient details given to evaluate the research design. Rutter[36] has reviewed the literature on this issue and concluded that

> The balance of evidence suggests that separation of mother and child in the neonatal period may have effects on maternal behavior which last a few months but that it is unusual for effects to persist for longer than that. . . . it is clear that both mothers and fathers can, and commonly do, develop strong attachments to their children in the absence of neonatal contact. (pp. 203–204)

Furthermore, the interpretation Klaus and Kennell gave to their findings is open to question. Thus, they reported that in home births, as contrasted to hospital deliveries, mothers show "unreserved elation" and appear to be in "a remarkable state of ecstasy"[25] (p. 46). But as Brazelton[5] pointed out, this may not be a sign of "bonding," but "signs of relief at having their autonomy intact" (p. 47). Lozoff[26] made the same point:

> The so-called "natural" childbirth and home deliveries in the United States . . . are the products of individuals struggling to control their own experience, in reaction against cultural patterns that place control in the hands of specialists. (p. 85)

Finally, as Rutter pointed out, the long-term effects that Klaus and Kennell reported "have generally applied to socially disadvantaged groups with many other problems"[36] (p. 203). In this regard, a recent study has reported that a significant positive maternal effect from immediate postnatal contact with the infant occurred in mothers with low social support systems.[23] To give a mother immediate and active contact with her newborn baby in the hospital involves more active positive contact with hospital staff than for a mother isolated from her infant. It may be that, for socially and economically deprived groups, it is this relationship with hospital personnel, accompanied by expressions of interest, encouragement, and reassurance, rather than the contact with the infant, that is important and helpful to the mother.

Several very recent reports, beyond those reviewed by Rutter, provide data that also challenge the neonatal "bonding" concept. Egeland and Vaughn[15] compared 32 infants identified as not receiving adequate maternal care in the first year of life (ratings of physical abuse, neglect, and failure to thrive) with a matched group of 33 infants receiving high-quality maternal care. No significant differences were found between the two groups in the paranatal factors making for mother-child separation after birth—prematurity, delivery complication, and medical problems requiring separation from the mother. Svejda and co-workers[39] compared 15 mothers following the usual postnatal routine with 15 mothers having extended immediate postnatal contact with their babies. No differences in maternal behavior were found between the two groups, using 28 discrete measures. The authors suggested that other studies with different findings did not control sufficiently for various contaminating variables. Minde and co-workers[30] studied the interaction of 32 mothers and their very low-birth-weight infants during the maternal visits to the premature nursery and during the infants' first three months at home, and reported that

> . . . our data showed no association between the type of initial

contact the mother had with her baby and her later activity pattern.

In summary, Egeland and Vaughn's conclusion[15] seems apt:

> There can be no doubt that any hospital procedure which makes the mother feel more comfortable or more competent to care for her new baby will be a positive influence on the development of the maternal bond. However, to imply that lack of contact between mothers and their newborns is indicative of a current failure to bond with the infant, or is predictive of later breakdowns in the mother-infant bond is a disservice to the millions of mothers and infants who have developed perfectly healthy bonds and attachments under the current hospital regimen. Finally, when parent-child bonds do break down, as in cases of abuse and neglect, researchers should look for multiple causes rather than pinpointing some very early event as the predisposing single trauma. Past experience with single causes (*e.g.*, anoxia in the 1950s) should keep us wary of assigning "blame" for the failure of bonds to early separations. (p. 84)

CRITIQUE OF LATER INFANCY BONDING CONCEPTS

As indicated above, the reactions of the 8-to-12-month-old infant in the Ainsworth Strange Situation are considered to reflect secure versus anxious attachment to the mother. This assumption can be questioned on several grounds. Firstly, there is the danger of transposing findings from artificial experimental settings to real life situations. In Bronfenbrenner's phraseology,[7]

> Much of American developmental psychology is the science of the behavior of children in strange situations with strange adults. (p. 3)

Similarly, McCall[28] warned that

> . . . the experimental method now dictates rather than serves the research questions we value, fund, and pursue; as a result the process of development as it naturally transpires in chil-

dren growing up in actual life circumstances has been largely
ignored. . . . What value is our knowledge if it is not relevant
to real children growing up in real families and in real neighborhoods?

And, referring specifically to attachment studies, Rutter[36] cautioned
about drawing conclusions from

. . . curious procedures involving mother, caretakers and
strangers not only going in and out of rooms every minute
for reasons quite obscure to the child but also not initiating
interactions in the way they might usually do. (p. 160)

Secondly, the infant's reaction to a stranger is a complex and variable
phenomenon influenced by a number of developmental and situational
factors. Differential response to parents versus strangers can be identified as early as two months, so that

. . . one must question our former idea of a linear model of
infant social relationships, with the mother-infant bond as the
primary one and all other relationships extending from it.[13]

Infants show positive affiliative responses to strangers as well as negative
reactions of wariness;[6] their responses are influenced by whether or not
the stranger towers over them,[46] and by whether the stranger is passive
or active in confronting the infant.[21] The infant's proximity-seeking behavior may serve different functions at different times and does not
appear

. . . to be a reliable index of preference for or attachment to
particular individuals.[20]

This variability in the infant's reactions to strangers has led some workers
to question the actual usefulness of the concept of stranger wariness.[34]
Finally, it is possible to interpret differential responses of the infant
to the Ainsworth Strange Situation or similar experimental procedures
as reflections of differences in temperamental characteristics rather than
secure versus anxious attachment. Waters[44] made this point emphati-
cally:

While a measure based on discrete behaviors may *look* like a

useful measure of looking, or distance interaction or attachment, it is more likely that the major consistent influence
across unselected instances of a discrete behavior will be the
ubiquitous dimensions of temperament.

We ourselves would certainly consider that the items of the infant's
behavior in the Ainsworth Strange Situation could be appropriately rated
under the temperamental categories of approach/withdrawal, adaptability, quality of mood, and intensity. Similarly, the items of behavior
described by Matas, Arend and Sroufe[29] in the free-play and problem-
solving style observations of a group of 24-month-old infants could also
be rated under the same four temperamental categories, plus persistence. Thus, the correlations found by these authors between earlier
ratings of these infants in the Ainsworth Strange Situation and their
behavioral style at 24 months could reflect consistency in temperament,
rather than the authors' interpretation of a relationship between quality
of attachment and later competence.

CONCLUSIONS

The 1910s and 1920s witnessed an explosion of scientific knowledge
in the field of nutrition. A number of vitamins were isolated, the amounts
required for healthy physical development determined, and the foods
that could supply these needs identified. Similar information on the role
of other chemicals such as calcium and iron salts, and the physiological
requirements for carbohydrates, fats, and proteins also became available.

With this knowledge available to them, mothers were able to provide
fully adequate diets for their infants' physical needs. The results in terms
of improved child health and development were highly salutary. Unfortunately, for a host of mothers in the 1920s this knowledge was distorted into categorical prescriptions of rigid dietary requirements on a
daily basis from birth onward. Infants who could not get their full quota
of vitamins, calcium, or iron even for a few days, because of illness or
other special circumstances, were presumed to have been inevitably affected with respect to their future physical health and development. The
anxiety and guilt this produced in mothers was enormous. Fortunately,
as the years passed, further research established that nutritional requirements were flexible and that the newborn or young infant who suffered
from inadequate food intake could compensate later without permanent
damage. With these insights, mothers began to relax their preoccupa-
tions over their children's daily diets. By the mid-1950s, as we interviewed

mothers in our longitudinal studies, we found them consistently knowledgeable as to their children's dietary requirements, but unconcerned over temporary variations or special idiosyncratic food preferences of their youngsters.

Perhaps we are going through a similar developmental sequence with regard to a child's psychological needs. We know a great deal about the importance of a positive parent-child relationship. We know a great deal about many of the specific factors that promote or deter such a relationship, and how these factors in the child and in the parent interact in a mutually influential developmental sequence.[11] But just as the child's nutritional requirements can be met successfully with a wide range of individual variation, so can his psychological requirements. Once mothers can appreciate this, that the neonate separated from his mother is not permanently damaged by this experience as such, that the child whose signals are not always easy to understand is not doomed to an unhealthy parent attachment, that the infant who appears "insecure" with strangers is not necessarily suffering from poor mothering, they can perhaps relax and actually become better mothers. As we put it recently:

> As we grow from childhood to maturity, all of us have to shed many childhood illusions. As the field of developmental studies has matured, we now have to give up the illusion that once we know the young child's psychological history, subsequent personality and functioning is ipso facto predictable. On the other hand, we now have a much more optimistic vision of human development. The emotionally traumatized child is not doomed, the parents' early mistakes are not irrevocable, and our preventive and therapeutic intervention can make a difference at all age-periods.[10]

REFERENCES

1. Ainsworth, M. et al. (1978). *Patterns of Attachment*. Hillsdale, NJ: Lawrence Erlbaum.
2. Beiser, H. (1964). Discrepancies in the symptomatology of parents and children. *Journal of American Academy of Child Psychiatry*, 3:457–468.
3. Bell, R. (1968). A reinterpretation of the direction of effects in studies of socialization. *Psychological Review*, 75:81–95.
4. Bowlby, J. (1951). *Maternal Care and Mental Health*. Geneva: World Health Organization.
5. Brazelton, B. (1976). (As cited in *Maternal Infant Bonding*, M. Klaus and J. Kennell, eds. St. Louis: C. V. Mosby.)

6. Bretherton, I. (1978). Making friends with one-year-olds: An experimental study of infant-stranger interaction. *Merrill-Palmer Quarterly*, 24:29–51.
7. Bronfenbrenner, U. (1974). Developmental research, public policy, and the ecology of childhood. *Child Development*, 45:1–5.
8. Bruch, H. (1954). Parent education or the illusion of omnipotence. *American Journal of Orthopsychiatry*, 24:723–732.
9. Chess, S. (1978). The plasticity of human development. *Journal of American Academy of Child Psychiatry*, 17:80-91.
10. Chess, S. (1979). Development theory revisited. *Canadian Journal of Psychiatry*, 24: 101–112.
11. Chess, S., Thomas, A. and Birch, H. (1959). Characteristics of the individual child's behavioral responses to the environment. *American Journal of Orthopsychiatry*, 29:791–802.
12. Clarke, A. M. and Clarke, A. D. B. (1976). *Early Experience: Myth and Evidence*. London: Open Books.
13. Connolly, K. (1972). Learning and the concept of critical periods in infancy. *Developmental Medicine and Child Neurology*, 14:705–714.
14. Dixon, S. et al. (1981). Early infant social interaction with parents and strangers. *Journal of American Academy of Child Psychiatry*, 20:32–52.
15. Egeland, B. and Vaughn, B. (1981). Failure of "bond formation" as a cause of abuse, neglect and maltreatment. *American Journal of Orthopsychiatry*, 51:78–84.
16. Fraiberg, S. (1977). *Every Child's Birthright: In Defense of Mothering*. New York: Basic Books.
17. Freud, S. (1949). *An Outline of Psychoanalysis*. New York: Norton.
18. Garbarino, J. (1980). Changing hospital childbirth procedures. *American Journal of Orthopsychiatry*, 50:588–597.
19. Greenspan, S. and Lourie, R. Developmental structuralist approach to the classification of adaptive and pathologic personality organization: Infancy and early childhood. *American Journal of Psychiatry*, 138:728.
20. Hale, D. (1980). Multiple functions of proximity seeking in infancy. *Child Development*, 51:636–645.
21. Horner, T. (1980). The methods of studying stranger reactivity in infants: A review. *Journal of Child Psychology and Psychiatry*, 21:203–219.
22. Kagan, J. (1976). Resilience and continuity in psychological development. In *Early Experience: Myth and Evidence*. A. M. Clarke and A. D. B. Clarke, eds. London: Open Books.
23. Kennell, J. (1981). Personal communication.
24. Klatskin, E., Jackson, E. and Witkin, L. (1956). The influence of degree of flexibility in maternal child care practices on early child behavior. *American Journal of Orthopsychiatry*, 26:79–93.
25. Klaus, M. and Kennell J. (1977). *Maternal-Infant Bonding*. St. Louis: C. V. Mosby.
26. Lozoff, B. (1976). (As cited in *Maternal Infant Bonding*, M. Klaus and J. Kennell, eds. St. Louis: C. V. Mosby.)
27. MacFarlane, J. (1964). Perspectives on personality consistency and change from the guidance study. *Vita Humana*, 7:115–126.
28. McCall, R. (1977). Challenges to a science of developmental psychology. *Child Development*, 48:333–344.
29. Matas, L., Arend, R. and Sroufe, L. (1978). Continuity of adaptation in the second year: The relationship between quality of attachment and later competence. *Child Development*, 49:547–556.

30. Minde, K. et al. (1980). Some determinants of mother-infant interaction in the premature nursery. *Journal of American Academy of Child Psychiatry,* 19:1–21.
31. Murphy, L. and Moriarty, A. (1976). *Vulnerability, Coping and Growth.* New Haven, CN: Yale University Press.
32. Orlansky, H. (1949). Infant care and personality. *Psychological Bulletin,* 46:1–48.
33. Raph, J. et al. (1968). The influence of nursery school on social interactions. *American Journal of Orthopsychiatry,* 38:144–152.
34. Rheingold, H. and Eckerman, C. (1973). Fear of the stranger: A critical examination. In *Advances in Child Development and Behavior,* H. Rees, ed. New York: Academic Press.
35. Rutter, M. (1972). *Maternal Deprivation Reassessed.* Middlesex, England: Penguin Books.
36. Rutter, M. (1981). *Maternal Deprivation Reassessed,* Second Edition. Middlesex, England: Penguin Books.
37. Sameroff, A. (1975). Early influences on development: Fact or fancy. *Merrill-Palmer Quarterly,* 20:275–301.
38. Schaffer, H. and Emerson, P. (1964). The development of social attachments in infancy. *Monographs of the Society for Research in Child Development,* 29:3, 72.
39. Svejda, M., Campos, J and Emde, R. (1980). Mother-infant "bonding": Failure to generalize. *Child Development,* 51:775–779.
40. Thomas, A. and Chess, S. (1977). *Temperament and Development.* New York: Brunner/Mazel.
41. Thomas, A. and Chess, S. (1980). *The Dynamics of Psychological Development.* New York: Brunner/Mazel.
42. Vaillant, G. (1977). *Adaptation to Life.* Boston: Little, Brown.
43. Waters, E., Wippman, J. and Sroufe, L. (1979). Attachment, positive affect and competence in the peer group. *Child Development,* 50:821–829.
44. Waters, E. (1978). The reliability and stability of individual differences in infant-mother attachment. *Child Development,* 49:483–494.
45. Watson, J. (1928). *Psychological Care of the Infant and Child.* New York: Norton.
46. Weintraub, M. and Putney, E. (1978). The effects of height on infants' social responses to unfamiliar persons. *Child Development,* 49:598–603.
47. White, B. (1975). *The First Three Years of Life.* Engelwood Cliffs, NJ: Prentice Hall.
48. Wolff, P. (1970). Critical periods in human cognitive development. *Hospital Practice,* 11:77–87.

4

Mother-to-Infant "Bonding"

M. Herbert and W. Sluckin

Department of Psychology, University of Leicester

Alice Sluckin

Leicestershire Child and Family Guidance Service

INTRODUCTION

The literature in such fields as social work, pediatrics and child psychiatry has been replete over many years, with reports on parent-child relationships and their importance for many aspects of the child's development. It is said that foolish or reprehensible child-rearing practices, particularly on the part of the mother, and distortions in the formation of the mother's attachment to her offspring are responsible for various unsatisfactory aspects of the child's physical and psychological development. Child abuse, both physical and emotional, is often considered to be associated etiologically with a failure on the part of the mother to become "bonded" to her child (e.g., Vesterdal, 1976); this in turn is linked to the postpartum separation of mother and child (e.g., Klaus and Kennell, 1976).

The reasons for the concern of pediatricians, child psychiatrists and social workers are many-sided, but arise not least out of important policy issues of a preventive nature. It is claimed that there is a much higher proportion of prematurity and neonatal disease in abused children than

Reprinted with permission from the *Journal of Child Psychology and Psychiatry*, 1982, Vol. 23, No. 3, 205–221. Copyright 1982 by the Association for Child Psychology and Psychiatry.

We should like to acknowledge the help of Dr. David P. Davies of the Department of Child Health, University of Leicester, in providing the initial stimulation for the writing of this paper.

in the normal population (Lynch and Roberts, 1976; Smith, 1975). One of the explanations put forward to account for this association is maternal rejection which arises out of failure, disruption or distortion of the mother-to-infant bonding process (see Brimblecombe et al., 1978; Vesterdal, 1976).

The family is much extolled as the bedrock of stable society. Stability within the family is rooted in the mutual attachment of parents and offspring. The nature and conditions of attachment of children to adults have received a great deal of attention in the last three or four decades (e.g., Bowlby, 1951, 1969). Initially there was a good deal of speculation about the facilitation of a "tie" of an infant to its mother, something having an important bearing on the child's future mental health. Concern was expressed in the concept of maternal deprivation and its pathogenic influence on the development of the child. Some conjectures about the unidimensionality of attachment behavior, the existence of a critical period in infant-to-mother attachment, an exclusive role for the mother in the formation of a bond and the dangers of separation have been modified in the face of growing empirical evidence (Bowlby, 1969; Rutter, 1972; Schaffer, 1977). The other attachments, those of adults to children, have been less extensively explored. This has not prevented the concept of mother-to-infant bonding (or its failure) from attaining some of the clinical significance and emotive connotations which in the early days were associated with the infant-to-mother attachment construct (e.g., Sugarman, 1977; Valman, 1980).

It is, of course, by no means true that the bond of adults to children has been altogether ignored by scientists. Parental behavior, and especially maternal behavior, has for a long time been arousing much interest. The determinants, both genetic and environmental, of the mother's attachment to her offspring have been investigated quite extensively in infra-human mammals (e.g., Rheingold, 1963). With regard to the human species, as Svejda et al. (1980, p. 775) observed, the last ten years has seen a growing interest in the possibility that the development of mother-to-infant attachment (assessed by specific actions indicating affection for the infant) is influenced by biological factors: the mother needs to be, as it were, bonded to her infant; her affection for her infant is treated by some writers as something she has to acquire over a limited span of time after the infant's birth (e.g., Klaus and Kennell, 1976).

Mother-to-infant attachment (usually referred to as bonding) is inferred in the literature from highly specific aspects of maternal behavior such as gazing, vocalizing, smiling, touching, fondling, face presentations and other actions. Not only do these activities show somewhat low intercorrelations but they do not have any necessary link with the concept of specific bonding. Most normal women have a predilection to smile, touch and tickle other people's babies when they come into contact with them, despite the fact that in no sense are they specifically bonded to them. Bonding implies a special relationship, an enduring, affectionate and responsible attachment to a child. Thus, individuals are much more likely to undergo self-sacrifice for members of their own families than they are for complete strangers. However, bonding is a difficult concept to operationalize. It is one thing to talk about caregiver–infant interactions, but quite another to infer special qualities of caregiver–infant attachment relationship. What is of great concern to practitioners is that in some circumstances (fortunately, rather rare) parents fail to become attached in any meaningful sense to their offspring and may overtly reject them. The antecedents and consequences of such failures are poorly understood.

The so-called "infant-elicited social behaviors" mentioned above, do not appear to be performed naturally by extremely rejecting parents (Herbert, 1974). Stern (1977) demonstrates that these separate behaviors are generally elicited together in one "co-ordinated package" spontaneously, and almost at a level of unawareness, in most caregivers. The mother performs a facial display while vocalizing and while gazing, and within the framework of a discrete head movement coupled with face presentation.

Stern (1977, p. 32) makes the point that the question "why do babies elicit these behaviors?" raises all the problematical issues of innateness versus learning. "Whenever we see a set of behavior that is probably used by all societies in a particular natural human situation, and which has had thousands of generations of evolutionary history to fashion an adaptive purpose, we wonder to what extent the acquisition is built upon some biologically innate base." It is only too easy, when practitioners, unfamiliar with the theoretical and methodological intricacies of studying attachment behavior, conceptualize such complex phenomena, to subscribe to "biological explanations" such as innate tendencies and critical sensitive (as opposed to merely sensitive) periods because things "look that way." Indeed, the *surmise* that mother-to-infant attachment in human beings is established as a result of the mother's exposure to, and contact with, her infant directly after delivery derives to a great extent from animal studies.

It is this issue to which this paper is addressed, as well as the related one of attempting to clarify the meaning of the term "bonding," a concept much more problematic than its usage by some practitioners would seem to imply. Indeed, we are particularly concerned to explore the practical consequences of the bonding hypothesis—its implications for assessment and treatment in social work and clinical settings.

Before considering any investigations, animal or human, it will be helpful to look further at the criteria by which judgments of attachment, or lack of attachment, are made. One criterion may, of course, be the mother's own report of her feelings towards her child. Thus, she might be adjudged to be attached to her child if she consistently, over a number of months and years, reports that she loves her child. However, her deeds may well be thought to be more important than her words, and so attachment would be largely assessed in terms of her actions. By this token a mother would be considered to be "bonded" to her child if she looked after it well, gave it much attention and showed affection for it in the form of "fondling, kissing, cuddling, and prolonged gazing" (Klaus and Kennell, 1976). Such measures of attachment are, of course, not always easy to quantify and they are obviously dependent to some degree upon the investigator's interpretations of observed behavior. Most deal simply with the amounts of physical contact with the baby and it is by no means self-evident that this has got anything to do with specific bonding. Appropriate scales of features of attachment are needed, and scoring must be done by observers without any knowledge of the extent of mother–infant contact in the early days of the child's life. The investigator must be on guard against disregarding overt signs of attachment when he/she had already formed the belief that a particular mother is not genuinely "bonded" to her child; for in such circumstances, it is tempting to reject verbal assurances of love, as well as acts normally indicating maternal attachment, as misleading. Clearly, the assessment of maternal attachment is more problematic than might appear on the face of it. This is the case even in studies of maternal behavior in animals.

MATERNAL ATTACHMENT IN INFRA-HUMAN MAMMALS

Maternal behavior is generally directed primarily towards the mother's own or adopted infant(s), not towards just any infant. How does this special relationship develop? It has been said that the mother's early exposure to an infant—exposure during a sensitive period—results in an attachment or bond to that infant. It has been argued that some animals, such as goats, share this with the human species (Klaus and Kennell, 1976). In the case of goats, such rapid learning to recognize and accept their young has been called "maternal imprinting" (Klopfer et al., 1964; Klopfer and Gamble, 1966; Klopfer and Klopfer, 1968), a phenomenon quite separate from classical, filial imprinting (see, for example, Sluckin [1979] on filial imprinting in animals and the human species).

Goats and sheep are species closely related to each other. In an early study, newborn kids and lambs were separated from their mothers soon after birth for varying periods of time (Collias, 1956). When the separation period was up to 45 minutes, the young in each of the limited number of cases investigated was accepted by its mother. When the separation period was longer, then in most cases the young were afterwards rejected (butted away), that is, they were treated like alien young. Another study, using a sizeable sample of newborn kids, indicated that five to ten minutes of contact soon after birth was enough for the mother to learn the identity of her own offspring (Herscher et al., 1958). In a later research at Cornell University, Herscher et al. (1963a) investigated experimentally the adopting of ewes and she-goats of strange lambs and kids; cross-species adoptions were also studied. All such adoptions could occur only after some days of enforced proximity, but it is highly significant that stable adoptions could in this way be established (Hersher et al., 1963b).

Before long, "maternal imprinting" in goats began to receive a good deal of attention from P. H. Klopfer and his co-workers at Duke University in North Carolina. Initially, it looked as if separation at birth of a kid from its mother for as little as one hour resulted in a rejection of the kid by its mother. As little as five minutes of contact after birth prevented rejection, even after three hours of separation subsequent to this short-duration contact. Since smell rather than vision mattered as far as the contact was concerned, Klopfer et al. (1964) were inclined to regard the mother's attachment as olfactory imprinting. Further and more detailed studies, however, led Klopfer and Gamble (1966) to conclude that maternal behavior in goats could not be considered as being essentially rooted in olfactory imprinting. Nevertheless, mother goats did appear to rely on smell for the recognition of their own young. It was further reported by Klopfer and Klopfer (1968) that an alien kid, substituted for the mother's own after parturition and allowed five minutes with the adoptive mother, would come to be treated by the mother as if it were her own offspring. The view that Klopfer later expressed was that in the goat, mother-to-infant bonds are "stable, specific, and rapidly formed." He pointed out at the same time that this is not universally true of mammals. Mother-to-infant "ties need be neither very specific, nor rapidly formed, nor yet stable" (Klopfer, 1971).

Later investigations of the behavior of goats showed that even in that species, this so-called maternal imprinting "may not occur as rapidly as previously reported" (Gubernick et al., 1979). Using both pure-bred and mixed-breed goats, the investigators found that "mothers given five minutes post-partum contact with their own kid generally failed to discriminate later between own and alien young, unless aliens had been kept with their own mother for more than eight hours." A further and detailed report (Gubernick, 1980) shows that a mother-goat will accept any alien kid, provided that that kid has not been for too long with another mother. This seems to suggest that acceptability of kids to a mother depends not so much on maternal imprinting as on the absence of "labels" put on them by other mother-goats; the "labels" that evoke rejection behavior in a mother are presumably olfactory, that is, smells of other mother-goats. What is still unknown is "how much time a kid needs to be with its mother for that kid to be rejected by another mother and to be recognised by its own mother" (Gubernick, 1980).

The most recent experimental study by Gubernick (1981) confirms the earlier finding, namely that "maternal labelling in goats appears to be based upon cues passed from the mother to her kid by licking and through mother's milk." By such means, mother-goats recognize young as their own and reject young with "labels" provided by other she-goats. It is this mechanism which would appear to account for the maternal "bond," rather than any maternal imprinting with their offspring.

Even if rapid olfactory imprinting had been found to occur in mother sheep and goats (and this is not the case), it would have been of very doubtful relevance to any possible mother-to-infant bonding in primates, including the human species. Ungulates are born in a herd where there is strong selection pressure for rapid mother-infant recognition. Primates are, generally speaking, more like nidicolous species. They also rely less on olfaction in communication than do other mammalian families. Above all, it is clear that the determination of the existence of any quick mother-to-newborn bonding in primates must rest on properly evaluated empirical evidence for any of the primate species in question. Such evidence for infra-human primates is, in fact, conspicuously lacking. Even those who believe in human mother-to-infant bonding during a critical postpartum period acknowledge that "in monkeys, a separation immediately after birth for one hour does not seem to affect the female's interest in being near her neonate" (Klaus and Kennell, 1976, p. 138).

MATERNAL ATTACHMENT IN THE HUMAN SPECIES

We have seen that the belief in the rapid "bonding" of the mother to her newborn infant cannot readily be based on an appeal to work with animals. Clearly, what is needed is empirical evidence obtained specifically from studies of human mothers' relationships to their offspring. There are various issues to disentangle in the rather confusing literature in this field. With regard to maternal behavior in general, and to bonding in particular, there are the separate questions of the time over which this takes place (e.g., in infancy only or later in life) and the variables (e.g., physical contact) which facilitate the development of bonding. Let us, therefore, examine such evidence as is available.

Although the advocacy of attaching or "bonding" mothers to their newborn infants nowadays is widespread, the number of empirical studies relevant to this notion is quite small. One of them is the work of Leifer et al. (1972), who set out to investigate whether maternal behavior would be deleteriously affected by a temporary separation of the mother from her newborn infant. Three groups of mothers were studied: (1) those of full-term babies; (2) those of premature babies placed in an incubator and unhandled by their mothers for up to 12 weeks; and (3) those of premature babies that were to some extent handled by their mothers from the start. Subsequent mothering was observed in all cases, and it was found that mothers in the three groups behaved substantially alike towards their infants in all respects relevant to good mothering. Nothing emerged from this study that definitely showed any lasting disruption of normal maternal behavior in the "separation" group.

Klaus et al. (1972) did detect some differences in mothering behavior between women who had extended contact as compared with those who had no extended contact with their newborn infants. At one month after birth the early-contact mothers spent more time in eye contact with their babies and fondled them more during feeding than the others. The information that was then lacking concerned differences between the two groups during subsequent months, and therefore it remained uncertain whether lack of lasting "bonding" could be inferred from the behavior of the "non-contact" mothers.

In an attempt to study maternal behavior over a longer period, Kennell et al. (1974) followed up one year later the mothers in the study just mentioned. The mothers were on this occasion interviewed and observed in a number of different situations. "Contact" mothers differed from "non-contact" mothers in their answers to interview questions, and were also more helpful during the physical examination of the baby. Mother-infant interactions in the two groups did not differ in most situations, including an important one of mother–infant play. In the light of these reported findings, it is difficult to understand how any firm conclusions could be drawn about "bonding" taking place exclusively during the first hours and days of life.

Other studies which have been quoted in support of the hypothesis of rapid bonding during an early sensitive period are equally inconclusive. Some are clinical studies, involving very small numbers of mothers, which have never been published in research-reporting journals. Others, e.g., Ringler et al. (1975), are concerned with children's speech development, where it could not be inferred that retardation was due to the restrictions of the postpartum mother–infant contact rather than to a host of other factors. What is clear is that when authors have claimed that mother-to-infant bonding occurred, or failed to occur, in the early hours and days after birth (Klaus and Kennell, 1976; Sugarman, 1977), evidence was entirely inadequate.

More recently, further investigations seemed at first to lend support to the bonding hypothesis. Thus, Carlsson et al. (1978) found that contact between mother and infant for up to two hours immediately after birth facilitated the mother's feeding activity four days later. Whether the longer-term consequence of this was stronger mother-to-infant attachment remained entirely unproven. In addition, Hales and his co-researchers (Hales et al., 1977) reported that mothers given skin-to-skin contact with their infants immediately after delivery displayed significantly more affectionate behaviors at 36 hours than did control mothers. These findings were not confirmed by De Chateau and Wiberg (1977). Twenty-two primiparous mothers given extra skin-to-skin and suckling contact with their infants after delivery differed at 36 hours from a control group of primiparous and multiparous mothers receiving routine care, on only four out of 35 measured variables. There were no significant differences in maternal affectionate behaviors. Although *en face* and encompassing behaviors tended to occur more often in extra-contact mothers, the trend was not significant.

Carlsson et al. (1979) investigated 50 mother–infant pairs in order to ascertain the effects of various amounts of contact between mother and child on the mother's later nursing behavior; they found that at six weeks after delivery the nursing behaviors of the extended-contact and limited-contact groups were indistinguishable. As the authors say, their results are "somewhat surprising" in view of the previous reports by Klaus, Kennell and their associates of "persistent changes in the interaction of the mother and child as a result of extended contact immediately after birth." Schaller et al. (in press) also report that whereas "mothers with extended body contact with their babies immediately after delivery showed more tactual contacts with their newborn when observed during the first week after parturition than mothers who had been exposed to ordinary hospital routine, this group difference could not be observed five weeks later."

Svejda et al. (1980) list several problems in the attempt to draw conclusions from the literature on the influence of early contact on maternal
behavior: the absence of a clear link between some observed maternal
behaviors and the attachment (bonding) construct; the inconsistency of
effects across studies; and the modest magnitude of previous findings.
Svejda and her colleagues, with painstaking attention to methodological
and procedural controls, tested the hypothesis that early and enhanced
mother-infant contact facilitates maternal attachment behavior. They
used a double-blind experimental design, random assignment of 30
mother-and-infant pairs to contact conditions and response indices appropriate to the attachment construct. Fifteen healthy primiparous
mothers had the infants for one hour at delivery and 90 minutes at each
feeding. Another 15 were kept to the usual hospital routine for newly
delivered mothers: brief contact at delivery and 30 minutes at each
feeding. In order to minimize a feeling of "specialness" in extra-contact
mothers, mothers who were not in the study but who shared a room
with these mothers had their infants longer at each feeding so that this
apparent difference in contact time would be eliminated. No differences
in maternal behavior were obtained on 28 discrete response measures
or on pooled sets of individual measures (affectionate, proximity-main-
taining, caretaking and miscellaneous response-types).

What we have, then, is a situation in which one of the few carefully
controlled investigations in this area of research, such as the one just
described together with the recent Swedish studies, fail to lend reliable
support to the bonding hypothesis. In addition, there are many indications in the literature (see De Chateau, 1980) for the view that the
mother's attachment to her infant has to do with a variety of factors
other than short-duration postpartum contact. Jones et al. (1980) found
that, while extra contact made no difference to subsequent mothering
behavior, the age of primiparous mothers did. These researchers reported that "mothers nineteen years of age and older demonstrated
significantly more maternal responsiveness toward their infants than did
mothers eighteen years and younger." Robson and Kumar (1980) noted
that "maternal affection was more likely to be lacking after delivery, if
the mother had had a forwater amniotomy and had, in addition, either
experienced a painful and unpleasant labor or been given more than
125 mg of pethidine." This is, of course, not an unexpected finding.
What is also not unexpected is that Robson and Kumar found that three
months after giving birth "a mother was more likely to express feelings
of dislike or indifference towards her baby if she was clinically depressed
at that time."

It is clear that there are many pitfalls to which the assessment of maternal attachment and its sequelae are liable. Social class, for example, appears to be a significant factor in studies of maternal behavior as a function of postpartum contact between mother and child (see Robson, 1981). It is difficult to draw conclusions about the influence (or lack of one) of early contact on maternal behavior when investigations fail to control this variable. The work of Kennell and of Klaus, which is seminal in this area, has been criticized as having limited generality, because the research sample was weighted fairly heavily in the direction of lower socioeconomic class. In their investigations, and in others dealing with underprivileged mothers, effects tend to be discovered which do not manifest themselves so clearly in studies of middle-class families.

With regard to the question of whether bonding only occurs during infancy, or whether it can occur later, the answer lies in the extensive use by society of adoption. This idea of making use of adoption seems somewhat paradoxical given the importance attached to bonding in the caring process. Not only is there no "blood bond" between adoptive mother and the child, but she has missed out vital weeks, months and sometimes years of exposure to the youngster. Not surprisingly, there is nothing to suggest that adoptive parents are in any way inferior to natural parents. Tizard (1977) reported a study of children who had been in care throughout their early years; they were followed up on leaving care. One group of children was adopted, another returned to their own families. It was found that the latter did less well than the adopted children, both in the initial stages of settling in and in their subsequent progress. The reason lay primarily in the attitudes of the two sets of parents: the adoptive group worked harder at being parents, possibly just because the child was not their own.

BONDING AND DISTURBED MOTHER-CHILD RELATIONSHIPS

As mentioned earlier in the paper, several authors have asserted that separation of the mother and infant for several weeks immediately after birth may damage irreversibly the subsequent mother–child relationship. Additionally, it has often been claimed that mothers prone to baby battering are mothers who have not been bonded to their babies soon after delivery. Cater and Easton (1980) set out to check this claim. They investigated 80 cases of child abuse with particular reference to the separation of the abusing parents from their newborn infants. Although early separation of parent and infant was found to be common in the families under investigation, combinations of other stresses and conflicts were also much in evidence. It is the latter that were thought to have predisposed mothers towards baby battering. The authors do not argue that lack of contact with newborn infants has definitely nothing to do with subsequent battering, but they strongly advocate that, for practical purposes, "other stress factors which impair parent–child relationships must also be given attention as important antecedents of non-accidental injury—for example, unstable domestic arrangements, and psychiatric disturbance and immaturity in the parents."

Gaines et al. (1978) studied 240 mothers, drawn from known-abuse, neglect and normal control populations. The multivariate analysis included 12 variables, of which six discriminated the abusing, neglecting and normal mothers at a high level of significance. Infant risk, determined on the basis of neonatal complications requiring hospitalization, was not a successful discriminator. According to the authors, "the hypothesized relationship between mother-neonate bonding and maltreatment was not supported."

Collingwood and Alberman (1979) carried out a study of 32 separate low-birthweight babies and 32 controls specifically aimed at identifying any long-term effects on the mother–child relationship following separation at birth. They state that "the lack of a connection in this study between disturbed mother–child relationship and duration of stay in special care baby units raises the possibility that factors other than low-birthweight and neonatal separation contribute to disturbed mother–child relationships" (p. 614).

Assuming that one could reliably diagnose a failure of bonding, i.e., a failure of mother–child attachment, how much would it contribute to initiating an appropriate plan of action in a clinical setting? The value of a dignoastic term lies in its descriptive functions and its implications for etiology, treatment and prognosis. A label without implications would be somewhat pointless. How appropriate, then, is the concept of maternal bonding as an unqualified descriptive term for maternal behavior? Bonding is frequently used in the pediatric and social work literature and at case reviews, in a manner that is suggestive of the reification of the concept; it is made almost to sound like a mechanical thing. If successful, the mother is "tied" figuratively to her offspring. This mechanical model seems to suggest an all-or-nothing phenomenon. Yet there is no evidence that caring is really like that; it seems more likely to involve dimensional continua of facets of loving and nurturance. Most of the clinical discussions of bonding fail to take into account the formidable methodological problems of specifying precisely what such a global term means or, indeed, of assessing the significance and inter-relatedness of those component behaviors thought to be indices of bonding.

Dunn and Richards (1977) set out in a longitudinal study of 77 mother–child pairs (from birth to five years) to see if a number of categories of behaviors that have been used as indices of affection did indeed intercorrelate. Correlations between measures were not high and they were unable to demonstrate a unitary attribute reflecting "warm" mothering. The analysis of early feeding interaction indicated that measures of maternal affectionate behavior do not co-vary in any simple way. The different facets of maternal style are associated with different infant and delivery factors; success and coordination of the feed, for instance, are affected by labor and delivery variables; total sucking, for example, is correlated with differences in the infant's reactivity (latency to cry on removal of teat) and not with the measurement of affectionate style and contact. Touching the baby—often used as an index of maternal feeling—did not correlate with the other measures of maternal "affection." The baby was a vital contributor to the early differences in mother–child interaction.

In the case of infant-to-mother attachment, Ainsworth (1969) recommends the use of multiple criteria to describe the way in which such behavior is organized and manifested. No less should be demanded for mother-to-child attachment. However, the specification of the behaviors describing bonding remains problematic; when it is applied in practice as if it described a unitary phenomenon (i.e., used as if it simply means that a mother loves a child and feels it belongs to her and she to it), then it is of limited value in anticipating the risk of parental abuse, to which it is so often linked. Mothers who feel little or no affection or sense of belonging towards their offspring have been known to care meticulously (some theorists would say by way of compensation) for their welfare. Mothers who love their children have also been known to batter their children in moments of desperation and in situations arising from varied causes. However, we possess no actuarial estimates, based on survey data, of how many indifferent mothers (or mothers initially separated from their babies) do not abuse their children. Prediction in this area is a difficult exercise.

Leiderman and Seashore (1975), in a follow-up of mothers of premature and full-term infants, looked at the separation–contact variable. They examined data on maternal attitudes 12 months after discharge from hospital, caretaking behavior 11 months after discharge and the baby's mental and motor development 15 months after discharge. Throughout a two-year period of observations, interviews and tests were conducted at staggered intervals which permitted frequent contact with most of the initial group of 66 families. The premature sample was divided into a separation and a contact group; the full-term babies served as a comparison group. The researchers found that the manipulation of the independent variable (separation–contact) had little long-term effect on the mother's subsequent behavior and attitudes, and almost no effect on the infant's behavior and test performance. Mothers who were allowed early contact with their babies did touch them more when assessed one year later, but the sex and birth order of the infant, the socioeconomic status of the family and the baby's behavior were even more potent determinants of maternal behavior. Even when all these factors were taken into consideration, only 40%, and in some cases much less, of the total variance in the mother's behavior is accounted for, leaving a lot of room for other variables not included in the study. Whiten (1977) has demonstrated, in his study of the effects of perinatal events, that it is extremely difficult to arrive at a sensitive and objective description of those features of mother–infant interaction which are important in terms of their significance or prominence in the everyday life of the mother and baby.

The global assessments of such independent variables as parental warmth, hostility, rejection and others which have figured in the indexing of bonding or its absence are too abstract and coarse to capture many of the subtle nuances of maternal behavior. They do not specify the variations in behavioral interactions between parents and infants which occur in *particular* situations, and which are necessary to define precise relationships between independent and dependent variables. Nor do they reflect the releasing effect of the child and his personality.

Dunn (1975) found continuities over time which she concludes are best described in terms of interactional styles rather than of exclusively maternal behavior. It was not possible to assume that a correlation between measures of maternal responsiveness is independent of infant characteristics. It is a point frequently overlooked by practitioners that measures of mother–infant interaction described in the literature refer to mother–infant relationship and not specifically to either mother– or infant behavior.

The notion of a sensitive period for the development of attachments (bonds) is supposedly an ethological explanation; it seems to suggest that bonding behavior is species specific and relatively uninfluenced by the previous experience and state of the mother or her expectations and cultural values. It is our strong impression that disproportionate weight is often given to the influence of these periods of separation, while the consideration of the influence of other potentially important variables tends to be neglected. Robson and Kumar (1980), in a prospective study of 112 primiparous and 41 multiparous women, found that approximately 40% of the former and 25% of the latter recalled that their predominant reactions when holding their babies for the very first time had been one of emotional indifference. For most women, these feelings of indifference dissipated within a few days. The following variables (in addition to factors mentioned earlier in this paper) were found to be associated with a delayed onset of maternal affection: separation from own father before the age of 11 years; "masculine" score on a projective test; lack of prior experience of looking after babies; higher negative self-reports about being pregnant and about somatic symptoms; and not perceiving the foetus as a person by 36 weeks ante-natally. At three months post-natally there was some association between early reported maternal feelings and the way a mother now said she felt about her baby. There was also a marked association between initial indifference and negative reports on an "attitude to baby scale" throughout the whole of the first postpartum year. There appeared to be no association, however, between initial maternal feelings for the neonate and later breast-feeding problems, maternal post-natal depression or reported maternal aggression towards the babies.

Of course, it could be argued that studies of normal samples may not be relevant to the considerations of the extreme deviant maternal behavior. This is unlikely to be picked up in any ordinary sized sample of the general population. There is a vast differences between the fantasy or impulse to batter one's child—not an uncommon one—and the actual realization of the impulse. And it could be argued that there is a world of difference between the patchy indifference of many mothers and the inclusive neglect, rejection and hostility of the relatively few who batter their infants; but these matters still await clarification. Nevertheless, given that factors such as the ones enumerated by Robson and Kumar (1980) are known to be important determinants of the mother's attitudes and actions, the emphasis on a sensitive period in mother–infant contact as a major independent variable producing "bonding" gives rise to several implications which need to be thought through.

PRACTICAL CONSEQUENCES OF THE "BONDING HYPOTHESIS": INTERVENTION/TREATMENT IMPLICATIONS

The notion that particular events at a critical time make a mother uniquely capable of caring (in various senses of the word) for her child raises some questions about the institutions of adoption and fostering, about hospital management of intensive-care units for premature babies and many other practical issues.

In our experience, a question often raised at case conference discussions is the irreversibility of early separations and the damage done to attachment systems. With regard to infant-to-mother attachment, an attitude of therapeutic nihilism has been created in the minds of many workers by the concept of fixed and irreversible attributes (e.g., the postulated link between early deprivation and the later delinquent behavior). Clarke and Clarke (1976), having reviewed the available evidence, come to the conclusion that, at present, valid scientific knowledge is still lacking; indeed, dogmatic statements about long-term effects of early experience are entirely misplaced. Nevertheless, they have been able to identify certain consistencies in the research findings; there is little reason to suppose that infant learning occurs more easily than later learning; and the long-term effects of short, traumatic incidents seem to be relatively slight, both in animals and in young human beings. The specific effects of a child's experience before seven months of age appear to be of a very short duration. Yet, in relation to mother-to-infant attachment, we now have a concept of a short sensitive period for the acquisition of long-lasting, complex, attitudinal and behavioral tendencies in adult females; as indicated earlier, there is no empirical evidence to support this.

Tredinnick and Fairburn (1980) conducted a nation-wide survey to look more closely at the practice of compulsorily *ordering* the removal of children from their mothers before or after birth. The practice is said to be on the increase in cases where other children in the family have been battered or killed. The local authority can apply for a place-of-safety order before birth, but a care order must be applied for within six weeks of birth. However, in some cases there has been failure to get a care order granted on a baby removed at birth. The authors are perturbed that in such cases "the bonding stage between mother and baby has been disallowed" and claim that the parents have been placed into a position of disadvantage "by denying the chance of 'bonding' and attachment experience now that we see more clearly how this starts off the good parenting sequence. . . ."

In the paper by Tredinnick and Fairburn (1980), and several others, runs the assumption that once a separation at birth has occurred, rehabilitation of the mother–child relationship can only be undertaken with difficulty. One social worker quoted goes as far as saying that once the baby has been removed from the mother and the "bonding process" is disrupted, adoption should take place as a matter of course. Looking at it from the point of view of the parents, the view is taken that by separating mother and child at birth, the ground is cut from under the parents' feet, "for they can justifiably argue that they have been allowed only limited bonding."

Tredinnick and Fairburn provide an excellent survey of some of the ethical or legal issues in this fraught area of decision-making. It is the opinion of the present authors that preventive child-care action and the rehabilitation of parent–child relationships is hindered rather than helped by introducing the bonding concept, in so far as it is tied to the critical period immediately after birth. Also, mother/baby units are suggested as the only viable method of rehabilitation, though it has been found that many referred mothers are unable or unwilling to cooperate within such settings. Adhering rigidly to the concept of "bonding failure" may interfere with the precise assessment of the mother's limitations —which, more often than not, have roots in her past (e.g., Frommer and O'Shea, 1973; Lynch and Roberts, 1977)—the intrinsic difficulties of temperament in the child (Herbert, 1981) and many other potentially significant contemporary controlling factors.

The problem for (say) the field social worker is that the pseudoexplanatory properties of the term "bonding" may inhibit the painstaking thought and analysis required when she is assessing a child in the context of a family with complex social and emotional problems in all of its members. Encountering what she perceives to be failure of bonding, the social worker is likely to link it etiologically to the child's difficulties and thereby be deterred from assessing precisely, in behavioral terms, where and when, and in what situations it occurs (Herbert, 1981). Fortunately, the literature on bonding does not seem to inhibit the use of fostering placements and adoption by social workers. Presumably, they work to an empirical assumption, based on past experience, that enduring bonds of love and concern develop in many of the surrogate parents who take on other people's offspring.

Of course, the hard-pressed social worker cannot afford to be as complacent as the scientist in risking Type II errors, i.e., denying relationships which actually exist, because of a cautious attitude to evidence. While it may be understandable that she errs on the side of making Type I errors (asserting relationships falsely) in a fraught area like child abuse, the implications of Type I errors may also be damaging to clients. Interventions which, at best, are ineffectual, at worst, harmful, may be the cost.

The practical consequences of the bonding concept for hospital policy have been both beneficial and harmful. In the U.K. and the U.S.A. more than 90% of all babies are separated after birth for at least brief periods. More prolonged separations are likely if the baby has to receive special care—an eventuality affecting some 14% of all British babies. With regard to the benign consequences, the policy ramifications of bonding may have mitigated the "costs" of the improved physical care by pediatricians of ill and low-birthweight infants, that cost being the separation of babies in intensive-care units. Mothers are encouraged to interact with their babies in many units. In the past, of course, maternity hospital routine tended to be rigid and mothers were separated from their infants for long periods—and not always for good reason. The bonding concept seems to have had the effect of humanizing maternity hospitals and has given mothers and fathers access to their babies (just as Bowlby's initial claims of irreversible damage, which he subsequently revised, brought about unrestricted visiting of children in hospital).

Among the less desirable effects of the bonding ideology is the attitude of those nurses who entertain rigid expectations of how a good mother should behave toward her baby. The emphasis on bonding could lead to the harassment of mothers who need time to adapt to their babies and who do not manifest the "correct" responses and responsiveness. Pressure tends to be counterproductive as, for example, happened at one time when maternity nurses became fervent advocates of breast-feeding; then, mothers who were not succeeding were made to feel failures and arrived home from hospital feeling depressed and resentful.

CONCLUSIONS

There appear to be no indications from animal studies, and seemingly no evidence from human studies, that directly support the theory that there is a brief optimal time after delivery during which the mother is able to form an attachment to her infant. Harlow (1971) suggests that mother-love in humans develops over a period of several months. Certainly, the notion of a critical period for the acquisition of a complex set of emotions, attitudes and behaviors in females must be unprecedented in the psychological literature on the human adult's behavior repertoire. Furthermore, it is difficult to comprehend the biological utility or social survival value of a situation in which difficulties of adjustment during the often exhausting, depressing days following labor and delivery had long-term consequences for the mother–child relationship. Dunn (1975) carried out a longitudinal study of 70 mother–baby pairs, the observations being recorded at various intervals over a 30-week time-span; apart

from demonstrating the extreme difficulty of basing predictions of future relationships on the early mother–infant interaction, Dunn concludes that the absence of a correlation between coordination measures
from the early feeds and the later consistent maternal measures "suggests
that the postpartum period, rather than being a sensitive period, may
be a time when the relationship between the mother and baby is buffered
against difficulties of adjustment" (p. 169).

She adds that it would make sense in adaptational terms if problems
of adjustment did not have long-term sequelae. Her findings suggest
that it may take three or four weeks for mother and infant to settle to
a characteristic pattern. Given the importance attached by some practitioners to finding ways of assessing mother–child relationships for potential difficulties such as child abuse, it may be more valid to look for
indices of adjustment at this later stage.

As Richards (1975) puts it: "The idea of separation does not in itself
constitute a psychological theory—it merely describes a particular state
of affairs" (p. 25). What we do know about the interactions of mothers
and their babies in the early postpartum days is that there is an immense
range of individual differences in their coordination and smoothness.
We still lack evidence about the long-term implications of these early
differences—for mother and baby pairs who remain together from birth
onwards, as well as for pairs separated for varying periods of time.
Without hard evidence about the former group it is not possible to be
sure whether qualitative differences in the early adjustment and interaction may have significant consequences for the evolving relationship,
even when mother and infant are not separated.

Although the cry for more research is a valid one, the difficulties of
testing the hypothesis that early separation has long-term consequences
are awesome. As mothers, these days, are not usually separated from
their neonates without justifiable reasons, it is almost impossible to make
up separation and nonseparation groups that are comparable in all other
respects.

Leiderman and Seashore (1975) comment on the implications for intervening in the cases of "at risk" premature infants. They do not deny
that separation in the newborn period may have an effect. But it is
probably nonspecific, acting through the family as a stress that creates
disequilibrium in the nuclear family structure. There was a suggestion
in their findings that some fathers could be affected, as were some
mothers, by the separation. The point being made by these authors is
that an allegedly ethological model of a sensitive period is not the most
parsimonious one for explaining the development of the mother-infant

relationship. "The specific behaviors that are acquired in the newborn period under conditions of high saliency, such as those in the newborn nursery, are, over time, supplemented and amended by the usual principles of learning. Thus, we would suggest that the most reasonable explanation for the maternal behaviors observed in this study is one that emphasizes cultural, social and experiential influences on the mother —influences that are modified according to well-known principles of social learning" (p. 230). The authors state that regardless of whether one adopts a learning theory or an ethological model, it should be apparent that an opportunity exists for rapid learning in the nursery during the newborn period. The nursery situation can therefore be utilized to encourage specific kinds of behavior, in both mothers and fathers, that might serve to enhance subsequent familial relationships and the cognitive development of the infant. Richards (1975, p. 26) comments on the extensive empirical evidence concerning the mother's self-confidence. As he puts it:

> The more contact she has, and perhaps even more importantly, the more responsibility she is allowed for the care of her child, the sooner the mother becomes self-confident and assured about her ability to look after the baby. Such a factor might be especially vital after the birth of a low-birth-weight baby because many mothers seem to feel that a premature birth implies a failure on their part to carry a pregnancy successfully, and their confidence is often particularly damaged. Another way in which separation could influence a mother is by giving her an implicit model of how she should care for the baby. If she does not see her baby for a day or so after delivery and then only at a brief feed each four hours (as is not unusual in American hospitals) the mother may then leave the hospital with the idea that this is the natural and expected pattern of the relationship which she should continue when she gets home. After all the hospital is run by pediatric and obstetric experts so it is reasonable for her to conclude that the pattern of contact laid down there is what modern science has "proved" to be best. Most mothers could hardly be expected to analyze the situation and conclude, as some social scientists have done, that the hospital routine is a product of the institutional structure and the convenience of doctors and nurses and has very little to do with the interest of either mother or baby.

We need to know a great deal more about the factors which are conducive to "normal" mothering in order to intervene most effectively in difficult situations. What we do know suggests that a pessimistic view of the irreversibility of early events or a nihilistic therapeutic stance with regard to mother-to-infant attitudes and behavior are both misplaced.

SUMMARY

The concept of maternal "bonding," i.e., rapid mother-to-neonate attachment, appears frequently in psychiatric, pediatric and social work discussions of childhood psychopathology and child abuse. "Bonding" is used as a diagnostic concept, and one which has to bear the weight of important explanatory, descriptive and predictive statements. In turn, it is related etiologically to postpartum contact and separations of mother and infant. The authors present a critical review of the concept, exploring its empirical basis, and the implications (logical and illogical) that flow from its application in practice. They conclude that the usage of the term "bonding" is often misleading, because of a tendency to reify and simplify attachment phenomena; in addition, there are no indications from animal investigations and no evidence from human studies which directly support the notion of a "sensitive period" in the formation of mother-to-infant attachments. They also describe the negative and pessimistic implications of using this concept in social work and clinical practice. Alternative ways of conceptualizing these early parent–child events are suggested.

REFERENCES

Ainsworth, M. D. S. (1969). Object relations, dependency and attachment: A theoretical review of the infant–mother relationship. *Child Development,* 40:969–1025.

Bowlby, J. (1951). *Maternal Care and Mental Health.* Geneva: World Health Organization.

Bowlby, J. (1969). *Attachment and Loss,* Vol. I. London: Hogarth Press.

Brimblecombe, F. S. W., Richards, M. P. M. and Robertson, N. R. C. (Eds.) (1978). *Separation and Special Care Baby Unit. Clinics in Developmental Medicine.* London: S.I.M.P.

Carlsson, S. G., Fagenberg, H., Horneman, G., Hwang, C.-P., Larsson, K., Rodholm, M., Schaller, J., Danielsson, B. and Gundewall, C. (1978). Effects of amount of contact between mother and child on the mother's nursing behavior. *Developmental Psychobiology,* 11:143–150.

Carlsson, S. G., Fagenberg, H., Horneman, G., Hwang, C.-P., Larsson, K., Rodholm, M., Schaller, J., Danielsson, B. and Gundewall, C. (1979). Effects of various amounts of contact between mother and child on the mother's nursing behavior: A follow-up study. *Infant Behavior Development,* 2:209–214.

Cater, J. I. and Easton, P. M. (1980). Separation and other stress in child abuse. *Lancet,* ii:972–974.

Clarke, A. M. and Clarke, A. D. B. (1976). *Early Experience: Myth and Evidence*. London: Open Books.

Collias, N. E. (1956). The analysis of socialization of sheep and goats. *Ecology*, 37:228–239.

Collingwood, J. and Alberman, E. (1979). Separation at birth and the mother–child relationship. *Developmental Medicine and Child Neurology*, 21:608–617.

De Chateau, P. (1980). Parent-neonate interaction and its long-term effects. In *Early Experiences and Early Behavior*, E. C. Simmel, ed. New York: Academic Press.

De Chateau, P. and Wiberg, B. (1977). Long-term effect on mother–infant behavior of extra contact during the first hours postpartum: Follow-up at three months. *Acta Paediatrica, Stockholm*, 66:145–151.

Dunn, J. F. (1975). Consistency and change in styles of mothering. In *Parent–Infant Interaction, CIBA Foundation Symposium*, Vol. 33, pp. 155–176. Amsterdam: Elsevier-Excerpta Medica—North Holland.

Dunn, J. B. and Richards, M. P. M. (1977). Observations on the developing relationship between mother and baby in the neonatal period. In *Studies in Mother–Infant Interaction,*. H. R. Schaffer, ed. London: Academic Press.

Frommer, E. A. and O'Shea, G. (1973). Antenatal identification of women liable to have problems in managing their infants. *British Journal of Psychiatry*, 123:149–156.

Gaines, R., Sandgrund, A., Green, A. H. and Power, E. (1978). Etiological factors in child maltreatment: A multivariate study of abusing, neglecting, and normal mothers. *Journal of Abnormal Psychology*, 87:531–540.

Gubernick, D. J. (1980). Maternal "imprinting" or maternal "labelling" in goats? *Animal Behavior*, 28:124–129.

Gubernick, D. J. (1981). Mechanism of maternal "labelling" in goats. *Animal Behavior*, 29:305–306.

Gubernick, D. J., Jones, K. C. and Klopfer, P. H. (1979). Maternal "imprinting" in goats? *Animal Behavior*, 27:314–315.

Hales, D. J., Lozoff, B., Sosa, R. and Kennell, J. H. (1977). Defining the limits of the maternal sensitive period. *Developmental Medicine and Child Neurology*, 19:454–461.

Harlow, H. F. (1971). *Learning to Love*. San Francisco: Albion.

Herbert, M. (1974). *Emotional Problems of Development in Children*. London: Academic Press.

Herbert, M. (1981). *The Behavioural Treatment of Problem Children: A Practice Manual*. London: Academic Press.

Hersher, L., Moore, A. U. and Richmond, J. B. (1958). Effect of postpartum separation of mother and kid on maternal care in the domestic goat. *Science*, 128:1342–1343.

Hersher, L., Richmond, J. B. and Moore, A. U. (1963a). Modifiability of the critical period for the development of maternal behavior in sheep and goats. *Behavior*, 20:311–320.

Hersher, L., Richmond, J. B. and Moore, A. U. (1963b). Maternal behavior in sheep and goats. In *Maternal Behavior in Mammals*, H. L. Rheingold, ed. New York: Wiley.

Jones, F. A., Green, V. and Krauss, D. R. (1980). Maternal responsiveness of primiparous mothers during the postpartum period: Age differences. *Paediatrica*, 65:579–584.

Kennell, J. H., Jerauld, R., Wolfe, H., Chester, D., Kreger, N., McAlpine, W., Steffa, M. and Klaus, M. H. (1974). Maternal behavior one year after early and extended postpartum contact. *Developmental Medicine and Child Neurology*, 16:172–179.

Klaus, M. H., Jerauld, R., Kreger, N., McAlpine, W., Steffa, M. and Kennell, J. H. (1972). Maternal attachment—importance of the first postpartum days. *New England Journal of Medicine*, 286: 460–463.

Klaus, M. H. and Kennell, J. H. (1976). Parent-to-infant attachment. In *Recent Advances in Paediatrics*, Vol. 5. D. Hull, ed. London: Churchill Livingstone.

Klopfer, P. H. (1971). Mother love: What turns it on. *American Scientist*, 59:404–407.

Klopfer, P. H., Adams, D. K. and Klopfer, M. S. (1964). Maternal imprinting in goats. *Proceedings of the National Academy of Science, U.S.A.*, 52:911–914.

Klopfer, P. H. and Gamble, J. (1966). Maternal imprinting in goats: The role of chemical senses. *Z. Tierpsychol,*. 23:588–592.

Klopfer, P. H. and Klopfer, M. S. (1968). Maternal imprinting in goats: Fostering of alien young. *Z. Tierpsychol,*. 25:862–866.

Leiderman, P. H. and Seashore, M. J. (1975). Mother–infant separation: Some delayed consequences. In *Parent-Infant Interaction. CIBA Foundation Symposium,* Vol. 33. Amsterdam: Elsevier-Excerpta Medica—North Holland.

Leifer, A. D., Leiderman, P. H., Barnett, C. R. and Williams, J. A. (1972). Effect of mother–infant separation on maternal attachment behavior. *Child Development,* 43:1203–1218.

Lynch, M. and Roberts, J. (1976). Child abuse—early identification in the maternity hospital. *Transactions 1st International Congress on Child Abuse and Neglect, Geneva.* Vol. 13, pp. 759–766.

Lynch, M. A., and Roberts, J. (1977). Predicting child abuse: Signs of bonding failure in the maternity hospital. *British Medical Journal,* 1:624–626.

Rheingold, H. L. (Ed.) (1963). *Maternal Behavior in Mammals.* New York: Wiley.

Richards, M. (1975). Early separation. In *Child Alive: New Insights into the Development of Young Children.* R. Lewin, ed. London: Temple Smity.

Ringler, N. M., Kennell, J. H., Jarvella, R., Novojosky, B. and Klaus, M. H. (1975). Mother-to-child speech at two years—effects of early postnatal contacts. *Behav. Paediat.,* 86:141–144.

Robson, K. M. (1981). A study of mothers' emotional reactions to their newborn babies. Unpublished Ph.D. dissertation, University of London.

Robson, K. M. and Kumar, R. (1980). Delayed onset of maternal affection after childbirth. *British Journal of Psychiatry,* 136:347–353.

Rutter, M. (1972). Parent–child separation: Effects on the children. *Journal of Child Psychology and Psychiatry,* 6:71–83.

Schaffer, H. R. (Ed.) (1977). *Studies in Mother–Infant Interaction.* London: Academic Press.

Schaller, J., Carlsson, S. G. and Larsson, K. (In press). Effect of extended post-partum mother–child contact on the mother's behavior during nursing. *Infant Behavior and Development.*

Sluckin, W. (1979). Imprinting and the young child. In *Modern Perspectives in the Psychiatry of Infancy,* J. G. Howells, ed. New York: Brunner/Mazel.

Smith, S. M. (1975). *The Battered Child Syndrome.* London: Butterworth.

Stern, D. (1977). *The First Relationship: Infant and Mother.* London: Fontana/Open Books.

Sugarman, M. (1977). Paranatal influence on maternal–infant attachment. *American Journal of Orthopsychiatry,* 47:407–421.

Svejda, M. J., Campos, J. J. and Emde, R. N. (1980). Mother–infant "bonding": Failure to generalize. *Child Development,* 51:775–779.

Tizard, B. (1977). *Adoption: A Second Chance.* London: Open Books.

Tredinnick, A. and Fairburn, A. (1980). Left holding the baby. *Community Care,* 310:22–25.

Valman, H. B. (1980). The first year of life: Mother–infant bonding. *British Medical Journal,* 280:308–310.

Vesterdal, J. (1976). Psychological mechanisms in child abusing parents. In *Child Abuse: Commission and Omission,* J. V. Cook and R. T. Bowles, eds. Toronto: Butterworth.

Whiten, A. (1977). Assessing the effects of perinatal events in the success of the mother–infant relationship. In *Studies in Mother–Infant Interaction,* H. R. Schaffer, ed. London: Academic Press.

5

A Chinese Perspective on Kohlberg's Theory of Moral Development

Dora Shu-Fang Dien

California State University, Hayward

This essay uses the Chinese culture as an example to underline the culturally specific contextual problems regarding Kohlberg's theory of moral development and to point to a new direction for cross-cultural research in this area. The Western view of man as an autonomous being who makes free and rational choices as a moral agent is clearly reflected in Kohlberg's stages of moral development as well as his methodology. The Confucian view of man as an integral part of an orderly universe with an innate moral sense to maintain harmony is quite different. Further, the preferred mode of resolving human conflict in China is reconciliation and collective decision making rather than individual choice, commitment, and responsibility as in the West. In the light of these fundamental differences in the two cultural traditions, an alternative to Kohlberg's theory is suggested.

Historian John Fairbank (1980), one of the West's leading authorities on China, recently observed that the Chinese "seem to be law-abiding without law" because the doctrine of Confucianism serving as a system of ethics "had the effect of producing a socialized people who had a sense of individual duties and limits. . . . China did not develop a doctrine of civil liberties and individual rights in the same way as the modern West," but they have a "profound moral sense of justice and proper conduct inherited from Confucianism" (p. 12). Such a fundamental dif-

Reprinted with permission from *Developmental Review*, 1982, Vol. 2, 331–341. Copyright 1982 by Academic Press, Inc.

ference between China and the West must have far-reaching implications of Kohlberg's theory of moral development when "the dilemmas presented to the subjects are designed to place obedience to authority and law in opposition to individual rights and human welfare" (Rosen, 1980, p. 66).

Based upon Piaget's (1965) conception of the moral judgment of the child, Kohlberg (1969) elaborated six stages of moral reasoning, from an obedience and punishment orientation to self-accepted moral principles, which are held to be developmentally fixed, invariant, and universal. This hierarchy of moral reasoning has been to a certain extent substantiated cross-nationally. However, "the rate and terminus of moral development is highly variable from one cultural setting to another. Individuals in highly industrialized settings seem to move through the lower stages at a more rapid rate and to achieve higher stages than do individuals in less industrialized and less urban settings" (White, Bushnell, and Regnemer, 1978, p. 59). Even within the United States, children of high socioeconomic background develop more rapidly along the sequence and are more likely to attain higher levels of moral judgment" (Hetherington & Parke, 1979, p. 613). As a matter of fact, Stage 4 (authority and social-order maintaining orientation) seems to be the dominant mode of moral reasoning among urban middle-class American adults (Rosen, 1980, p. 67). Kohlberg acknowledges that Stage 6 (conscience or principle orientation) is a rare occurrence; probably only 5% of American adults ever achieve this level (Rosen, 1980, p. 93). Nevertheless, he continues to assert that the "principled morality" based upon our conception of justice is a "culturally universal" stage of moral judgment (Kohlberg, 1980, p. 74) and that "justice is a naturalistic virtue, emerging in children (at differing rates and with differing points of final equilibration) in all cultures as a result of their interaction with other persons and with social institutions" (Fowler, 1980, p. 130).

This assertion of the universality of the stage sequence has been severely criticized by Simpson (1974) as well as Kurtines and Grief (1974). The latter even recommended the wholesale abandonment of Kohlberg's theory. Nevertheless, most researchers have accepted the validity of at least the earlier stages while finding the upper half or third of the stages problematic (Murphy and Gilligan, 1980). What has been overlooked is that even though the stage progression at the lower levels has been found cross-culturally, there may still be qualitative differences in the responses classified within the same stage. Gorsuch and Barnes (1973), for example, found in their study of the Black Caribs of British Honduras that the respondents "seemed to express a real concern with helping others, as concern seldom found in stage 2s in the United States. They were concerned not because of a moral norm within the culture, but because they could reasonably expect to have the favor returned to them. Another element that made these 2s distinctive was that the possible violations of norms were not perceived as a live option because group pressure would be immediately applied" (p. 297). The authors further pointed out that because of a strong collectivistic orientation in their culture, some respondents could not relate to the dilemmas at all. They therefore suggested that "these moral dilemmas were insufficient to catch the nuances of this culture's thinking, and might also imply that a different set of 'stages' or typologies of moral reasoning might be developed in collectivistically oriented cultures" (p. 298). The present author believes that even among the so-called "collectivistic" societies, there may be enough diversity to warrant closer scrutiny into the culturally specific contextual differences. We will use the Chinese culture as an example to highlight this point and to suggest a new approach to this area of research.

TWO CONCEPTIONS OF MORALITY

The Judeo-Christian religious tradition holds that God is the creator of all things and that the act of creation is not something that God had to do but rather it was a completely free act. Furthermore, man is said to be made in the image of God, therefore, he "somehow possesses a freedom which resembles the freedom by which God creates." Thus the idea that man has freedom of self-determination is inherent in this tradition, though "the Bible always assumes that the fulfillment of divine commands will work for man's Good" (Grisez and Shaw, 1974, p. xi).

Greek philosophers, on the other hand, developed conceptions for judgments of moral good and moral evil, of right and wrong, based upon reasoning in accordance with the requirement of human nature. Rationality became the key to the definition of morality in Western philosophy. Thus when animals act instinctively to save human lives, they are not seen as acting morally. By the same token, the undesirable behaviors of the insane, senile, or brain damaged are not considered immoral because they lack the moral reasoning faculty (Sapontzis, 1980).

Deriving from these two traditions is the idea that man is an autonomous being, free to make his own choices and to determine his own destiny. As a moral agent, he has to take the responsibility for his actions. Existential philosophers in the West believe that while freedom characterizes the human condition, it brings with it the anguish of taking the responsibility for making individual choices (Sartre, 1966) and the feeling of overwhelming loneliness while doing so (Moustakas, 1961). We admire indomitable individuals who fulfill their human condition by exercising their responsibility for making decisions according to their beliefs and principles.

Despite his claim for universality, Kohlberg's six-stage hierarchy that progresses from an obedience and punishment orientation to a conscience or principle orientation clearly reflects this cultural ideal. Simpson (1974) believes that "Kohlberg's stage 6s are not functioning independently of their socialization; they have been very thoroughly socialized into the company of intellectual elites who value and practice analytic, abstract, and logical reasoning" (p. 95). In a study of forms of intellectual and ethical development during the college years at Harvard, Perry (1968) also identified a developmental progression from reliance on authority to individual choice, commitment, and responsibility, and he attributed this to the impact of our liberal arts education. Thus, the conclusions drawn by Perry may suggest a cultural bias in the formulation of Kohlberg's scheme.

In China, the Confucian conception of morality has been the cultural ideal held by the educated elite but it permeates through the lower classes "because of a constant 'trickling down' and a constant, centuries-long process of indoctrination of the lower classes by the elite" (Eberhard, 1971, p. ix). This is most effective through public education as we can see in Taiwan. Although Socialist China has rejected Confucianism as archaic and feudalistic, there are strong similarities between Maoist and Confucian conception of man, in particular, the importance of character molding and the minimizing of any distinction between a private and a public domain (Munro, 1977). Thus in reality, we find close resemblance between the observed behaviors of school children in Taiwan (Wilson, 1970) and those on mainland China (Kessen, 1975).

The Confucians believe that there is a "common principle of order running through heaven, earth, and human society" (Munro, 1969, p. 39). They see the universe as moral, with a design exhibiting justice and goodness. It is man's responsibility to interpret the signals of nature's way and act accordingly. Rules of conduct are integrally parallel to the ways of nature; therefore, morality is absolute and universal. This view has dominated the Chinese value system for such a long time that the belief that "society cannot function unless the individual relinquishes some of his freedoms" has become one of the three major organizing principles of the Chinese society (Eberhard, 1971, p. 1). The individual is expected to subordinate his own identity to the interest of the group.

As part of the scheme of things, human beings are believed to be born with certain innate moral tendencies whose preservation and cultivation insure a harmonious social order. Ignoring the proper rules of conduct results in chaos. The most important of these moral tendencies is *jen*. The character *jen* combines the symbol for man and the symbol for two, and is pronounced exactly like the word for man. It has been variously translated as "love," "benevolence," "human-heartedness," "man-to-manness," "sympathy," and "perfect virtue." It is basically the deep affection for kin rooted in filial piety and extended through the family circle to all men. Confucius said, "The man of *jen* is one who, desiring to develop himself, develops others, and in desiring to sustain himself, sustains others. To be able from one's own self to draw a parallel for the treatment of others; that may be called the way to practice *jen*" (Welty, 1973, pp. 143–144). This tendency is innate and instinctual. It is illustrated in *Mencius*, a Confucian classic, by "an adult who 'all of a sudden' sees a child about to fall into a well and immediately experiences alarm and distress." He would spontaneously reach out to rescue the child. Acting morally is therefore a natural inclination and is judged by the "ease" with which the action occurs and the "joy" one derives from such an action (Munro, 1969, p. 68).

The Confucian ideal is a sage, a man who, through long study and self-discipline, has "developed humanness or love (*jen*); it gave a man an almost mystical empathy for his fellow men, and an acute sensitivity to all the delicately balanced forces at work in the universe" (Wright, 1964, pp. vii–viii). He is one who has attained the highest wisdom and understanding of justice to judge human affairs, taking into consideration all the aspects of a given situation. This ideal terminus for moral development which emphasizes spontaneous feelings, intuition, and synthesis, certainly contrasts with Kohlberg's stage 6 which strives for analytical thinking, individual choice, and responsibility. The process of development is also seen as a gradual accumulation of knowledge and wisdom rather than progressing along a sequence of qualitatively different stages.

These two differing views of man and morality are closely related to the preferred mode of resolving human conflict in the respective cultures. A comparison of these two modes will bring to light the cultural embeddedness of Kohlberg's moral dilemmas.

MODES OF RESOLVING CONFLICTS

In the West, social order and the rights of individuals are under the protection of an elaborate set of laws. However, laws cannot fully take into account all the complexity of human situations. Sometimes one has to violate a law in order to fulfill a higher moral principle, but justice must be done no matter how noble the deed may be. Thus we have the story of John Brown who violated the law in his attempt to liberate the slaves in the American South and was executed. He knowingly made his choice and accepted the consequence. We can only admire his lofty spirit and self-sacrifice. In the story of Billy Budd, the Captain had to execute a perfectly good man who was provoked into killing an evil superior. We know how painful the Captain must have felt in making that decision, yet we understand his commitment to uphold the law. This mode of making individual choices and taking individual responsibilities is part of the individual orientation that characterizes the Americans in contrast to the group orientation of the Chinese (Hsu, 1970).

The Chinese emphasize harmonious interdependent social existence. Therefore, the preferred mode of resolving conflict is reconciliation rather than choice and commitment as in the West. The concept of justice in this context is based upon the proper weighing of *ch'ing* (human sentiments or feelings), *li* (reason), and *fa* (law). The Confucians have always argued against control by penal law on three grounds. First, universally applied laws would undermine the natural distinctions be-tween the noble and mean, leading to chaos. Second, laws cannot cover all possible circumstances. It is therefore better to have good officials decide each case, taking into consideration any unique circumstances. Third, law controls through fear of punishment and this may result in people becoming contentious in their attempt to evade the law rather than changing their attitudes and behaviors (Munro, 1969, p. 111).

Although China today, in its new efforts at Westernization, is working toward developing a more comprehensive legal system, the traditional mode of conciliatory resolution has persisted. This is evidenced by a recent trial conducted in Shanghai, which was tellingly described as a "busybody" divorce trial by a Western observer (Beecher, 1979).

This case involves a 35-year-old woman who filed a divorce suit against her 39-year-old husband because of a domestic dispute which stemmed from her desire to separate her household from that of her in-laws. Her purpose was to gain more personal freedom and exclusive attention from her husband, but the husband could not go along, undoubtedly because of his filial feelings. A court hearing was held after numerous investigations and attempts at conciliation had failed. At the trial there were no lawyers. Instead, representatives of the couple's Neighborhood Committee and of their respective workplaces were called upon to report on their efforts at reconciliation and their evaluations of the case. The hearing was held before a judge and two assistants called "people's assessors." There was heavy pressure against the breakup because the couple had a child. The general consensus was that as both parties had a college education, began their marriage with romantic love, and, above all, loved their child deeply, they therefore could have a good marriage if they tried harder. A compromise was reached and the judge concluded, "In our society we should have unity in the family. After mediation today, both agreed to try reconciliation. And both offered some self-criticism. You have also agreed on some family matters. I should like to point out that in our Socialist country men and women enjoy equality. This is stipulated in the First Article in the Marriage Law. When anything goes wrong you should discuss it together. Take her temperament as an example. When you fly into a rage, you're very bad tempered. And he's very obstinate. . . . If you quarrel with each other very often your work will suffer" (p. 7).

In this instance we not only see the importance of reconciliation, but also the primacy of the collective over the individual. This approach was carried to the extreme during the Cultural Revolution, as Ruth Sidel (1973) reported: "When there are quarrels within or between families, the leaders gather everyone together and study how Mao's thought applies to the problem. Everyone participates—aged people, "little Red Guards" (children), and workers. An entire building might participate" (p. 29).

THE CULTURAL EMBEDDEDNESS OF KOHLBERG'S MORAL DILEMMAS

In order to identify the developmental process of moral judgment, Kohlberg devised a series of moral dilemmas suitable for children 10 to 16 years of age, in which the protagonist must choose between alternative actions either in conformity with rules and authority or in accordance with the needs and welfare of others contrary to the requirements of the former. The subject is questioned as to whether the protagonist should have taken such an action and why. Based upon the form of reasoning behind his/her responses, he/she is placed at one of the six stages of moral development from "obedience and punishment" orientation to "conscience or principle" orientation (the description of the stages can be found in numerous textbooks on child or human development). The following is one of the dilemmas:

> Joe is a 14-year-old boy who wanted to go to camp very much. His father promised him he could go if he saved up

the money for it himself. So Joe worked hard at his paper route and saved up the $40 it cost to go to camp and a little more besides. But just before camp was going to start, his father changed his mind. Some of his friends decided to go on a special fishing trip, and Joe's father was short of the money it would cost. So he told Joe to give him the money he had saved from the paper route. Joe didn't want to give up going to camp, so he thought of refusing to give his father the money.

Should Joe refuse to give his father the money or should he give it to him? Why? (Duska and Whelan, 1975, p. 121)

If this story were to be used in China, one would of course question whether Chinese subjects could really understand the meaning of going to camp or going on a fishing trip in the lives of these individuals. But more importantly, one must examine the significance of the father–son relationship in the context of the subject's culture. Under the Confucian precept regarding filial piety, the son is expected to obey parental orders and to make sacrifices for the happiness of his parents. What choice does the child in the story have?

In conducting cross-cultural research, Kohlberg and others do make an effort to revise some of the stories to be appropriate for the culture in question. For example, the Heinz dilemma involving a druggist was changed in the following way to be used in a village in Taiwan:

A man and his wife had just migrated from the high mountains. They started to farm but there was no rain and no crops grew. No one had enough food. The wife got sick from having little food and could only sleep. Finally she was close to dying from having no food. The husband could not get any work and the wife could not move to another town. There was only one grocery store in the village, and the storekeeper charged a very high price for the food because there was no other store and people had no place else to go to buy food. The husband asked the storekeeper for some food for his wife, and said he could pay for it later. The storekeeper said, "No, I won't give you food unless you pay first." The husband went to all the people in the village to ask for food but no one had food to spare. So he got desperate and broke into the store to steal food for his wife.

Should the husband have done that? Why? (Kohlberg, 1980, pp. 29–30)

Although the setting and the characters are appropriate enough for the village, the situation still seems highly contrived. When one compares this with a real-life situation described by Margery Wolf (1968), one wonders if such a heartless village storekeeper could actually exist. Wolf witnessed the owner of a village store, Mr. Ng, trying to collect a bad debt from a neighbor in the presence of Mr. Ng's wife who tends the store most of the time.

> Mr. Ng was saying angrily to his wife, "You think that everyone is of good heart and just give things to them."
>
> Mrs. Ng, looking anxiously at her husband's rising color, answered, "Well, they said they would give me the money after they sold the pig. How could I know that they wouldn't give it to me?"
>
> Mr. Ng gave his wife a look of utter scorn and, turning his attention to the hapless debtor, a Mrs. Lim, he continued, "You all come here and get things and don't give me any money, but when I go buy all these things I have to give money. How can I go along like this? I have to go and borrow money so that I can buy things for the store!"
>
> Some of the on-lookers exchanged skeptical glances over this statement. Mr. Ng did not seem to notice and warmed to his subject. "How can I borrow money and then lend it to other people? That's what it amounts to. And that is no way to do business."
>
> Mrs. Lim answered, soothingly, "Now, Ng, your temper is thin, but my son is not a bad person. It is just that we have no money. The money we got from the pig had to go to people we borrowed money from and we still owe them more money. My poor son is the only one earning money in our family and he has to feed us all. We have to borrow a little each month just to have enough to eat. He only makes NT$700 a month and you can't feed six people on that."
>
> Several of the loungers began at this point to calculate just how much money would be needed to feed a family the size of Mrs. Lim's, and the consensus of opinion was that her son's income was indeed not up to the job. Mr. Ng did not join in these interesting calculations but continued to rub his head and make frustrated comments about the store, debtors, fate, etc. He finally growled at the group in general, "Oh, this store! This store just can't give people food if they don't give it money!"

Mrs. Lim smiled at him sympathetically, and said, "Well, if you had a store in the city, you could do things that way, but not in the country. In the country you have to let people have things whether they have money or not. I know it is hard on you, but you just have to do it that way."

Several members of the group agreed with Mrs. Lim and informed Mr. Ng of it (pp. 20–21).[1]

In this story we see how a village storekeeper needs to let poor villagers shop on credit with no specified terms. As Mrs. Lim said, "In the country you have to let people have things whether they have money or not. I know it is hard on you, but you just have to do it that way." In such a village the storekeeper in Kohlberg's dilemma would appear to be quite a villain. One wonders if he is really comparable to the druggist in Heinz' dilemma. The situation described by Wolf also brought out the use of public opinion for arbitration. A dilemma for a single individual in the West may be perceived as a problem to be discussed openly in the social setting in China. In Kohlberg's methodology, the subject is asked to make an either–or choice between two major alternatives; he/she is not given the option of proposing a solution. Rest (1979) carried it even further by constructing a multiple-choice instrument and thereby forcing the respondent to select one of a set of given choices. Such a method precludes the culturally characteristic approach of reconciliation through public discussion in China.

A NEW DIRECTION

In short, built into Kohlberg's methodology as well as the scheme of his developmental theory is the prevailing Western conception of man as an autonomous being, free to make choices and determine his destiny. Conflicting claims need to be adjudicated by law, yet obedience to such man-made laws may compete with other principles governing individual rights and human welfare. The choice of action is ultimately left to the individual who must take the responsibility for his action. One is ideally socialized to develop fully one's rational faculty so that one may arrive at well-reasoned decisions. Applying this theory to a culture which emphasizes harmony, reconciliation, collective decision making, and cultivation of sensitivity to the balancing forces in human affairs does not help us see and trace the development of that society's most important characteristic features.

---

[1] Reprinted, with permission of the publisher, from Wolf (1968).

The Chinese commonly use the phrase *pu-tung-shih* to refer to a child, meaning the child does not understand human affairs. What we need to look at is the process by which the child acquires this understanding. Anthropologist Harumi Befu (1977) has pointed out that norms of reciprocity and rules of exchange govern social interaction in every society, but these rules may be more salient in some societies than others. He has studied the ubiquitous gift-giving custom in Japan and related it to the concepts of *on* and *giri* which imply a strong moral compulsion to return a favor (Befu, 1967, 1974). One does not, of course, wish to maintain that there are not very important differences between Japanese and Chinese social systems, but in this regard, at least, there are interesting similarities. Although the present author knows of no comparable analysis of the Chinese society, the importance of establishing "connections" in China is a well-known fact. The rules of exchange are complex and unspecified. Furthermore, as objects of exchange, there are instrumental resources as well as expressive ones Moral maturity in such a society may well mean an ability to make a judgment based upon an insight into the intricate system of cultural norms of reciprocity, rules of exchange, various available resources, and the complex network of relationships in a given situation. The learning process involved cannot be easily conceptualized by existing learning theories. Youniss' (1978) new interpretation of Piaget's notion of social knowledge offers some promise.

According to this interpretation, the child is motivated to seek regularity in his interaction with others. He eventually finds it in two general methods of interpersonal relations. One is the relations of constraint, that is, "one person's imposition of rules or ideas on another without equal reciprocity," and the other is the relations of cooperation that involves reciprocity and collaboration. The former leads to heteronomous knowledge whereas the latter leads to the development of rational and autonomous thought. This interpretation can account for the general finding of a basically two-stage distinction in cross-cultural studies. However, the mature stage is one that is subject to cultural variation in meaning. In addition, Youniss seems to think that rational and autonomous thought develops through the cognitive process of mathematical–logical abstraction. This may well be true in the West. If White's (1972) characterization of Western mode of thinking as being "lineal/sequential/either-or" and the Eastern mode as being "multi-level/ integrated/simultaneous" has any validity, a different process of abstraction would need to be considered in the case of the Chinese.

In conclusion, the present analysis casts strong doubt as to the applicability of Kohlberg's theory of moral development cross-culturally even within the lower levels. A two-stage theory based upon Youniss' (1978) interpretation of Piaget's conception of moral development with attention paid to cultural variation in the definition of moral maturity as well as to the developmental process offers an alternative for future exploration.

REFERENCES

Beecher, W. (1979). A "busybody" divorce trial in China. *The San Francisco Sunday Examiner and Chronicle*, Aug. 26, 2.

Befu, H. (1967). Gift-giving and social reciprocity in Japan, an exploratory statement. *France-Asia/Asia* 188:161–177.

Befu, H. (1974). Power in exchange: Strategy of control and patterns of compliance in Japan. *Asian Profile*, 2:601–622.

Befu, H. (1977). Social exchange. *Annual Review of Anthropology*, 6:255–281.

Duska, R. and Whelan, M. (1975). *Moral Development: A Guide to Piaget and Kohlberg*. New York: Paulist Press.

Eberhard, W. (1971). *Moral and Social Values of the Chinese: Collected Essays*. Chinese Materials and Research Aids Service Center.

Fairbank, J. K. (1980). China: The center of the world. *China: Advertising Supplement to the San Francisco Examiner*, Sept. 7, 12–14.

Fowler, J. (1980). Moral stages and the development of faith. In *Moral Development, Moral Education, and Kohlberg: Basic Issues in Philosophy, Psychology, Religion, and Education*. B. Munsey, ed., pp. 130–160. Birmingham, AL: Religious Education Press.

Gorsuch, R. L. and Barnes, M. L.(1973). Stages of ethical reasoning and moral norms of Carib youths. *Journal of Cross-Cultural Psychology*, 4:283–301.

Grisez, G. and Shaw, R. (1974). *Beyond the New Morality: The Responsibility of Freedom*. Indiana: University of Notre Dame Press.

Hetherington, E. M. and Parke, R. D. (1979). *Child Psychology: A Contemporary Viewpoint*. New York: McGraw-Hill.

Hsu, F. L. K. (1970). *Americans and Chinese: Reflections on Two Cultures and Their People*. New York: Doubleday.

Kessen, W. (Ed.) (1974). *Childhood in China*. New Haven: Yale University Press.

Kohlberg, L. (1969). Stage and sequence: The cognitive-developmental approach to socialization. In *Handbook of Socialization Theory and Research*. D. A. Goslin, ed., pp. 347–380. Chicago: Rand McNally.

Kohlberg, L. (1980). Stages of moral development as a basis for moral education. In *Moral Development, Moral Education, and Kohlberg: Basic Issues in Philosophy, Psychology, Religion, and Education*. B. Munsey, ed., pp. 15–98. Birmingham, AL.: Religious Education Press.

Kurtines, W. and Grief, E. (1974). The development of moral thought: Review and evaluation of Kohlberg's approach. *Psychological Bulletin*, 81:453–470.

Moustakas, C. E. (1961). *Loneliness*. New York: Prentice-Hall.

Munro, D. J. (1969). *The Concept of Man in Early China*. Stanford: Stanford University Press.

Munro, D. J. (1977). *The Concept of Man in Contemporary China*. Ann Arbor: The University of Michigan Press.

Murphy, J. M. and Gilligan, C. (1980). Moral development in late adolescence and adulthood: A critique and reconstruction of Kohlberg's theory. *Human Development*, 23:77–104.

Perry, W. G., Jr. (1968). *Forms of Intellectual and Ethical Development in the College Years: A Scheme*. New York: Holt, Rinehart & Winston.

Piaget, J. (1965). *The Moral Judgment of the Child*. (M. Gabain, trans.) New York: The Free Press. (Originally published, 1932.)

Rest, J. R. (1979). *Development in Judging Moral Issues*. Minneapolis: The University of Minnesota Press.

Rosen, H. (1980). *The Development of Sociomoral Knowledge: A Cognitive-Structural Approach*. New York: Columbia University Press.

Sapontzis, S. F. (1980). Are animals moral beings? *American Philosophical Quarterly*, 17:45–52.

Sartre, J. (1966). *Of Human Freedom*. W. Baskin, ed. New York: Philosophical Library.

Sidel, R. (1973). *Women and Child Care in China*. Baltimore, MD: Penguin Books.

Simpson, E. L. (1974). Moral development research: A case study of scientific cultural bias. *Human Development*, 17:81–106.

Welty, P. T. (1973). *The Asians: Their Heritage and Their Destiny*. Philadelphia: Lippincott.

White, C. B., Bushnell, N. and Regnemer, J. L. (1978). Moral development in Bahamian school children: A 3 year examination of Kohlberg's stages of moral development. *Developmental Psychology*, 14:58–65.

White, J. (1972). *The Highest State of Consciousness*. Garden City, N.Y.: Doubleday.

Wilson, R. W. (1970). *Learning to Be Chinese: The Political Socialization of Children in Taiwan*. Cambridge, MA: MIT Press.

Wolf, M. (1968). *The House of Lim*. Englewood Cliffs, N.J.: Prentice-Hall.

Wright, A. F. (1964). *Confucianism and Chinese Civilization*. New York: Atheneum.

Youniss, J. (1978). Dialectical theory and Piaget on social knowledge. *Human Development*, 21:234–247.

6

New Maps of Development: New Visions of Maturity

Carol Gilligan

Graduate School of Education, Harvard University

Two modes of moral reasoning are distinguished in boys' and girls' discussion of moral dilemmas: one oriented to justice and rights, one to care and response. These different modes are associated with different forms of self-definition and reflect different images of relationships. The contrasting images of hierarchy and web derive from childhood experiences of inequality and interdependence which give rise to the ideals of justice and of care. The representation of these two lines of development and their interplay yields a new mapping of human growth.

That development is the aim of a liberal education seems clear until we begin to ask what is a liberal education and what constitutes development. The current spirit of reappraisal in the field of education stems in part from the fact that some old promises have failed and new practices must be found if the vision of education for freedom and for democracy is to be realized or sustained. But this current reappraisal in the field

Reprinted with permission from the *American Journal of Orthopsychiatry*, 1982, Vol. 52, No. 2, 199–212. Copyright 1982 by the American Orthopsychiatric Association, Inc.

Presented, in earlier versions, to the National Academy of Education, October 1981, and to the Conference on Adolescent Development and Secondary Schooling, Wisconsin Center for Education Research, November 1981. Research was supported by grant R03-MH31571 from the National Institute of Mental Health and grant G790131 from the National Institute of Education. Portions of this paper are contained in a full-length work, *In a Different Voice: Psychological Theory and Women's Development*, by Carol Gilligan, Harvard University Press, 1982.

of education finds its parallel in the field of developmental psychology where a similar reassessment is taking place, a reassessment that began in the early 1970s when developmental psychologists began to question the adulthood that formerly they had taken for granted and when the exclusion of women from the research samples from which developmental theories were generated began to be noticed as a serious omission and one that pointed to the exclusion of other groups as well. Thus, if the changing population of students, particularly the larger number of adults and especially of adult women entering postsecondary education, has raised a series of questions about the aims of education and the nature of educational practice, the study of adulthood and of women has generated a new set of questions for theorists of human development.

To ask whether current developmental theories can be applied to understanding or assessing the lives of people who differ from those upon whose experience these theories were based is only to introduce a problem of far greater magnitude, the adequacy of current theories themselves. The answer to the initial question is in one sense clear, given that these theories are used repeatedly in assessing the development of different groups. But the question asked in such assessment is how much like the original group is the different group being assessed. For example, if the criteria for development are derived from studies of males and these criteria are then used to measure the development of females, the question being asked is how much like men do women develop. The assumption underlying this approach is that there is a universal standard of development and a single scale of measurement along which differences found can be aligned as higher and lower, better and worse. Yet, the initial exclusion of women displays the fallacy of this assumption and indicates a recognition of difference, pointing to the problem I wish to address. While I will use the experience of women to demonstrate how the group left out in the construction of theory calls attention to what is missing in its account, my interest lies not only in women and the perspective they add to the narrative of growth but also in the problem that differences post for a liberal educational philosophy that strives toward an ideal of equality and for a developmental psychology that posits a universal and invariant sequence of growth. In joining the subjects of morality and women, I focus specifically on the questions of value inherent in education and in developmental psychology, and indicate how the lives of women call into question current maps of development and inform a new vision of human growth.

The repeated markings of women's experience as, in Freud's terms, "a dark continent for psychology"[5] raises a question as to what has shadowed the understanding of women's lives. Since women in fact do not live on a continent apart from men but instead repeatedly engage with them in the activities of everyday life, the mystery deepens and the suggestion emerges that theory may be blinding observation. While the disparity between women's experience and the representation of human development, noted throughout the psychological literature, has generally been seen to signify a problem in women's development, the failure of women to fit existing models of human growth may point to a problem in the representation, a limitation in the conception of the human condition, an omission of certain truths about life. The nature of these truths and their implications for understanding development and thinking about education are the subjects of this paper.

CONSTRUCTION OF RELATIONSHIPS AND THE CONCEPT OF MORALITY

Evidence of sex differences in the findings of psychological research comes mainly from studies that reveal the way in which men and women construct the relation between self and others. While the differences observed in women's experience and understanding of relationships have posed a problem of interpretation that recurs throughout the literature on psychoanalysis and personality psychology, this problem emerges with particular clarity in the field of moral judgment research. Since moral judgments pertain to conflicts in the relation of self to others, a difference in the construction of that relationship would lead to a difference in the conception of the moral domain. This difference would be manifest in the way in which moral problems are seen, in the questions asked which then serve to guide the judgment and resolution of moral dilemmas. While the failure to perceive this difference has led psychologists to apply constructs derived from research on men to the interpretation of women's experience and thought, the recognition of this difference points to the limitation of this approach. If women's moral judgments reflect a different understanding of social relationships, then they may point to a line of social development whose presence in both sexes is currently obscured.

THEORIES OF MORAL DEVELOPMENT

This discussion of moral development takes place against the background of a field where, beginning with Freud's theory that tied superego formation to castration anxiety, extending through Piaget's study of boys' conceptions of the rules of their games, and culminating in

Kohlberg's derivation of six stages of moral development from research on adolescent males, the line of development has been shaped by the pattern of male experience and thought. The continual reliance on male experience to build the model of moral growth has been coupled with a continuity in the conception of morality itself. Freud's observation that "the first requisite of civilization is justice, the assurance that a rule once made will not be broken in favour of an individual,"[4] extends through Piaget's conception of morality as consisting in respect for rules[16] and into Kohlberg's claim that justice is the most adequate of moral ideals.[12] The imagery that runs through this equation of morality with justice depicts a world comprised of separate individuals whose claims fundamentally conflict but who find in morality a mode of regulating conflict by agreement that allows the development of life lived in common.

The notion that moral development witnesses the replacement of the rule of brute force with the rule of law, bringing isolated and endangered individuals into a tempered connection with one another, then leads to the observation that women, less aggressive and thus less preoccupied with rules, are as a result less morally developed. The recurrent observations of sex differences that mark the literature on moral development are striking not only in their concurrence but in their reiterative elaboration of a single theme. Whether expressed in the general statement that women show less sense of justice than men[5] or in the particular notation that girls, in contrast to boys, think it better to give back fewer blows than one has received,[16] the direction of these differences is always the same, pointing in women to a greater sense of connection, a concern with relationships more than with rules. But this observation then yields to the paradoxical conclusion that women's preoccupation with relationships constitutes an impediment to the progress of their moral development.

THE MORAL JUDGMENTS OF TWO ELEVEN-YEAR-OLDS

To illustrate how a difference in the understanding of relationships leads to a difference in the conceptions of morality and of self, I begin with the moral judgments of two 11-year-old children, a boy and a girl who see in the same dilemma two very different moral problems. Demonstrating how brightly current theory illuminates the line and the logic of the boy's thought while casting scant light on that of the girl, I will show how the girl's judgments reflect a fundamentally different approach. I have chosen for the purposes of this discussion a girl whose moral judgments elude current categories of developmental assessment, in order to highlight the problem of interpretation rather than to exemplify sex differences per se. My aim is to show how, by adding a new line of interpretation, it becomes possible to see development where previously development was not discerned and to consider differences in the understanding of relationships without lining up these differences on a scale from better to worse.

The two children—Amy and Jake—were in the same sixth grade class at school and participated in a study[8] designed to explore different conceptions of morality and self. The sample selected for study was chosen to focus the variables of gender and age while maximizing developmental potential by holding constant, at a high level, the factors of intelligence, education, and social class that have been associated with moral development, at least as measured by existing scales. The children in question were both bright and articulate and, at least in their 11-year-old aspirations, resisted easy categories of sex-role stereotyping since Amy aspired to become a scientist while Jake preferred English to math. Yet their moral judgments seemed initially to confirm previous findings of differences between the sexes, suggesting that the edge girls have on moral development during the early school years gives way at puberty with the ascendance of formal logical thought in boys.

The dilemma these children were asked to resolve was one in the series devised by Kohlberg to measure moral development in adolescence by presenting a conflict between moral norms and exploring the logic of its resolution. In this particular dilemma, a man named Heinz considers whether or not to steal a drug, which he cannot afford to buy, in order to save the life of his wife. In the standard format of Kohlberg's interviewing procedure, the description of the dilemma itself—Heinz's predicament, the wife's disease, the druggist's refusal to lower his price—is followed by the question, should Heinz steal the drug? Then the reasons for and against stealing are explored through a series of further questions, conceived as probes and designed to reveal the underlying structure of moral thought.

Jake

Jake, at 11, is clear from the outset that Heinz should steal the drug. Constructing the dilemma as Kohlberg did as a conflict between the values of property and life, he discerns the logical priority of life and uses that logic to justify his choice:

> For one thing, a human life is worth more than money, and
> if the druggist only makes $1000, he is still going to live, but

if Heinz doesn't steal the drug, his wife is going to die. [*Why
is life worth more than money?*] Because the druggist can get a
thousand dollars later from rich people with cancer, but Heinz
can't get his wife again. [*Why not?*] Because people are all
different, and so you couldn't get Heinz's wife again.

Asked if Heinz should steal the drug if he does not love his wife, Jake
replies that he should, saying that not only is there "a difference between
hating and killing," but also, if Heinz were caught, "the judge would
probably think it was the right thing to do." Asked about the fact that,
in stealing, Heinz would be breaking the law, he says that "the laws have
mistakes and you can't go writing up a law for everything that you can
imagine."

Thus, while taking the law into account and recognizing its function
in maintaining social order (the judge, he says, "should give Heinz the
lightest possible sentence"), he also sees the law as man-made and therefore subject to error and change. Yet his judgment that Heinz should
steal the drug, like his view of the law as having mistakes, rests on the
assumption of agreement, a societal consensus around moral values that
allows one to know and expect others will recognize "the right thing to
do."

Fascinated by the power of logic, this 11-year-old boy locates truth in
math which, he says, is "the only thing that is totally logical." Considering
the moral dilemma to be "sort of like a math problem with humans," he
sets it up as an equation and proceeds to work out the solution. Since
his solution is rationally derived, he assumes that anyone following reason would arrive at the same conclusion and thus that a judge would
also consider stealing to be the right thing for Heinz to do. Yet he is also
aware of the limits of logic; asked whether there is a right answer to
moral problems, he says that "there can only be right and wrong in
judgment," since the parameters of action are variable and complex.
Illustrating how actions undertaken with the best of intentions can even-
tuate in the most disastrous of consequences, he says

> . . . like if you give an old lady your seat on the trolley, if you
> are in a trolley crash and that seat goes through the window,
> it might be that reason that the old lady dies.

Theories of developmental psychology illuminate well the position of
this child, standing at the juncture of childhood and adolescence, at what
Piaget described as the pinnacle of childhood intelligence, and beginning
through thought to discover a wider universe of possibility. The moment

of preadolescence is caught by the conjunction of formal operational thought with a description of self still anchored in the factual parameters of his childhood world, his age, his town, his father's occupation, the substance of his likes, dislikes, and beliefs. Yet as his self-description radiates the self-confidence of a child who has arrived, in Erikson's terms, at a favorable balance of industry over inferiority—competent, sure of himself, and knowing well the rules of the game—so his emergent capacity for formal thought, his ability to think about thinking and to reason things out in a logical way, frees him from dependence on authority and allows him to find solutions to problems by himself.

This emergent autonomy then charts the trajectory that Kohlberg's six stages of moral development trace, a three-level progression from an egocentric understanding of fairness based on individual need (stages one and two), to a conception of fairness anchored in the shared conventions of societal agreement (stages three and four), and finally to a principled understanding of fairness that rests on the free-standing logic of equality and reciprocity (stages five and six). While Jake's judgments at 11 are scored as conventional on Kohlberg's scale, a mixture of stages three and four, his ability to bring deductive logic to bear on the solution of moral dilemmas, to differentiate morality from law, and to see how laws can be considered to have mistakes, points toward the principled conception of justice that Kohlberg equates with moral maturity.

Amy

In contrast, Amy's response to the dilemma conveys a very different impression, an image of development stunted by a failure of logic, an inibility to think for herself. Asked if Heinz should steal the drug, she replies in a way that seems evasive and unsure:

> Well, I don't think so. I think there might be other ways besides stealing it, like if he could borrow the money or make a loan or something, but he really shouldn't steal the drug, but his wife shouldn't die either.

Asked why he should not steal the drug, she considers neither property nor law but rather the effect that theft could have on the relationship between Heinz and his wife. If he stole the drug, she explains.

> . . . he might save his wife then, but if he did, he might have to go to jail, and then his wife might get sicker again, and he

couldn't get more of the drug, and it might not be good. So, they should really just talk it out and find some other way to make the money.

Seeing in the dilemma not a math problem with humans but a narrative of relationships that extends over time, she envisions the wife's continuing need for her husband and the husband's continuing concern for his wife and seeks to respond to the druggist's need in a way that would sustain rather than sever connection. As she ties the wife's survival to the preservation of relationships, so she considers the value of her life in a context of relationships, saying that it would be wrong to let her die because, "if she died, it hurts a lot of people and it hurts her." Since her moral judgment is grounded in the belief that "if somebody has something that would keep somebody alive, then it's not right not to give it to them," she considers the problem in the dilemma to arise not from the druggist's assertion of rights but from his failure of response.

While the interviewer proceeds with the series of questions that follow Kohlberg's construction of the dilemma, Amy's answers remain essentially unchanged, the various probes serving neither to elucidate nor to modify her initial response. Whether or not Heinz loves his wife, he still shouldn't steal or let her die; if it were a stranger dying instead, she says that "if the stranger didn't have anybody near or anyone she knew," then Heinz should try to save her life but he shouldn't steal the drug. But as the interviewer conveys through the repetition of questions that the answers she has given are not heard or not right, Amy's confidence begins to diminish and her replies become more constrained and unsure. Asked again why Heinz should not steal the drug, she simply repeats, "Because it's not right." Asked again to explain why, she states again that theft would not be a good solution, adding lamely, that, "if he took it, he might not know how to give it to his wife, and so his wife might still die." Failing to see the dilemma as a self-contained problem in moral logic, she does not discern the internal structure of its resolution; as she constructs the problem differently herself, Kohlberg's conception completely evades her.

Instead, seeing a world comprised of relationships rather than of people standing alone, a world that coheres through human connection rather than through systems of rules, she finds the puzzle in the dilemma to lie in the failure of the druggist to respond to the wife. Saying that "it is not right for someone to die when their life could be saved," she assumes that if the druggist were to see the consequences of his refusal to lower his price, he would realize that "he should just give it to the wife and then have the husband pay back the money later." Thus she considers the solution to the dilemma to lie in making the wife's condition more salient to the druggist or, that failing, in appealing to others who are in a position to help.

Just as Jake is confident the judge would agree that stealing is the right thing for Heinz to do, so Amy is confident that, "if Heinz and the druggist had talked it out long enough, they could reach something besides stealing." As he considers the law to "have mistakes," so she sees this drama as a mistake, believing that "the world should just share things more and then people wouldn't have to steal." Both children thus recognize the need for agreement but see it as mediated in different ways: he impersonally through systems of logic and law, she personally through communication in relationship. As he relies on the conventions of logic to deduce the solution to this dilemma, assuming these conventions to be shared, so she relies on a process of communication, assuming connection and believing that her voice will be heard. Yet while his assumptions about agreement are confirmed by the convergence in logic between his answers and the questions posed, her assumptions are belied by the failure in communication, the interviewer's inability to understand her response.

MEASURING MORAL DEVELOPMENT: ASSESSING DIVERSE PERCEPTIONS

While the frustration of the interview with Amy is apparent in the repetition of questions and its ultimate circularity, the problem of interpretation arises when it comes to assessing her development. Considered in the light of Kohlberg's conception of the stages and sequence of moral development, her moral judgments are a full stage lower in moral maturity than those of the boy. Scored as a mixture of stages two and three, they seem to reveal a feeling of powerlessness in the world, an inability to think systematically about the concepts of morality or law, a reluctance to challenge authority or to examine the logic of received moral truths, a failure even to conceive of acting directly to save a life or to consider that such action, if taken, could possibly have an effect. As her reliance on relationships seems to reveal a continuing dependence and vulnerability, so her belief in communication as the mode through which to resolve moral dilemmas appears naive and cognitively immature.

Yet her description of herself conveys a markedly different impression. Once again, the hallmarks of the preadolescent child depict a child secure in her sense of herself, confident in the substance of her beliefs, and sure of her ability to do something of value in the world. Describing herself at 11 as "growing and changing," Amy says that she "sees some things differently now, just because I know myself really well now, and I know a lot more about the world." Yet the world she knows is a different world from that refracted by Kohlberg's construction of Heinz's dilemma. Her world is a world of relationships and psychological truths, where an awareness of the connection between people gives rise to a recognition of responsibility for one another, a perception of the need for response. Seen in this light, her view of morality as arising from the recognition of relationship, her belief in communication as the mode of conflict resolution, and her conviction that the solution to the dilemma will follow from its compelling representation seem far from naive or cognitively immature; rather, her judgments contain the insights central to an ethic of care, just as Jake's judgments reflect the logic of the justice approach. Her incipient awareness of the "method of truth," central to nonviolent conflict resolution, and her belief in the restorative activity of care, lead her to see the actors in the dilemma arrayed not as opponents in a contest of rights but as members of a network of relationships on whose continuation they all depend. Consequently her solution to the dilemma lies in activating the network by communication, securing the inclusion of the wife by strengthening rather than severing connection.

But the different logic of Amy's response calls attention to a problem in the interpretation of the interview itself. Conceived as an interrogation, it appears as a dialogue that takes on moral dimensions of its own, pertaining to the interviewer's uses of power and to the manifestations of respect. With this shift in the conception of the interview, it immediately becomes clear that the interviewer's problem in hearing Amy's response stems from the fact that Amy is answering a different question from the one the interviewer thought had been posed. Amy is considering not *whether* Heinz should act in this situation (*Should* Heinz steal the drug?) but rather *how* Heinz should act in response to his awareness of his wife's need (Should Heinz *steal* the drug?). The interviewer takes the mode of action for granted, presuming it to be a matter of fact. Amy assumes the necessity for action and considers what form it should take. In the interviewer's failure to imagine a response not dreamt of in Kohlberg's moral philosophy lies the failure to hear Amy's question and to see the logic in her response, to discern that what from one perspective appears to be an evasion of the dilemma signifies in other terms a recognition of the problem and a search for a more adequate solution.

Thus in Kohlberg's dilemma these two children see two very different moral problems—Jake a conflict between life and property that can be resolved by logical deduction, Amy a fracture of human relationship that must be mended with its own thread. Asking different questions that arise from different conceptions of the moral domain, they arrive at answers that fundamentally diverge, and the arrangement of these answers as successive stages on a scale of increasing moral maturity calibrated by the logic of the boy's response misses the different truth revealed in the judgment of the girl. To the question, "What does he see that she does not?", Kohlberg's theory provides a ready response, manifest in the scoring of his judgments at a full stage higher than hers in moral maturity; to the question, "What does she see that he does not?", Kohlberg's theory has nothing to say. Since most of her responses fall through the sieve of Kohlberg's scoring system, her responses appear from his perspective to lie outside the moral domain.

Yet just as Jake reveals a sophisticated understanding of the logic of justification, so Amy is equally sophisticated in her understanding of the nature of choice. Saying that "if both the roads went in totally separate ways, if you pick one, you'll never know what would happen if you went the other way," she explains that "that's the chance you have to take, and like I said, it's just really a guess." To illustrate her point "in a simple way," she describes how, in choosing to spend the summer at camp, she

> . . . will never know what would have happened if I had stayed here, and if something goes wrong at camp, I'll never know if I stayed here if it would have been better. There's really no way around it because there's no way you can do both at once, so you've got to decide, but you'll never know.

In this way, these two 11-year-old children, both highly intelligent, though perceptive about life in different ways, display different modes of moral understanding, different ways of thinking about conflict and choice. Jake, in resolving the dilemma, follows the construction that Kohlberg has posed. Relying on the theft to avoid confrontation and turning to the law to mediate the dispute, he transposes a hierarchy of power into a hierarchy of values by recasting a conflict between people into a conflict of claims. Thus abstracting the moral problem from the interpersonal situation, he finds in the logic of fairness an objective means of deciding who will win the dispute. But this hierarchical or-dering, with its imagery of winning and losing and the potential for violence which it contains, gives way in Amy's construction of the di-lemma to a network of connection, a network sustained by a process of communication. With this shift, the moral problem changes from one of unfair domination, the imposition of property over life, to one of unnecessary exclusion, the failure of the druggist to respond to the wife.

This shift in the formulation of the moral problem and the concomitant change in the imagery of relationships are illustrated as well by the responses of two eight-year-olds who participated in the same study[8] and were asked to describe a situation in which they weren't sure of the right thing to do:

> *Jeffrey* (age 8): When I really want to go to my friends and my mother is cleaning the cellar, I think about my friends, and then I think about my mother, and then I think about the right thing to do. [*But how do you know it's the right thing to do?*] Because some things go before other things.

> *Karen* (age 8): I have a lot of friends, and I can't always play with all of them, so everybody's going to have to take a turn, because they're all my friends. But like if someone's all alone, I'll play with them. [*What kind of things do you think about when you are trying to make that decision?*] Um, someone all alone, loneliness.

While Jeffrey sets up a hierarchical ordering in thinking about the conflict between desire and duty, Karen describes a network of relationships that includes all of her friends. Both children deal with the issues of exclusion and priority created by choice, but while Jeffrey thinks about what goes first, Karen focuses on who is left out.

MORAL JUDGMENT AND SELF-DESCRIPTIONS

In illustrating a difference in children's thinking about moral conflict and choice, I have described two views that are complementary rather than sequential or opposed. In doing so, I go against the bias of developmental theory toward ordering differences in a hierarchical mode. This correspondence between the order of developmental theory and that manifest in the boys' responses contrasts with the disparity between the structure of theory and that manifest in the thought of the girls. Yet, in neither comparison does one child's thought appear as precursor of the other's position. Thus, questions arise about the relation between these perspectives; what is the significance of these differences, and how do these two modes of thinking connect? To pursue these questions, I return to the eleven-year-olds and consider the way they describe themselves.

[*How would you describe yourself to yourself?*]

Jake: Perfect. That's my conceited side. What do you want—any way that I choose to describe myself?

Amy: You mean my character? [*What do you think?*] Well, I don't know. I'd describe myself as, well, what do you mean?

[*If you had to describe the person you are in a way that you yourself would know it was you, what would you say?*]

Jake: I'd start off with eleven years old. Jake [last name]. I'd have to add that I live in [town] because that is a big part of me, and also that my father is a doctor because I think that does change me a little bit, and that I don't believe in crime, except for when your name is Heinz . . . that I think school is boring because I think that kind of changes your character a little bit. I don't sort of know how to describe myself, because I don't know how to read my personality. [*If you had to describe the way you actually would describe yourself, what would you say?*] I like corny jokes. I don't really like to get down to work, but I can do all the stuff in school. Every single problem that I have seen in school I have been able to do, except for ones that take knowledge, and after I do the reading, I have been able to do them, but sometimes I don't want to waste my time on easy homework. And also I'm crazy about sports. I think, unlike a lot of people, that the world still has hope. . . . Most people that I know I like, and I have the good life, pretty much as good as any I have seen, and I am tall for my age.

Amy: Well, I'd say that I was someone who likes school and studying, and that's what I want to do with my life. I want to be some kind of a scientist or something, and I want to do things, and I want to help people. And I think that's what kind of person I am, or what kind of person I try to be. And that's probably how I'd describe myself. And I want to do something to help other people. [*Why is that?*] Well, because

> I think that this world has a lot of problems, and I think that
> everybody should try to help somebody else in some way, and
> the way I'm choosing is through science.

In the voice of the 11-year-old boy, a familiar form of self-definition appears, resonating to the schoolbook inscription of the young Stephen Daedalus ("himself, his name and where he was")[10] and echoing the descriptions that appear in *Our Town*,[18] laying out across the coordinates of time and space a hierarchical order in which to define one's place. Describing himself as distinct by locating his particular position in the world, Jake sets himself apart from that world by his abilities, his beliefs, and his height. Although Amy also enumerates her likes, her wants, and her beliefs, she locates herself in relation to the world, describing herself through actions that bring her into connection with others, elaborating ties through her ability to provide help. To Jake's ideal of perfection against which he measures the worth of himself, Amy counterposes an ideal of care against which she measures the worth of her activity. While she places herself in relation to the world and chooses to help others through science, he places the world in relation to himself as it defines his character, his position, and the quality of life.

CONCLUSIONS

As the voices of these children illuminate two modes of self-description and two modes of moral judgment, so they illustrate how readily we hear the voice that speaks of justice and of separation and the difficulty we encounter in listening to the voice that speaks of care and connection. Listening through developmental theories and through the structures of our educational and social system, we are attuned to a hierarchical ordering that represents development as a progress of separation, a chronicle of individual success. In contrast, the understanding of development as a progress of human relationships, a narrative of expanding connection, is an unimagined representation. The image of network or web thus seems more readily to connote entrapment rather than an alternative and nonhierarchical vision of human connection.

This central limitation in the representation of development is most clearly apparent in recent portrayals of adult life, where the insistent focus on self and on work provides scanty representation of an adulthood spent in the activities of relationship and care. The tendency to chart the unfamiliar waters of adult development with the familiar markers of adolescent separation and growth leads to an equation of development with separation; it results in a failure to represent the reality of connection both in love and in work. Levinson,[15] patterning the stages of adult development on the seasons of a man's life, defined the developmental process explicitly as one of individuation, yet reported his distress at the absence of friendships in men's lives. Vaillant,[17] deriving his account of adaptation to life from the lives of the men who took part in the Grant study, noted that the question these men found most difficult to answer was, "Can you describe your wife?" In this light, the observation that women's embeddedness in lives of relationship, their orientation to interdependence, their subordination of achievement to care, and their conflicts over competitive success leave them personally at risk in mid-life, though generally construed as a problem in women's development, seems more a commentary on our society and on the representation of development itself.

In suggesting that the consideration of women's lives and of adulthood calls attention to the need for an expansion in the mapping of human development, I have pointed to a distinction between two modes of self-definition and two modes of moral judgment and indicated how these modes reflect different ways of imagining relationships. That these modes are tied to different experiences may explain their empirical association with gender, though that association is by no means absolute. That they reflect different forms of thought—one relying on a formal logic whose development Piaget has described, the other on a narrative and contextual mode of thought whose development remains to be traced—indicates the implication of this distinction for psychological assessment and education.

The experiences of inequality and of interdependence are embedded in the cycle of life, universal because inherent in the relationship of parent and child. These experiences of inequality and interdependene give rise to the ethics of justice and care, the ideals of human relationship—the vision that self and other will be treated as of equal worth, that despite differences in power, things will be fair; the vision that everyone will be responded to and included, that no one will be left alone or hurt. The adolescent, capable of envisioning the ideal, reflects on the childhood experiences of powerlessness and vulnerability and conceives a utopian world laid out along the coordinates of justice and care. This ability to conceive the hypothetical and to construct contrary-to-face hypotheses has led the adolescent to be proclaimed a "philosopher,"[11] a "metaphysician par excellence."[9] But the representation of the adolescent's moral philosophy in the literature of developmental psychology has been limited to the portrayal of changes in the conception of justice that supports the adolescent's claim to equality and the separation of other and self. My own work[7] has expanded this description by identifying two different moral languages, the language of rights that protects separation and the language of responsibilities that sustains connection. In dialogue, these languages not only create the ongoing tension of moral discourse, but also reveal how the dynamics of separation and attachment in the process of identity formation relate to the themes of justice and care in moral growth. This expanded representation of identity and moral development allows a more complex rendering of differences, and points to the need to understand and foster the development of both modes.

The old promise of a liberal education, of an education that frees individuals from blinding constraints and engenders a questioning of assumptions formerly taken for granted remains a compelling vision. But among the prevailing assumptions that need to be questioned are the assumptions about human development. The lives of women, in pointing to an uncharted path of human growth and one that leads to a less violent mode of life, are particularly compelling at this time in history and thus deserve particular attention. The failure to attend to the voices of women and the difficulty in hearing what they say when they speak has compromised women's development and education, leading them to doubt the veracity of their perceptions and to question the truth of their experience. This problem becomes acute for women in adolescence, when thought becomes reflective and the problem of interpretation thus enters the stream of development itself. But the failure to represent women's experience also contributes to the presentation of competitive relationships and hierarchical modes of social organization as the natural ordering of life. For this reason, the consideration of women's lives brings to the conception of development a much needed corrective, stressing the importance of narrative modes of thought and pointing to the contextual nature of psychological truths and the reality of interdependence in human life.

The process of selection that has shadowed this vision can be seen in Kohlberg's reading of Martin Luther King's letter from the Birmingham jail,[11] since Kohlberg extracted King's justification for breaking the law in the name of justice but omitted the way in which King's vision of justice was embedded in a vision of human connection. Replying to the clergy who criticized his action, King not only offered a justification of his action but also defended the necessity for action, anchoring that necessity in the realization of interdependence:

> I am in Birmingham because injustice is here. I cannot sit idly
> by in Atlanta and not be concerned about what happens in

Birmingham. Injustice anywhere is a threat to justice everywhere. We are caught in an inescapable network of mutuality, tied in a single garment of destiny. Whatever affects one directly, affects all indirectly.

Thus, like Bonhoeffer,[1] who stated that action comes "not from thought but from a readiness for responsibility," King tied his responsiveness to a caring that arises from an understanding of the connection between people's lives, a connection not forged by systems of rules but by a perception of the fact of relationship, a connection not freely contracted but built into the very fabric of life.

The ideals of a liberal democratic society—of freedom and equality—have been mirrored in the developmental vision of autonomy, the image of the educated man thinking for himself, the image of the ideal moral agent acting alone on the basis of his principles, blinding himself with a Rawlsian "veil of ignorance," playing a solitary Kohlbergian game of "moral musical chairs." Yet the developmental psychologists who dared, with Erikson,[3] to "ask what is an adult," immediately began to see the limitations of this vision. Erikson himself has come increasingly to talk about the activity of caretaking and to identify caring as the virtue and strength of maturity.[2] When integrated into a developmental understanding, this insight should spur the search for the antecedents of this strength in childhood and in adolescence. Kohlberg,[13] turning to consider adulthood, tied adult development to the experiences of "sustained responsibility for the welfare of others" and of the irreversible consequences of choice. The resonance of these themes of maturity to the voice of the 11-year-old girl calls into question current assumptions about the sequence of development and suggests a different path of growth.

The story of moral development, as it is presently told, traces the history of human development through shifts in the hierarchy of power relationships, implying that the dissolution of this hierarchy into an order of equality represents the ideal vision of things. But the conception of relationships in terms of hierarchies implies separation as the moral ideal—for everyone to stand alone, independent, self-sufficient, connected to others by the abstractions of logical thought. There is, then, a need to represent in the mapping of development a nonhierarchical image of human connection, and to embody in the vision of maturity the reality of interdependence. This alternate vision of the web of connection is the recognition of relationship that prevents aggression and gives rise to the understanding that generates response.

REFERENCES

1. Bonhoeffer, D. (1953). *Letters and Papers from Prison.* New York: Macmillan.
2. Erikson, E. (1976). Reflections on Dr. Borg's life cycle. *Daedalus,* 105:1–29.
3. Erikson, E. (1970). Reflections on the dissent of contemporary youth. *Daedalus,* 99:154–176.
4. Freud, S. (1929). Civilization and its discontents. In *Standard Edition of the Complete Psychological Works of Sigmund Freud,* Vol. XXI, J. Strachey, ed. London: Hogarth Press, 1961.
5. Freud, S. (1926). The question of lay analysis. In *Standard Edition of the Complete Psychological Works of Sigmund Freud,* Vol. XX, J. Strachey, ed. London: Hogarth Press, 1961.
6. Freud, S. (1925). Some physical consequences of the anatomical distinction between the sexes. In *Standard Edition of the Complete Psychological Works of Sigmund Freud,* Vol. XIX, J. Strachey, ed. London: Hogarth Press, 1961.
7. Gilligan, C. (1982). *In a Different Voice: Psychological Theory and Women's Development.* Cambridge, MA: Harvard University Press.
8. Gilligan, C., Langdale, S. and Lyons, N. (1982). The Contribution of Women's Thought to Developmental Theory: The Elimination of Sex-Bias in Moral Development Theory and Research. Final report to the National Institute of Education, Washington, D.C.
9. Inhelder, B. and Piaget, J. (1958). *The Growth of Logical Thinking from Childhood to Adolescence.* New York: Basic Books.
10. Joyce, J. (1916). *A Portrait of the Artist as a Young Man.* New York: Viking Press, 1956, p. 15.
11. King, M., Jr. (1964). *Why We Can't Wait.* New York: Harper and Row.
12. Kohlberg, L. (1981). *The Philosophy of Moral Development.* San Francisco: Harper and Row.
13. Kohlberg, L. (1973). Continuities and discontinuities in childhood and adult moral development revisited. In *Life-Span Developmental Psychology: Personality and Socialization,* P. Baltes and K. Schaie, eds. New York: Academic Press.
14. Kohlberg, L. and Gilligan, C. (1971). The adolescent as a philosopher: The discovery of the self in a post-conventional world. *Daedalus,* 100:1051–1086.
15. Levinson, D. (1978). *The Seasons of a Man's Life.* New York: Knopf.
16. Piaget, J. (1932). *The Moral Judgment of the Child.* New York: Free Press, 1965.
17. Vaillant, G. (1977). *Adaptation to Life.* Boston: Little, Brown.
18. Wilder, T. (1938). *Our Town.* New York: Coward-McCann.

Part II

INFANCY STUDIES

The consensus in developmental theory that the infant has human characteristics from the moment of birth onward and that these play an active role in a continuous interactional process with the parents receives additional specific support and elaboration in this year's contributions.

Field and her colleagues report evidence of the neonate's ability to discriminate and imitate adult expressions of happiness, sadness, and surprise, a finding which would have been greeted with utter disbelief 20 years ago. She rejects the explanation of an innate releasing mechanism or fixed action pattern which would have been favored by traditional ethological theory. Instead, her explanation is based on a view of the perceptual and intersensory competence of the newborn child.

Crockenberg and Smith report a careful study of the causal links between young infant irritability and maternal contact and responsiveness, an issue which has generated contradictory reports in the literature. Their findings are specific and clear-cut, and highlight the multiple factors involved in the mother-infant interaction in the elaboration of this temperamental characteristic of the child.

Johnson and his co-workers describe the result of a survey of maternal perceptions of emotion in their own infants in a large sample of mothers. The findings provide valuable normative data, emphasize that mothers perceive a number of discrete emotions in their infants, even very early in life, and indicate some meaningful age trends. The authors also offer a number of possible alternative explanations for their results. Such maternal perceptions must influence the course of the mother-infant relationship, and further exploration of the dynamics of these perceptions should be a fruitful area for research.

Meares and his associates investigated the manner in which a mother comes to attribute personality traits to her newborn infant. They used the mother's ratings on the Broussard and Hartner Scale, which the originators of the Scale assumed to reflect the mother's "fantasies," rather than the child's actual characteristics. On the contrary, the data of Meares and his associates indicated that the mother's rating was influenced not only by subjective factors but also by a fine observation of the infant's behavior.

The Ainsworth Strange Situation procedure has been taken by many psychologists to provide a strategy for assessing the character of the child's attachment to the mother and to have predictive value for the infant's subsequent functioning. Lamb and his co-workers go beyond this experimental model to study the infant's behavior in this test situation when the father is involved, to compare the findings when the mother is part of the test procedure, and to explore the correlation of their findings with the child's sociability with strangers. They were surprised to find that the security of infant-father attachment, as rated by the Ainsworth test, was more closely related to infant sociability than the security of infant-mother attachment, which indicated that the meaning of this test and the factors influencing the results are more complex than many have considered. As the authors say, "There is clearly a need for more research on cultural and temperamental influences on the patterns of infant-parent interaction in the Strange Situation."

Finally, Thompson and Lamb report on the relationship of stranger sociability to temperament and social experience during the second year. They found a stronger relationship to temperament, especially fearfulness, than to dimensions of prior social experience. Their results emphasize the need to consider the functional influence of temperament (as well as other variables) in assessing the meaning of an infant's reactions to strangers, such as in the Ainsworth Strange Situation procedure.

7

Discrimination and Imitation of Facial Expressions by Neonates

Tiffany M. Field, Robert Woodson, Reena Greenberg, and Debra Cohen

Department of Pediatrics and Psychology, Mailman Center for Child Development, University of Miami Medical School

Human neonates (average age, 36 hours) discriminated three facial expressions (happy, sad, and surprised) posed by a live model as evidenced by diminished visual fixation on each face over trials and renewed fixations to the presentation of a different face. The expressions posed by the model, unseen by the observer, were guessed at greater than chance accuracy simply by observing the face of the neonate, whose facial movements in the brow, eyes, and mouth regions provided evidence for imitation of the facial expressions.

Facial expressions of emotions such as happiness, sadness, and surprise have been observed in the very young infant (1) and in several cultures (2). Because of their early appearance and their apparent universality, these basic facial expressions may reflect innate processes (3). We have investigated whether neonates can discriminate and imitate these facial expressions. Projected photographs of facial expressions are discriminated as early as 3 months of age in a visual habituation paradigm (4). The young infant is also physically capable of reproducing these expressions; all but one of the discrete facial muscle actions of adults have been identified in the neonate (5). Although a debate continues on what processes may be involved (6), imitations of facial movements such as lip

Reprinted with permission from *Science*, 1982, Vol. 218, No. 8, 179–181. Copyright 1982 by the American Association for the Advancement of Science.

protrusion, mouth widening, and tongue thrusting have been reported for 12- to 21-day-old babies (7). We now have evidence for both the discrimination and imitation of facial expressions at an even younger age, shortly after birth.

In this study, a series of three facial expressions (happy, sad, and surprised) were modeled by an adult for 74 neonates (mean age, 36 hours) (8). The model held the neonate upright with the newborn's head supported in one hand and torso in the other hand. The two faces were separated by approximately 10 inches. The neonate's visual fixations on the adult's face and the neonate's facial movement patterns were recorded by an observer who stood behind the model in order to see the infant's face but remained unaware of the expression being modeled. Split-screen videotaping of the neonates' and model's faces provided checks on the reliability of coding by observer and face presentation by model (9).

To sustain alertness and to elicit the neonate's visual fixations on the model's face, the model provided vestibular stimulation (two deep knee bends) and auditory stimulation (two tongue clicks) prior to each trial. The model then fixed a happy, sad, or surprised expression on her face. Three series of trials or one series for each face were presented in a counter-balanced Greco-Latin-square order to control for state change effects. Face 1 was sustained in a fixed position until the infant looked away from the model's face, at which time the model reelicited the neonate's visual fixation with vestibular and auditory stimulation. Face 1 trials were repeated until the neonate looked at that face for less than 2 seconds. Face 2 and face 3 trials were then presented according to the same procedure (Fig. 1).

For each trial, the observer coded on a paper grid (i) total time per trial; (ii) predominant target and pattern of neonatal visual fixation per trial on the model's eyes, mouth, or alternately on the eyes and mouth; (iii) the presence of specific mouth movements of the neonate, including widening of the lips (as in a happy face), tight and somewhat protruded lips (pouting or sad face), wide opening of the mouth (as in a surprise face), or tongue protrusion; (iv) presence or absence of eye widening (as in a surprise face); (v) presence of relaxed or furrowed brow (as in happy or sad face, respectively); and (vi) observer's guess as to which expression was being modeled.

Because we used a trials-to-criterion procedure yielding a different number of trials per expression per infant (range, 4 to 15; mean, 5.8), the number of trials during which these movements occurred was converted to the proportion of the total number of trials presented for each

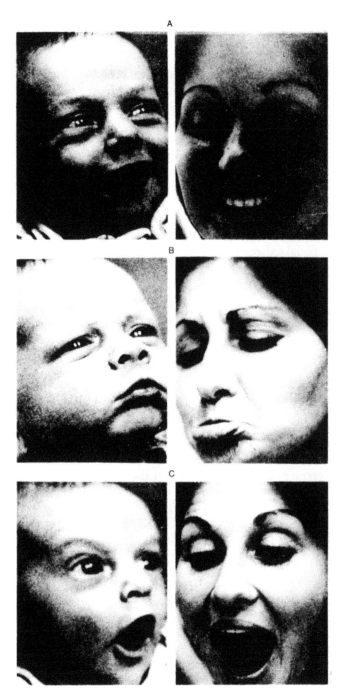

Figure 1. Sample photographs of a model's happy, sad, and surprised expressions and an infant's corresponding expressions.

facial expression. For the same reason, the trials were divided in thirds (early, middle, and late) for analyses of the visual habituation data. Repeated measures analyses of variance were then conducted with the order of trials (3) as a between-subjects measure and the facial expressions modeled (3) as a repeated measure. There were no significant effects of order of trials or type of facial expression in the habituation-dishabituation. Visual fixations significantly decreased from the middle to late trials [mean decrease, 11.9 seconds, $F(2, 142) = 5.49. P < .005$] and significantly increased from the late trials of the facial expression to the early trials of the subsequent expression [mean, 8.1 seconds, $F(2, 142) = 5.81. P < .005$]. Thus, the visual habituation and dishabituation of the facial stimuli suggest that neonates can discriminate at least these three basic facial expressions (10).

The neonate visually fixated the mouth region and alternately looked at the mouth and eye regions for a greater proportion of the trials than the eye region, irrespective of the facial expression being modeled (11). The neonate's alternating fixations on the mouth and the eye region occurred during a greater proportion of the surprise expression trials than for the other facial expressions [$F(2, 142) = 4.74. P < .01$]. Fixations on the mouth region occurred for a greater proportion of trials during happy and sad than surprised expressions [$F(2, 142) = 3.26. P < .05$]. The model's surprise expression featured salient eye and mouth positions (both widened), whereas the happy and sad expressions were characterized primarily by mouth positions—widening of the lips for the happy expression and tightened, protruding lips for the sad expression (Fig. 1). These differential visual fixation patterns suggest that the neonate can perceive distinctive features of these facial expressions: of the mouth in happy and sad faces, and of both the mouth and eyes in the surprise expression.

Figure 2 depicts the proportion of trials on which differential mouth movements were observed during the different face trials. Because of the problem posed by different baseline frequencies, the distributions of each behavior were analyzed separately across the different expressions modeled (7). There were no differences in the proportion of trials that tongue protrusion occurred as a function of different facial expressions ($P > .05$). However, widened eyes and wide mouth opening occurred for a greater proportion of surprise than other face trials [$F(2, 142) = 3.97, P < .05$ and $11.49, P < .001$, respectively]. Lip widening occurred more frequently during happy face trials [$F(2, 142) = 3.41, P < .05$], and tightened-mouth-protruding lips [$F(2, 142 = 3.41, P < .05$] and furrowed brow [$F(2, 142) = 10.16, P < .001$] occurred more

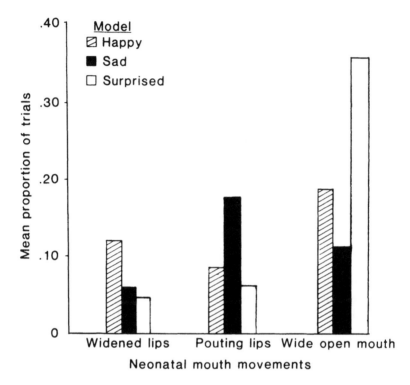

Figure 2. Mean proportion of trials during which different neonatal mouth movements occurred as a function of facial expression modeled. Mouth movements include widened lips (as in a happy expression), pouting lips (sad), and wide open mouth (surprised). Proportions do not total 100 because these discrete movements occurred predominantly during the middle trials (approximately 39 percent of the trials).

frequently during sad expression trials. Comparison of the occurrence of these facial movements across the expressions for which those movements would not be expected (omitting the imitative expression movements corresponding to the modeled expressions) yielded no significant differences. This finding provides additional support for the notion that the neonate's facial movements that simulate those of the model are attributable to imitation. An analysis of early, middle, and late trials data for these expressions revealed that a greater proportion of these expressions occurred during the middle trials [$F(2, 142) = 5.29, P < .01$], suggesting that these were not arousal responses or fixed action patterns (12).

Analyses of the observer's guesses included only those data for each subject's first series of trials. The chance probability of correctly guessing the facial expression would be 33 percent. The surprise facial expressions were correctly guessed 76 percent of the trials, at a significantly greater than chance level ($\chi^2_{(24)} = 65.23$, $P < .001$). Surprise expressions were correctly guessed more often than happy (58 percent) or sad expressions (59 percent). However, the happy ($\chi^2_{(23)} = 35.76$, $P < .05$) and sad expressions ($\chi^2_{(24)} = 38.41$, $P < .05$) were also correctly guessed. The surprise expression featured two salient features in two regions (eyes and mouth). When the infant reproduces both of these features, the probability of an accurate guess by the observer was increased.

These results suggest that the neonate is capable of discriminating at least these three different facial expressions. Ensuring that the infant was alert and using a trials-to-criterion habituation procedure so that each infant could process the information at his own pace may have facilitated the demonstration of facial discriminations.

The imitative expressions provide support for Meltzoff and Moore's data (7) on imitative gestures by 12- to 21-day-old infants. They suggested three potential underlying mechanisms: shaping of the response by the model, an innate releasing mechanism, and the neonate's capacity to integrate visual and proprioceptive information. Consistent with their conclusions, the videotapes of the model's behaviors suggest that shaping or reinforcing the neonate's responses did not occur. Although "fixing" a face is not easy and may produce some muscle movement, there were no discernible movements on the model's face. That these imitations might be based on an innate releasing mechanism or fixed action pattern is also unlikely (13) given the organization and lack of stereotypy of the infants' differential responses to these three different facial expressions. Instead, we favor the view of Meltzoff and Moore (7) that there is an innate ability to compare the sensory information of a visually perceived expression (as evidenced in this study by their ability to discriminate the facial expressions) with the proprioceptive feedback of the movements involved in matching that expression (as manifested by their differential responses to the facial expressions).

REFERENCES

1. Hiatt, S. W., Campos, J. J. and Emde, R. N.(1979). *Child Development*, 50:1020. Izard, C. E., Heubner, R. R., Risser, D., McGinness, C. G. and Dougherty, L. M. (1980). *Developmental Psychology*, 16:132.
2. Darwin, C. (1872). *The Expression of the Emotions in Man and Animals*. London: Murray. Ekman, P. and Friesen, W. V. (1971). *Journal of Personality and Social Psychology*, 17:124.

3. Izard, C. E. (1971). *Face of Emotion*. New York: Appleton-Century-Crofts. Tomkins, S. S. and McCarter, R. (1964). *Perceptual Motor Skills*, 18:119.
4. Young-Brown, G., Rosenfeld, H. M. and Horowitz, F. D. (1977). *Child Development*, 48:555; La Barbera, J., Izard, C., Vietze, P. and Parisi, S. (1976). *ibid.*, 47:535.
5. Oster, H. and Ekman, P. (1978). *Minnesota Symposium of Child Psychology*, 11:231.
6. Anisfeld, M. (1979). *Science*, 205:214; Masters, J. C., *ibid.*, p. 215; Jacobson, S. W. and Kagan, J., *ibid.*, p. 215; Meltzoff, A. N. and Moore, M. K., *ibid.*, p. 217.
7. Meltzoff, A. N. and Moore, M. K. (1977). *ibid.*, 198:75.
8. All infants were full term (mean, 39.4 weeks), of normal birth weight (mean, 3296 g), and experienced an uncomplicated vaginal delivery with a minimum of obstetric medication and no general anesthesia. Two different adults served as models.
9. Reliability figures are based on the tapes of 12 infants and calculated by Kappa [J. J. Bartko and W. T. Carpenter, *Journal of Nervous and Mental Disease*, 163:307 (1976)]: total time per trial (.97); predominant pattern visual fixation (.91); mouth position (.82); eye position (.86); brow position (.83); and guess (.76).
10. Mean ($\pm$ standard deviation) fixation times (in seconds); early trials, 12.4 $\pm$ 9.7; middle trials, 16.2 $\pm$ 11.2; and late trials, 4.3 $\pm$ 2.9.
11. Mean proportion of trials with fixations on eyes: .13 (happy model), .15 (sad), and .23 (surprise); on mouth: .32 (happy), .40 (sad), and .23 (surprised); and on both eyes and mouth: .23 (happy), .29 (sad), and .45 (surprised).
12. As Meltzoff and Moore (7) have suggested, if each infant's response to one expression is compared with his response to another similar expression demonstrated by the same adult at the same distance from the infant and under the same conditions, and if differential imitation occurs, it cannot be attributed to a mere arousal of activity by a human face.
13. S. W. Jacobson's data [*Child Development*, 50:425 (1979)] suggest that a fixed action pattern mechanism may explain the matching behavior demonstrated by Meltzoff and Moore (7). Although A. P. Burd and A. E. Milewski (paper presented at the biennial meeting of the Society for Research in Child Development, Boston, 2 to 5 April, 1981) were unable to replicate Jacobson, this failure may be due to subtle differences in procedure relating to infant state or position of the eliciting stimulus.

8

Antecedents of Mother-Infant Interaction and Infant Irritability in the First Three Months of Life

Susan B. Crockenberg

University of California, Davis

Perrin Smith

Sutter Memorial Hospital, Sacramento

This research investigated the relationship of infant and mother characteristics to the development of infant temperament and mother-infant interaction during the first three months of life. Fifty-six mothers and their low-risk newborn infants participated in the research. Maternal questionnaires were administered prenatally and Neonatal Behavioral Assessments were administered in the early postnatal period; mother-infant interaction was observed at one and three months. Data were analyzed using hierarchical multiple regression techniques. The results indicate that neonatal irritability shows some consistency when time to calm is the criterion; that observed fussing and crying is associated not with neonatal irritability, but with unresponsive maternal attitudes and behavior; that initial irritability is associated with greater responsiveness to female than to male infants; and that

Reprinted with permission from *Infant Behavior and Development*, 1982, Vol. 5, 105–119.

This investigation was funded through the Agricultural Experiment Station, University of California, Davis. The authors thank Nancy Adams for her careful and sensitive data collection, Shirley Feldman and Mary Rothbart for their responses to an earlier draft of this paper, and Jody Bargones, Michael Birkman, Jennifer Davis, Christine Eaton, Sheryl Flocchini, Karen McCluskey, Lynn Sinnott, Kathy Shadburn and Arlene Yuki for their contributions to the project. Special recognition is given to Curt Acredolo for his assistance in data analyses and to the families who participated in the project.

by 3 months, antecedent mother and infant characteristics contribute significantly to the prediction of observed mother behavior. Findings are discussed in terms of a transactional model of development.

The first three months after birth have been identified as a period during which mother and infant establish patterns of reciprocal interaction. Inappropriate interaction during that time has been associated with later developmental difficulties (Ainsworth & Bell, 1969; Sander, 1969, 1975). At issue in this study are the characteristics of infants and mothers which influence the nature of their interaction during those early months. Of particular interest are the potential effects of an irritable infant temperament on the evolving mother-infant relationship, and alternately, the effects of mother-interaction patterns on subsequent infant irritability.

Infant Irritability

In their classic study of infant temperament, Thomas, Chess, and Birch (1968) identified an infant temperament type characterized by irregular biological functioning, frequent negative mood, slowness to adapt to change, and responses of high intensity. Infants exhibiting such characteristics were labeled "difficult." Since those characteristics were based on descriptions of babies during the first three months of life, it was suggested that they reflected inborn infant responses rather than environmentally induced behaviors.

Subsequent research on the consistency of infant temperament, and specifically on infant irritability, has produced conflicting data. Moss (1967) reported low but significant continuity in infant fussing and crying between three weeks and three months. Bell and Ainsworth (1972), however, reported no consistency in observed fuss/cry frequency over the first six months of life, and concluded that maternal behavior should be recognized as the primary determinant of infant irritability over the first year of life. Subsequently, Sameroff, Krafchuk, and Bakow (1978) found no relationship between newborn irritability as measured by the Neonatal Behavioral Assessment Scale (Brazelton, 1973) and observed fussing and crying or rated temperament at 4 months.

Basic to the issue of consistency in infant irritability is the appropriateness of the measures employed. Total fuss/cry frequencies are inevitably confounded by the length of time before a mother responds to her infant's cries. Bell and Ainsworth (1972) recognized this problem and thus distinguished between maternal unresponsiveness and infant crying for their within-quarter correlations. Maternal unresponsiveness was the length of time before a mother intervened in a fuss/cry episode, while infant irritability was the amount of crying *after* intervention (time to calm). Unfortunately, their between-quarter correlations included only maternal unresponsiveness and total fuss/cry; time to calm was not considered. While time to calm is undoubtedly influenced by mother's soothing skill, such a measure is less confounded by mother behavior than is the total amount of fussing (which is confounded by both time to intervene and soothing skill) and it is therefore more likely to assess infant temperament. This research will address the measurement issue by including both total fuss/cry frequency and time to calm as outcome temperament measures, and analyzing their mother and infant antecedents.

Infant Irritability and Maternal Behavior

There is considerable case-study, anecdotal, and clinical support for the view that early infant irritability is associated with maladaptive patterns of caretaking, including withdrawal, hostility, uninvolvement, and unresponsiveness (Aleksandrowicz & Aleksandrowicz, 1975; Bennett, 1976; Brazelton, 1962; Prechtl, 1963; Thomas, Chess, & Birch, 1968; Yarrow, 1965). More systematic large-scale studies, however, have produced conflicting results.

Moss (1967) examined the relationship between infant irritability and maternal contact at three weeks and again at three months in a sample of 30 first-born babies. At three weeks, infant irritability correlated with maternal contact .68 for females and .20 for males. But at three months, the correlation was .54 for females, − .47 for males. Moss suggests that boys are less consolable, mothers are less reinforced for their responsiveness and, over time, decrease their responsiveness toward their male babies. However, cross-lagged correlations between infant irritability at three weeks and maternal contact at three months, which would provide evidence in support of that hypothesis, were not provided.

In contrast, Bell and Ainsworth (1972) assert that low maternal responsiveness produced high subsequent infant crying, rather than the reverse. Twenty-six middle-class, white mother-infant pairs were observed at three-week intervals during the first year of life. Correlations were computed between infant crying and maternal unresponsiveness (time to intervene), both within- and between-quarters. First quarter crying did not correlate significantly with maternal unresponsiveness in the subsequent quarter, while maternal unresponsiveness in the first (and successive quarters) was significantly related to infant crying in each following quarter. A recent critique of that study (Gewirtz & Boyd, 1977) argues that Bell and Ainsworth's results are suspect because, among other problems, antecedent and concurrent variables not included in the analyses may have contributed to the behavior outcome (infant fussing and crying) to an unknown extent. It is argued, therefore, that their conclusions about the origins of infant irritability and maternal unresponsiveness based on those data must be viewed somewhat skeptically.

That skepticism is supported by Dunn's (1975) study of 70 mother-infant pairs followed from the first 10 days through 30 weeks, in which long crying times and a high frequency of crying bouts at one age were associated with decreased maternal touching on later ages. Similarly, Campbell (1979) reported that mothers of six babies assessed as "difficult" at 4 months continued to be in contact with them less at 8 months, when the infants were no longer perceived as difficult. Unfortunately, infant temperament ratings at 4 months, like observed crying, may themselves be affected by mother behavior, thereby confounding the causal direction of that relationship. Further, the one study which assessed infant temperament during the newborn period (Bakow, Sameroff, Kelly, & Zax, 1973) found no relationship between early infant irritability and maternal behavior at 4 months.

In sum, the research is contradictory with respect to the causal links between infant irritability and maternal contact and responsiveness. Methodological differences in the research may explain the discrepant results. The reviewed studies used different measures of infant irritability and maternal behavior, and observed infants and mothers at different intervals after birth. Moreover, responsiveness to an infant's irritability may depend on sex of infant, parity, and on maternal attitudes toward caretaking.

Maternal Characteristics and Maternal Behavior

A mother's attitude toward spoiling has been suggested as a likely influence on her responsiveness to infant crying by both Bell and Ainsworth (1972), and Dunn (1977). In a similar vein, Tulkin and Cohler (1973) reported that middle-class mothers who believed in reciprocity spent more time in face-to-face contact, responded more to vocalizations and crying, played more frequently with their infants, and restricted the child's behavior less when their infants were 10 months old.

Dunn (1977) noted also that parity affected mother behavior. In her research, she found that mothers of first babies tended to stick more closely to preset feeding schedules, and their babies cried more. Newborn feeding studies (Thoman, Barnett, & Leiderman, 1977; Thoman, Barnett, Leiderman, & Turner, 1970) support the view that the less experienced mothers of first-borns are less responsive to their infants' cues. Nonetheless, mothers of first-borns spent more time feeding their infants and stimulated them more—a finding replicated by 3-month-old infants (Jacobs & Moss, 1976; Lewis & Kreitzberg, 1979).

The recognition that both mother and infant characteristics correlate with subsequent mother and infant behavior and interaction is consistent with a transactional model of development (Bell, 1974; Sameroff, 1975; Sander, 1975). From a transactional perspective, the characteristics of infants and caretakers exert a mutual and reciprocal influence, yielding unique patterns of behavior. Methodologically, a transactional model requires independent measures of infant and mother behavior over time and analytical procedures which allow infant and mother effects to be considered simultaneously.

The present research has employed such a method in order to address the following questions:

1) Does neonatal irritability predict subsequent time to calm, thereby providing evidence of an irritability temperament dimension?
2) Does neonatal irritability influence maternal responsiveness and contact, and is the effect different for male and female, first-born and later-born infants?
3) Do parity and maternal attitudes about spoiling and responsiveness influence maternal contact and responsiveness to crying, and thereby infant fussing and crying?
4) Does a combination of infant and mother predictors significantly increase the predictability of mother and infant outcome measures?

METHOD

Subjects

Fifty-four Caucasian and two Asian-American mothers (37 primiparous, 19 multiparous) were contacted through prenatal groups or obstetricians, or in the hospital following the birth of their child.[1] The

---

[1] Of the 19 multiparous mothers, 18 had one child other than the target infant, one had two other children. There were no differences in questionnaire responses related to before and after administration of the questionnaire.

mothers ranged in age from 19 to 35 years, with 79% in the 21–30 year bracket. One half of the families, excluding the five student families, were middle-class as indicated by their placement in the first, second, and third levels of Hollingshead's (1965) occupational code; the remaining families were working-class. All families were intact.

There were 28 males and 28 females in the sample of infants, balanced by birth order. All infants were carried to term, above the 10th percentile for gestational growth, with no physical anomalies. There were 51 vaginal and five C-section deliveries.[2] All mothers and infants were in good physical condition when they left the hospital and were considered low-risk.

Procedures

Maternal questionnaire.—A 34-item questionnaire was developed to assess a variety of maternal attitudes, beliefs, and expectations (Smith, Note 3). As a means of identifying homogenous sets of items reflecting attitudes of responsiveness and flexibility, the attitude questionnaire responses of 95 pregnant or recently delivered women (including study participants) were subjected to a principal components factor analysis with a quartimax rotation. Of the four major factors which emerged, two were clearly centered around responsiveness (responsiveness to crying and responsiveness to night crying), while one was clearly a flexibility factor. Exact factor scores were then computed for each factor by summing the weighted standard scores of the three or four items having the highest loadings on each. These three factor scores were then summed to create the general index of responsiveness/flexibility.

Neonatal Behavioral Assessment Scale (NBAS).[3]—Instructions for administering and scoring the exam were followed exactly as described in Brazelton (1973), except that the pin prick aversive stimulus was eliminated. The assessments were made in the infant's homes on the fifth and tenth days following birth. Scores from the peak of excitement, rapidity of buildup, and irritability items were combined in an irritability

---

[2] There were no significant *t*-test differences between infants delivered vaginally and those delivered by Caesarian-section.

[3] The principal investigator and a postgraduate researcher were trained by Suzanne Dixon, University of California, San Diego Medical School. Two testers administered Brazelton assessments to newborn infants until they achieved 100% agreement within two levels and 90% agreement within one level prior to data collection. The results of the full Brazelton Assessment are available from the first author.

cluster,[4] and averaged across the two administrations as suggested by Kaye (1978). In view of the low day-to-day reliability reported for this cluster by Kaye (1978) and others, special care was taken to assess infants when they were well-fed and initially asleep as called for by test directions. In addition, only one test score was used if any *three* of the following conditions occurred: If the tester noted this was not the infant's best performance; if the mother indicated the baby's performance on the exam was atypical; if the testing conditions varied markedly from recommended conditions; or if the infant's scores on the two exams differed sharply. This procedure resulted in an irritability cluster score based on one examination for five infants and significant across-day reliability for the remaining infants, $r(51) = .38$, $p < .01$. Mean irritability for the entire sample was 5.54, $s.d. = 1.13$.

Mother-infant observations.—Four-hour home visits, including approximately 3½ hours of observation time, were made when infants were 1-month and 3-months old. Observations were scheduled for a time when a mother would be alone with her baby except for other children in the family. The baby would likely be awake and at least one feeding period would occur. Before each observation, the observer chatted with the mother to find out how the baby was doing, what sort of feeding and sleeping schedule the baby was on, and if anything unusual had occurred that day or the night before which might be expected to influence the baby's irritability.

A 10-second-observe, 10-second-record time sampling schedule was used, with both mother and infant behavior recorded in each interval. Within each 10-second interval category, use was mutually exclusive. Four assistants were each trained to use these categories by observing five or more pilot families. Interobserver reliability was established prior to the one-month observation and again preceding the three-month observation. Occurrence agreement was calculated by dividing the number of instances coders agreed on the use of a specific category for a specific interval by the sum of agreements plus disagreements for that

---

[4]An irritability item cluster was considered preferable to a consolability cluster because neither the consolability nor the self-quieting items can be scored if the infant fails to become irritable during the exam. In such instances, the third item in that cluster, hand to mouth, which may exhibit some short-term reliability but bears only a tenuous conceptual relationship with the outcome variables in this research, would constitute the cluster score. Moreover the irritability cluster does not suffer from the same deficiencies attributed to the total fuss/cry measure because, unlike mothers, testers are reasonably uniform in the amount of time they allow an infant to try before intervening.

category. Occurrence agreement for category use was .90 (range .83–1.00). Although in some cases observers had previously administered either Brazelton examinations or maternal questionnaires, those data were not available to them at the time of the observations.

Mother and infant observation categories.—Table 1 presents the observed mother behaviors and infant states, and the raw mean frequencies and standard deviations for those categories.

To insure that Involved Contact reflected a qualitative aspect of the mother-infant relationship, instances of mother behavior judged as in-

TABLE 1
Mother Behavior and Infant State Categories

Mother Behavior	Description	$\bar{x}$ [b] 1 mo.	3 mo.	s.d. 1 mo.	3 mo.
No contact[a]	No physical, visual or vocal contact between mother and infant	41.29	96.59	38.83	58.97
Routine contact[a]	Caretaking (bathing, feeding, etc.) or holding without vocal, visual or tactile stimulation	22.39	24.71	22.43	18.71
Involved contact	All caretaking and non-caretaking contact with additional vocal, visual or tactile stimulation	116.09	178.93	57.13	55.07
Eye contact[a]	Smiling/eye contact between infant and mother	36.51	58.34	22.67	28.48
Time to intervene	Average number of seconds from onset of crying until mother responds	23.09	22.24	22.24	30.10
Infant State	**Description**				
Fuss/cry	Frequency of 10-second fuss and cry intervals	75.41	60.89	44.02	32.64
Alert	Frequency of 10-second alert intervals (infant is awake and neither fussing nor drowsy)	193.57	327.25	88.36	63.84
Sleep/drowsy[a]	Frequency of 10-second sleep/drowsy intervals	340.52	227.30	104.92	78.18
Time to calm	Average time to calm after intervention in fuss and cry episodes	43.48	32.54	22.28	19.31

[a]Observed but not included in subsequent analyses.

[b]For mother contact categories, mean raw frequencies are for behaviors which occurred while the infant was alert.

appropriate or insensitive were deleted from the Involved Contact total. Examples of deleted behavior included speaking impatiently to a slow-feeding baby, speaking harshly when a baby grabbed the mother's hair, and continuing to jiggle or bounce a baby roughly after she had indicated distress at such treatment. Instances of such behavior were too infrequent to allow construction of a category of insensitive or inappropriate mothering, however.

RESULTS

To determine the degree of consistency in mother and infant behavior, correlations were calculated both within and between observations. Correlations of infant variables were partialled for total intervals observed. Correlations of mother variables were calculated for raw frequencies and also partialled for intervals alert.

With respect to the infant variables, within-observation correlations between total fuss/cry and time to calm were significant at both observations, $r(56) = .48, p < .001, r(56) = .39, p < .01$. Only time to calm was consistent over time, $r(56) = .31, p < .01$.

Mother variables of involved contact and time to intervene were negatively correlated within one- and three-month observations, $r(56) = -.26, p < .05$, and $r(56) = -.34, p < .005$, respectively. There was no substantial effect of partialling intervals alert. For correlations across observations, involved contact was significantly correlated over time, although the degree of relationship was considerably lower using raw data, $r(56) = .24, p < .05$, and $pr(55) = .52, p < .001$. Apparently, much of the observed consistency in mother behavior during the first three months is a function of the infant's availability for interaction. Time to intervene was not consistent over time, although one-month time to intervene negatively predicted three-month involved contact, $r(56) = -.24, p < .05$, and $pr(55) = -.32, p < .01$.

Multivariate Analyses of Infant Irritability and Maternal Contact and Responsiveness

The influence of neonatal irritability and maternal characteristics on subsequent infant state (total fuss/cry and time to calm), and on observed mother contact and time to intervene was examined through hierarchical multiple regressions (analyses of partial variance, Cohen & Cohen, 1975). Extensive partialling of control and other variables, and the order of variable inclusion reduced confounding of infant temperament effects.

Such a model provides a conservative test of temperament effects since any predictability temperament shared with other variables is attributed to those variables as they are entered earlier in the regression equation. Moreover, entry of interactions, selected on the basis of previous research, allowed us to investigate possible mediating effects of infant sex and parity on the impact of infant irritability.

Predictors of infant state.—Total intervals were first extracted as a potential covariate of fuss/cry. Parity, sex, and type of feeding (bottle or breast) were then entered as control variables. For one-month infant variables, these were followed by the maternal attitude factor and then by neonatal irritability. The entry of three selected interactions completed the analyses. For three-month infant variables, the control variables were followed first by maternal attitude *and* one-month mother behavior (with time alert at one-month included as a covariate) and then by neonatal irritability, 1-month infant state, and the selected interactions.

The only significant predictor of 1-month time to calm was neonatal irritability, $pr = .29, F(1, 50) = 4.54, p < .05$. There were no significant predictors of one-month fuss/cry. The results of the three-month infant state variables are summarized in Table 2. Again, neonatal irritability was the strongest predictor of time to calm. Babies who were irritable during the neonatal period took longer to calm at both observations. At 3 months, first-born babies took longer to calm also, possibly because their mothers were less experienced, and hence less skillful in calming them, or alternately because first-born infants took longer to recover from the trauma of birth.

Only parity and maternal attitude significantly predicted total fussing and crying. First-born infants and those whose mothers were less responsive anf flexible in their expressed attitudes fussed and cried more at 3 months. A post hoc analysis of partial variance revealed that the relationship between maternal attitude and three-month fussing and crying was significant, even after neonatal irritability and one-month infant state were extracted prior to maternal attitude, $pr = -.28, F(1, 49) = 4.08, p < .05$. In addition, although time to intervene correlated with total fuss/cry within observations $r(56) = .43, p < .005, r(56) = .33, p < .025$, the latter correlation was no longer significant when maternal attitude was partialled from the regression.

Predictors of mother behavior.—Intervals alert was extracted first as a potential covariate of mother contact. Parity, sex, and type of feeding

TABLE 2
Predictors of Three-Month Infant State[a]

Predictors	Fuss/Cry				Time to Calm			
	pr	R^2 increase	d.f.	F	pr	R^2 increase	d.f.	F
Covariate								
Intervals observed[b]	.15	.022	1,54	1.23	—	—	—	—
Control Variables								
Parity	−.27	.071	1,53	4.18*	−.28	.079	1,54	4.63*
Sex	.25	.057	1,52	3.51	.13	.016	1,53	<1
Feeding	.12	.012	1,51	<1	.23	.046	1,52	2.81
Mother & Infant Variables								
Attitude	−.28	.065	1,50	4.18*	−.14	.017	1,51	1.05
Time to intervene-1	.08	.005	1,49	<1	.11	.011	1,50	<1
Neonatal irritability	.03	.001	1,48	<1	.40	.135	1,49	9.48***
Infant state-1[c]	−.05	.002	1,47	<1	.18	.021	1,48	1.53
Interactions								
Sex × parity	−.28	.058	1,46	3.79	−.07	.003	1,47	<1
Parity × irritability	.05	.002	1,45	<1	.23	.036	1,46	2.61
Sex × irritability	.13	.019	1,44	<1	.09	.005	1,45	<1
Total	R=.56	R^2=.31	11,44	1.83	R=.61	R^2=.37	10,45	2.64**

Note: Variables were entered one at a time in the order listed. Partial correlations have all prior variables extracted. Significance levels are based on the increase in R^2 for each variable at entry.

[a]Three infants were identified as atypically irritable due to shots or mild colds. The group average was substituted for those infants.

[b]Included only for fuss/cry.

[c]One-month fuss/cry and one-month time to calm, respectively.

*p < .05; **p < .025; ***p < .005

were extracted as control variables, followed by maternal attitude and then, for the 1-month behaviors, neonatal irritability and the selected interactions. For the 3-month behaviors, the model remained the same except that intervals alert and mother behavior at 1 month were entered prior to neonatal irritability and the one-month infant state measure.

The results reveal that covariate and control variables account for all the significant predictors of one-month mother behavior. Involved contact is predicted by time alert, $pr = .76$, $F(1, 54) = 75.54$, $p < .0001$; parity, $pr = -.39$, $F(1, 53) = 9.37$, $p < .005$; breast-feeding, $pr = .28$, $F(1, 51) = 4.20$, $p < .05$; and sex x parity, $pr = .35$, $F(1, 48) = 6.91$, $p < .025$. To investigate this interaction, means for the sex/parity groups were compared. Second-born females experienced significantly less involved contact than all other groups. There were no significant predictors of 1-month time to intervene.

Table 3 presents the multiple regression analyses for three-month mother behavior. Congruent with 1-month results, time alert and parity continued to predict involved mother contact. In addition, however, mothers with responsive and flexible attitudes engaged in more involved contact and responded more quickly when their infants cried. And despite the significant positive relationship between irritability and involved mother contact, mothers were more responsive to high irritable female babies than to high irritable male babies. As a means of assessing the sex by irritability interaction, the Johnson-Neyman technique for determin-

TABLE 3
Predictors of Three-Month Mother Behavior

Predictors	Involved Contact				Time to Intervene			
	pr	R^2 increase	d.f.	F	pr	R^2 increase	d.f.	F
Covariate								
Intervals alert-3[a]	.33	.11	1,54	6.61**	—	—	—	—
Control Variables								
Parity	−.45	.18	1,53	13.19****	.02	.000	1,54	<1
Sex	.07	.004	1,52	<1	−.05	.002	1,53	<1
Feeding	.21	.033	1,51	2.45	.00	.000	1,52	<1
Mother Variables								
Attitude	.33	.074	1,50	6.12**	−.37	.139	1,51	8.29***
(Intervals alert-1)[a]	−.09	.005	1,49	<1	—	—	—	—
Mother behavior-1[b]	.46	.127	1,48	12.90****	.10	.009	1,50	<1
Infant Variables								
Neonatal irritability	.33	.051	1,47	5.67*	−.26	.059	1,49	3.67
Infant state-1	−.10	.005	1,46	<1	−.20	.032	1,48	2.04
Interactions								
Sex × parity	.13	.007	1,45	<1	.01	.000	1,47	3.30
Parity × irritability	.03	.000	1,44	<1	.27	.055	1,46	3.60
Sex × irritability	−.06	.001	1,43	<1	.32	.072	1,45	5.12*
Total	R=.77	R^2=.59	12,43	5.22****	R=.61	R^2=.37	10,45	2.63**

Note: Variables were entered one at a time in the order listed. Partial correlations (pr) have all prior variables extracted. Significance levels are based on the increase in R^2 for each variable at entry.

[a]Included only for involved contact.

[b]One-month involved contact and one-month time to intervene, respectively.

*$p < .05$; **$p < .025$; ***$p < .01$; ****$p < .001$

ing critical regions was employed (Kerlinger & Pedhozor, 1973). It was found that for irritability scores greater than one standard deviation above the mean (very high irritability levels), time to intervene scores were significantly higher for males than for females.

Post hoc analyses in which maternal attitude was entered into the analyses of partial variance prior to parity showed no reduction in the predictive value of parity, and suggest that differences in mother behavior associated with parity are not a function of the measured attitudinal differences.

In sum, by three months after birth, both mother and infant variables predicted observed mother-infant interaction. The multiple Rs were highly significant, even when one-month mother behavior was excluded, and entered variables accounted for 37 and 59% of the variance of involved contact and time to intervene outcome measures.

In view of the unexpectedly high predictive value of the time alert variable, hierarchical multiple regressions were again employed. At one-month, time alert was significantly predicted by type of feeding, $p = -.28$, $F(1, 51) = 4.43$, $p < .05$ (breast-fed infants were less alert); and by neonatal irritability, $pr = -.35$, $F(1, 49) = 6.86$, $p < .025$. Three-month time alert was predicted only by a sex x irritability interaction, $p = -.36$, $F(1, 44) = 6.65$, $p < .025$. Using the Johnson-Neyman technique, it was found that for irritability scores greater than or equal to .26 standard deviations above the mean, females were significantly more alert than males.

DISCUSSION

Infant Irritability

To investigate the possible effect of infant irritability on mother-infant interaction, irritability must be measured independently of the mother during the neonatal period, and should exhibit some stability. In this study, infant irritability showed definite consistency over time when time to calm after intervention was the criterion. Infants assessed as more irritable during the first 10 days of life took longer to calm at both observations. Apparently, initial physiological differences give rise to individual differences in degree of irritability that are consistent, at least through the first 3 months after birth. In striking contrast, but consistent with earlier research (Sameroff, Krafchuk & Bakow, 1978), newborn irritability failed to predict the total amount of fussing and crying at either observation. These findings support the view that the total amount of time an infant fusses and cries may be an inappropriate measure of infant temperament and hence an inappropriate validity criterion for the Neoatal Behavioral Assessment Scale.

Bell & Ainsworth (1972) proposed that mothers' beliefs about spoiling determined their responsiveness or unresponsiveness to their babies' fuss and cry signals and, thereby, the amount of time the babies were observed to fuss and cry. That is precisely the finding of this study. Both maternal attitudes of unresponsiveness and inflexibility, and the actual time it took a mother to respond to fuss/cry signals predicted the amount of time an infant fussed and cried at 3 months. Moreover, that the cross-time correlation of initial maternal attitude and subsequent fussing and crying remained significant after all covariate, control, and infant variables were partialled, directly addresses Gewirtz & Boyd's (1977) criticism of Bell and Ainsworth's analyses. That finding, in conjunction with the absence of the relationship between neonatal irritability and total fuss/cry, and the positive correlation between time to intervene and total fuss/cry (reduced to nonsignificance when maternal attitude is extracted) suggests that by three months, the confounded within-observation relationship between time to intervene and infant fussing and crying is most likely a function of mother behavior.

Noteworthy also is the absence of significant predictors of 1-month fussing and crying, a finding which may reflect the high level of non-hunger fussing apparent in 4-week old infants (Emde, Gaensbauer, & Harmon, 1976). Those researchers suggest that the elevated fussiness of all babies at that age makes it unlikely that "variations in mothering play a major role in its emergence, maintenance, or decline" (p. 84).

Infant Irritability and Maternal Responsiveness

That mothers respond differently to irritable infants as a function of their sex is apparent in the three-month data: Mothers of irritable females responded more quickly to fuss/cry signals than mothers of irritable males. This pattern of differential responsiveness is similar to Moss' (1967) finding of high maternal contact for females, and low maternal contact for males at three months. Further, it suggests that irritable male infants may be at risk for later aberrations in development. It is noteworthy in this context that early irritability in males has been associated with subsequent reduced social interest in others (Bell, Weller, & Waldrop, 1971).

Why should mothers of irritable females be particularly responsive? Possibly, mothers empathize with female infants by virtue of their shared sex. Or, mothers may respond to the sexual stereotype that girls require protection. Alternately, mothers may be more responsive to irritable female infants because of some characteristic of the infants themselves. Moss (1967) suggested that the most irritable females were less irritable than the most irritable males, and that moderate irritability attracted mothers to their infants without wearing them down. Although male and female infants in this study differed neither in initial irritability, nor in subsequent time to calm, the five most irritable infants were all males. Since differences in responsiveness were most apparent at very high irritability levels, Moss' explanation is plausible. In addition, however, infant girls may have been more attractive, despite their irritability, by virtue of their greater alertness. By 3 months, irritable males were the least alert group, irritable females the most. This pattern of correlates lends credence to the view that the amount of alert time is a behavioral index of the infant's maturational status (Emde et al., 1976; Parmelee, Wenner, & Schulz, 1964), and suggests further that the female's alertness may compensate for her irritability.

Emde et al. (1976) indicate that the coincidental decline in fussiness and the onset of smiling between two and three months after birth is associated with parental delight, and a sense that the infant is truly human. An alert infant is available for reciprocal interaction, and for smiling and eye contact, and thereby provides a mother with tangible reward for the extraordinary effort she expends in caring for her baby (Robson, 1967). A mother deprived of this reward may feel less delight and less emotional involvement with her infant, particularly if he is also fussy and difficult to soothe. The irritable male infants in this study fit this pattern: By three months, they have less responsive mothers in comparison with the more alert, though irritable, female babies. It should be noted, however, that as a group irritable infants are more likely to experience involved contact with their mothers, and there is no evidence that this relationship holds to a greater extent for females than males. At least at three months, then, withdrawal of mothers from their irritable male infants appears limited to the rapidity with which they respond to crying.

Covariate, Control and Attitudinal Predictors of Mother Contact

Much to our surprise (in view of our effort to observe babies during awake periods), the amount of time infants were alert during the observation was initially the strongest predictor of involved mother contact. In addition to affirming the likely effect of infant maturational status on the mother-infant interaction, that finding offers a new perspective on the absence of correlation between maternal attitude and one-month involved contact. At 4 weeks, infants as a group have just significantly increased the amount of time they are alert (Emde et al., 1976), and we would expect individual variation in time alert to be large for that reason. It follows that the influence of maturational variables should be proportionally greater at 1 month than at 3 months; and alternately, that the influence of mother variables should be more apparent at 3 months. That pattern is apparent in the present data.

Also worth noting is that the infant's status as a first- or later-born, included as the control variable parity, predicts the type of maternal contact he is likely to enjoy. Congruent with other studies (Jacobs & Moss, 1976; Lewis & Kreitzberg, 1979), later-born infants experience less involved contact with their mothers than do first-born infants, though not less responsiveness to their fussing and crying. Consistent with Lamb's (1977) findings, our observations suggest that the lower contact and responsiveness of multiparous mothers is often a direct consequence of their interaction with another child in the family. Observers noted that when multiparous mothers were out of contact, they were frequently diapering, feeding, toilet-training or retrieving an older child. When they were in contact with their babies, they were frequently reading or talking to an older child. That parity continued to predict mother contact after maternal attitude was extracted from the equation is additional evidence that it is the reality of caring for two children simultaneously, rather than parity-linked attitudes, which determines the nature of the mother-infant interaction for those pairs.

In summary, this study indicates that:

1. Neonatal irritability shows consistency when time to calm is the outcome variable,
2. Observed fussing and crying is associated *not* with neonatal irritability, but with unresponsive maternal attitudes and behavior,
3. Initial irritability is associated with greater responsiveness to female infants relative to male infants, possibly because they are more alert and potentially more rewarding to their mothers,
4. A likely maturational characteristic, time alert, is a strong predictor of mother contact,
5. Parity and maternal attitudes also predict maternal contact,
6. By three months, antecedent mother *and* infant characteristics contribute significantly to the prediction of observed mother behavior.

More generally, this research is consistent with the theoretical position that the process of development is a complex transaction of organism and environment most appropriately investigated with methods that consider multiple factors over time (Sameroff, 1975).

REFERENCES

Ainsworth, M. D. S. and Bell, S. M. V. (1969). Some contemporary patterns of mother-infant interaction in the feeding situations. In *Stimulation in Early Infancy*, J. A. Ambrose, ed. London: Academic Press.

Aleksandrowicz, M. K. and Aleksandrowicz, D. R. (1975). The molding of personality: A newborn's innate characteristics in interaction with parent's personalities. *Child Psychiatry and Human Development*, 5:231–241.

Bakow, H., Sameroff, A., Kelly, P. and Zax, M. (1973). Relations between newborn behavior and mother-child interaction at 4 months. Paper presented at the biennial meetings of the Society for Research in Child Development, Philadelphia, March.

Bell, R. (1974). Contributions of human infants to caregiving and social interaction. In *The Effect of the Infant on Its Caregivers*. M. Lewis and L. Rosenblum, eds. New York: John Wiley and Sons.

Bell, R., Weller, G. and Waldrop, M. (1971). Newborn and preschooler: Organization of behavior and relations between periods. *Monographs of the Society for Research in Child Development*, 36.

Bell, S. and Ainsworth, M. (1972). Infant crying and maternal responsiveness. *Child Development*, 43:1171–1190.

Bennett, S. L. (1976). Infant caretaker interactions. In *Infant Psychiatry: A New Synthesis*, C. N. Rexford, L. W. Sander and T. Shapiro, eds. New Haven, CT: Yale University Press.

Brazelton, T. B. (1962). Crying in infancy. *Pediatrics*, 29:579–588.

Brazelton, T. (1973). *Clinics in Developmental Medicine: Neonatal Behavioral Assessment Scale*. Philadelphia, PA: J. B. Lippincott Co.

Campbell, S. (1979). Mother-infant interaction as a function of maternal ratings of temperament. *Child Psychiatry and Human Development*, 10:67–76.

Cohen, J. and Cohen, P. (1975). *Applied Multiple Regression/Correlation Analysis for the Behavioral Sciences*. Hillsdale, NJ: Lawrence Erlbaum Associates.

Dunn, J. F. (1975). Consistency and change in styles of mothering. CIBA Foundation Symposium 33 (new series), *Parent-Infant Interaction*. New York: Associated Scientific Publishers.

Dunn, J. (1977). *Distress and Comfort*. Cambridge, MA: Harvard University Press.

Emde, R., Gaensbauer, T. and Harmon, R. (1976). *Emotional Expression in Infancy*. New York: International Universities Press.

Gewirtz, J. and Boyd, E. (1977). Does maternal responding imply reduced infant crying? A critique of the 1972 Bell & Ainsworth report. *Child Development*, 48:1200–1207.

Hollingshead, A. (1965). *Two Factor Index of Social Position*. New Haven, CT: Yale Station.

Jacobs, B. S. and Moss, H. A. (1976). Birth order and sex of siblings as determinants of mother-infant interaction. *Child Development*, 47:315–322.

Kaye, K. (1978). Discriminating among normal infants by multivariate analysis of Brazelton scores: Lumping and smoothing. *Monographs of the Society for Research in Child Development*, 43:60–80.

Kerlinger, F. N. and Pedhazor, E. J. (1973). *Multiple Regression in Behavioral Research*. New York: Holt, Rinehart, & Winston.

Lamb, M. (1977). The effects of ecological variables on parent-infant interaction. Paper presented at the biennial meetings of the Society for Research in Child Development, New Orleans, March.

Lewis, M. and Kreitzberg, V. S. (1979). Effects of birth order and spacing on mother-infant interactions. *Developmental Psychology*, 15:617–625.

Moss, H. (1967). Sex, age, and state as determinants of mother-infant interaction. *Merrill-Palmer Quarterly*, 13:19–36.

Parmelee, A., Wenner, W. and Schulz, H. (1964). Infant sleep patterns from birth to 16 weeks of age. *Journal of Pediatrics*, 65:576–582.

Prechtl, H. F. R. (1963). The mother-child interaction in babies with minimal brain damage. In *Determinants of Infant Behavior* (Vol. 12), B. M. Foss, ed. New York: Wiley, 1963.

Robson, K. S. (1967). The role of eye-to-eye contact in maternal-infant attachment. *Journal of Child Psychology and Psychiatry*, 8:13–25.

Sameroff, A. (1975). Early influences on development: Fact or fancy. *Merrill-Palmer Quarterly*, 21:267–294.

Sameroff, A. J., Krafchuk, E. E. and Bakow, H. A. (1978). Issues in grouping items from the Neonatal Behavioral Assessment Scale. *Monographs of the Society for Research in Child Development*, 43:46–59.

Sander, L. W. (1969). The longitudinal course of early mother-child interaction: Cross-case comparison in a sample of mother-child pairs. In *Determinants of Infant Behavior* (Vol. 4), B. M. Foss, ed. New York: Wiley.

Sander, L. W. (1975). Infant and caretaking environment: Investigation and conceptualization of adaptive behavior in a system of increasing complexity. *Explorations in Child Psychiatry*, E. J. Anthony, ed. New York: Plenum Press.

Smiht, P. Unpublished Master's thesis, University of California, Davis, 1978.

Thoman, E. B., Barnett, C. R. and Leiderman, P. H. (1971). Feeding behaviors of newborn infants as a function of parity of the mother. *Child Development*, 42:1471–83.

Thoman, E. B., Barnett, C. R., Leiderman, P. H. and Turner, A. M. (1970). Neonate-mother interaction: Effects of parity on feeding behavior. *Child Development*, 41:1103–1111.

Thomas, A., Chess, S. and Birch, H. G. (1968). *Temperament and behavior disorders in children*. New York: New York University Press.

Tulkin, S. and Cohler, B. (1973). Childrearing attitudes and mother-child interaction in the first year of life. *Merrill-Palmer Quarterly*, 19:95–106.

Yarrow, L. W. (1965). An approach to the study of reciprocal interactions in infancy: Infant-caregiver pairs in foster care and adoption. Paper presented at the biennial meeting of the Society for Research in Child Development, Minneapolis.

PART II: INFANCY STUDIES

9

Maternal Perception of Infant Emotion From Birth Through 18 Months

**William F. Johnson, Robert N. Emde,
and Betty Jean Pannabecker**

University of Colorado Health Sciences Center

Craig R. Stenberg

University of Denver

Margaret H. Davis

Denver, Colorado

This study reports on maternal perceptions of emotion in their own infants. Concurrent and retrospective estimates of emotion onset were obtained from 597 mothers of infants who varied in age from 1 through 18 months. Information was also obtained about the frequency with which mothers perceived emotions in themselves and in their infants. Unexpectedly, a substantial number of emotions were reported in young infants. During the first three postnatal infant months, a majority of mothers reported the presence of five of the 11 emotion categories studied (interest, joy, surprise, anger, and distress).

Reprinted with permission from *Infant Behavior and Development*, 1982, Vol. 5, 313–322.
Robert Emde is supported by Research Scientist Award #K05 MH 36808 and NIMH Project Grant #2 R01 MH 22803. Special thanks are due to James Sorce, Joseph Campos, and members of the Developmental Psychobiology Research Group for constructive criticism and to Judith Thorpe and Leola Schultz for technical assistance.

Another study of 26 mothers of newborns found similar results concerning the prevalence of perceived emotions. Age trends and possible explanations for the high frequency of perceived emotions in early infancy are discussed. An important issue is to what extent mothers relied on infant behaviors and to what extent they made use of contextual cues.

Recent experimental and theoretical investigations of infant development have recognized the importance of emotional variables in infancy (Sroufe, 1979), particularly in caregiving decisions (Campos, Goldsmith, Svejda, & Stenberg, 1981, in press). Building upon the pioneering work of Ekman (Ekman, Friesen, & Ellsworth, 1972), Tompkins (1962, 1963), and Izard (1971, 1972, 1977) which demonstrated cross-cultural recognizability of discrete emotional expressions in the adult, infancy researchers have examined a variety of interrelated topics. For example, investigators have demonstrated the specificity of infant facial displays (Hiatt, Campos, & Emde, 1979; Izard, Huebner, Risser, McGinnes, & Dougherty, 1980; Oster & Ekman, 1978), the capacity of mothers to distinguish discrete emotion signals (Emde, Kligman, Reich, & Wade, 1978), and the impact of maternal emotions on the infant (Sorce & Emde, 1981; Sorce, Emde, & Klinnert, 1981).

This paper reports on a largely untapped source of information about mother-infant emotional life: maternal perceptions of their own infants' emotional expressions. It provides normative, descriptive data about maternal reports which may be of heuristic value for further research and theorizing. As compared with laboratory judgments of behavior, mothers are biased in unknown ways, but their perceptions include some of the most extensive sampling possible. In their day-to-day observations, mothers are likely to encounter a wide range of emotions in varying contexts; they attend to more than facial expressions; they are also likely to be present during unusual occurrences of meaningful behavior.

Furthermore, mothers' reports of their infants' emotions have ecological validity. Although mothers may be influenced by their own feelings and see them reflected in their infants, we believe the mothers' reports are meaningful because they represent perceptions that may influence caregiving. Finally, because of extensive time sampling, maternal reports may provide information relevant to the age of onset of infant emotional expressions which cannot be easily obtained in the laboratory.

METHOD

Survey Instrument

The Survey instrument was designed for mothers and consisted of: (a) a page of identifying information including questions about age, race, education, and parity; (b) an emotion onset questionnaire; and (c) two versions of the differential emotions scale II (DES-II) (Izard, 1972; Izard, Dougherty, Bloxom, & Kotsch, unpublished manuscript), one pertaining to infant emotions over the previous week and one pertaining to maternal emotions over the previous week.

The onset questionnaire had 11 questions about particular emotions in the form of: "Does your baby show ——?" with yes or no as possible answers. If a mother responded positively, she was requested to estimate the month in which she first noticed the relevant emotion in her child. This resulted in two types of onset data: (a) Concurrent: The presence or absence of an emotion at the time of the survey, (b) Retrospective: The estimate of the month of onset for those infant emotions reported as present. Mothers were asked about the onset of the following emotions: interest, joy, surprise, anger, contempt, fear, shyness, guilt, disgust, distress, and sadness.[1]

The DES-II consists of 30 words referring to 10 different emotions identified by Izard's differential emotions theory (Izard, 1977). Three of the 30 words refer to each of the 10 emotions. The DES-II has been found to be a reliable and valid instrument for measuring adult emotions (Izard, Dougherty, Bloxom, & Kotsch, unpublished manuscript). This is the first time that the DES-II has been used to rate infant behavior although maternal responses to a picture rating task asking them for the emotions being displayed in selected still photographs of 3½-month-old infants (Emde et al., 1978) fell into categories similar to those described by Izard. For this reason, we felt that the DES-II could also be used to accurately assess infant emotions as well.

Mothers were asked to read the DES-II and answer, by means of a 5-point frequency scale, how often over the past week they had observed each emotion in their infants (version one) and in themselves (version two). The frequency scale included the categories "rarely or never," "occasionally," "moderately often," "quite often" and "very often"; these were later assigned ordinal values from 1 to 5, respectively.

---

[1]The 10 emotional categories of the DES include all those used to construct our onset questionnaire except for the category of sadness. The DES includes "sadness" under the category of "distress"; however, we felt that for infancy "distress" might have a different connotation than "sadness" and that its onset was worth inquiring about separately.

Since we consider that our sample of mothers may have arisen from a population different from that upon which the DES-II was validated, we subjected the mothers' self-reports to factor analysis. This showed that the 30 items of the DES as the mothers applied them to themselves factored into seven of the 10 emotion categories set forth by Izard. An eighth factor, joy and distress, was bipolar, thus accounting for nine of Izard's a priori categories (Fuenzalida, Emde, Pannabecker, & Stenberg, 1981). This factor structure closely approximated the results found by Izard.

Initially we intended to carry out the entire survey through face-to-face interviews in "well baby clinic" settings. However, after several months of data collection we realized that mailed questionnaires would greatly increase our ability to reach a large number of mothers. Since a statistical comparison revealed no differences between these approaches, we made progressively greater use of mailed surveys to complete our data collection. All data were collected during a year's time.

Sample

A total of 597 questionnaires were completed. Three hundred and three were from face-to-face interviews (100% return) and 294 were from mailed surveys (66% response for the 448 sent). Eight questionnaires were discarded by the computer according to prearranged criteria for uncovering marked within-case discrepancies between DES-II data and onset data. In these instances questionnaire responses were words with "occasionally" or "moderately often" for at least two emotion categories despite the recording of "no emotion present" in the onset portion of the questionnaire for the same emotions. The resulting number of 589 was the basis for all data analysis.

A mean of 32.6 mothers responded for each infant month from one to 18 months of age. Ninety-seven percent of the mothers were married and 87% were Caucasian, 9% Hispanic, 3% Black, and 1% Indian or Oriental. Sixty percent of the mothers were housewives, and the mean grade level achieved was 14.3 years with a range from 8 to 21 years. Fathers were similarly well-educated with a mean grade level of 15.2 years. Of the infants, 56% were firstborn and 53% were male.

Results

As can be seen from Tables 1 and 2, mothers report a number of emotions in their very young infants. Since there were no differences between the individual months of each age quarter, the data in Tables

TABLE 1*
Presence of Emotions: Concurrent

Infant Quarter	I	II	III	IV	V	VI
(months)	1–3	4–6	7–9	10–12	13–15	16–18
	Percent of Mothers Indicating Emotion Was Present					
Interest	99	100	100	100	100	100
Joy	95	100	100	100	100	100
Surprise	74	95	94	94	99	100
Anger	84	93	95	96	93	99
Distress	68	74	76	73	78	71
Fear	58	75	69	78	84	90
Shyness	9	41	66	75	88	89
Sadness	34	40	53	61	62	58
Disgust	22	28	31	40	44	49
Contempt	16	15	21	29	36	28
Guilt	0	3	10	31	49	49

* Actual N's vary somewhat from 589 because not all questionnaires contained complete information about each emotion.

TABLE 2*
Onset of Emotions: Retrospective

Infant Quarter	I	II	III	IV	V	VI
	Percent of All Mothers (N=589) Indicating The Particular Emotion Onset During Each Quarter					
Interest	85	12	2	1	0	0
Joy	83	13	3	1	0	0
Surprise	61	26	7	5	1	0
Anger	51	26	11	10	11	11
Distress	66	16	7	7	2	2
Fear	46	23	14	12	3	2
Shyness	14	36	25	19	4	2
Sadness	33	29	17	17	3	1
Disgust	20	33	18	19	8	2
Contempt	27	25	17	28	3	0
Guilt	3	11	21	45	13	7

* Actual N's vary somewhat from 589 because not all questionnaires contained complete information about each emotion.

1 and 2 were grouped by three-month intervals to produce the six "quarters" reported.

As shown in Table 1, interest, joy, surprise, anger, distress, and fear (6 of the 11 emotion categories) were perceived to be present by a majority of mothers of infants in the first age quarter. These are distinct from the remaining five emotions—shyness, sadness, disgust, contempt, and guilt—which are recorded as present in their infants by ⅓ or fewer of mothers of first quarter infants.

Table 1 also indicates some general patterns of onset among the 11 emotions. Interest, joy, surprise, and anger are observed by ¾ or more of the mothers of the youngest grouping of infants (quarter one); furthermore, well over 90% of mothers had seen their older infants express these emotions. This is in contrast to the onset patterns for sadness, disgust, contempt, and guilt, where even among the mothers of the oldest infants in the study, less than ⅔ reported these emotions.

Distress and fear exhibit a third onset pattern, being reported present in about ⅔ of the youngest infants but showing only modest increases in frequency of reporting throughout the age period under study. Distress was observed by 68% of mothers of infants in the sixth quarter. Fear exhibits a gradual age change in frequency of observation; it was recorded as present in 58% of the youngest babies and in 90% of the oldest subsample.

The onset pattern demonstrated by shyness is unlike that for the other emotions. Very few babies (9%) in the youngest age grouping were thought to be exhibiting shyness but the frequency with which mothers recognized this emotion in their infants increased dramatically over the next four quarters (41, 66, 75, and 88%, respectively), finally leveling off in the last quarter with almost 90% of mothers observing shyness in their children.

Table 2 presents the second kind of onset data—the retrospective estimates of the month of onset for those emotions which mothers reported seeing in their infants. In other words, it answers the following question: For those mothers reporting particular emotional expressions, when did they first see them?

While this provides more information than was true for simple presence-or-absence judgments, there are inherent difficulties in interpretation. Parental memory becomes a factor to be reckoned with, and a mother's estimate can only include responses less than the age of her baby, leading to clumping of the data toward the early age intervals. Despite these difficulties it can be seen that Table 2, in general, reproduces the age trends evident in Table 1.

Of those mothers perceiving certain emotions, a majority responded that interest, joy, surprise, anger, and distress had their onset in their infant's first quarter. These five emotions were also those that a majority of mothers of first quarter infants had observed as present (as per Table 1). Fear, the sixth emotion seen by a majority (58%) of mothers of first quarter infants, was reported by slightly under 50% of the whole sample as having its onset in the baby's first quarter. Table 2 also reveals that over 80% of all mothers saw interest and joy as first occurring by 3 months of age; over 75% saw surprise and anger as occurring by 6 months. The onset of shyness is generally attributed to the second and third quarters. There is considerable scatter as mothers estimate the onset of sadness, disgust, contempt, and guilt.

Mean infant and maternal DES scores were calculated for the entire sample (N = 589), and were used as a basis for comparing maternal and infant emotional levels. Interestingly, mothers perceived more of a number of emotions in their infants than they perceived in themselves (more interest, joy, surprise, anger, fear, and shyness; $p < .001$ in each instance). On the other hand, they perceived more distress ($p < .001$) and guilt ($p < .01$) in themselves than in their infants. The differences between perceptions of maternal and infant disgust were not significant; however, discriminations among these low frequency emotions were probably impossible because of basement scaling effects.

In spite of these differences between maternal and infant overall DES values there were ordinal similarities across the emotion categories. For both mothers and infants, the hedonically-positive emotions, namely interest, joy, and surprise, had the highest DES values and were thus seen to occur most frequently. Anger was the negative emotion mothers reported most often in themselves and in their infants. Fear and shyness were seen less often and the other emotions were infrequently reported in either mothers or their children.

Maternal and infant DES scores for each infant age quarter were also compared by means of t-tests (Table 3). This analysis revealed an interesting phenomenon during early infancy. For four emotions (interest, joy, surprise and shyness) there is a cross-over pattern evident in the t-scores of the first two quarters. That is, mothers of the youngest infants reported that they felt these emotions more frequently than they observed them in their infants; whereas in the second quarter and thereafter the situation was reversed, with the infant perceived as expressing these same four emotions more frequently. Fear comes close to exhibiting the same cross-over phenomenon. The first quarter t-score of 0.0 indicates that mothers perceived this emotion as occurring equally fre-

TABLE 3
t-Values of Maternal vs. Infant DES Scores
For Each Quarter (N = 589)

Emotion	I	II	III	IV	V	VI
Interest	-0.61^{ns}	3.93***	5.55***	2.80**	3.63***	4.39***
Joy	-3.51***	6.15***	10.45***	8.89***	8.63***	8.17***
Surprise	-4.61***	2.72**	1.85^{ns}	1.23^{ns}	1.77^{ns}	2.16*
Anger	4.05***	5.28***	1.12^{ns}	3.73***	5.29***	4.12***
Distress	-9.23***	-7.95***	-8.62***	-7.04***	-6.72***	-5.70***
Fear	0.00^{ns}	2.77**	2.46*	2.88**	1.53^{ns}	2.65**
Shyness	-2.42*	2.19*	5.66***	9.00***	5.51***	5.06***
Sadness	NOT ONE OF THE 10 DES CATEGORIES					
Disgust	-1.57^{ns}	-0.84^{ns}	-4.36***	-1.65^{ns}	-2.97**	-0.55^{ns}
Contempt	-3.61***	-3.11**	-3.02**	-2.79**	-2.55*	-1.55^{ns}
Guilt	-6.46***	-8.59***	-9.77***	-6.17***	-4.64***	-3.77***

ns	=	non—significant
*	=	$p < .05$
**	=	$p < .01$
***	=	$p < .001$

quently in themselves and in their infants during this time period. It is significant to note that in the second quarter and thereafter, however, mothers perceived this emotion as occurring significantly more frequently in their babies than in themselves. Anger is unique in that it is the only emotion for which mothers reported its occurrence more frequently in their infants throughout the age span under study. Values for distress, disgust, contempt, and guilt suggest that these emotions are consistently perceived as being more frequent in mothers themselves than in their infants.

In order to specify the extent of correspondence between maternal perceptions of her own emotions and those in her infant, correlations between maternal and infant DES values are calculated for each emotion. For the sample as a whole correlations ranged between $+0.19$ for guilt and $+0.42$ for anger and surprise; the mean correlation was $+0.34$. Correlations were not altered substantially when the sample was partialed according to infant sex or age, maternal parity, or maternal employment status.

In other analyses, primiparous mothers did not differ significantly from multiparous mothers in their estimates of emotion onset. The sex of the infant was not found to affect either maternal or infant DES for any of the emotions. The same was true for maternal education and job status.

DISCUSSION

The finding that mothers perceived a substantial number of emotions in their young infants (as per Tables 1 & 2) was not expected by our multidisciplinary team of investigators. Based on previous work (Emde, 1980; Emde, Gaensbauer, & Harmon, 1976) we had thought that most mothers would see interest, joy, and distress in their young babies but not surprise, anger, and fear. For the latter emotions, we had rarely observed the characteristic patterned responses of facial expression and/or related motoric behaviors before three postnatal months. An examination of the data by monthly intervals during early infancy revealed this finding to be consistent.

Because even mothers of 1-month-old infants reported observing a number of emotions in their infants, we undertook an additional study of newborns to see if mothers would perceive a similar number of emotions if they had even less time to interact with their infants. Twenty-six mothers of newborns were contacted during their lying-in period and were given the study questionnaire, which they were instructed to take home and fill in when their infants were 1-week-old. The demographic characteristics of these mothers differed somewhat from those of the whole study population in that they tended to be younger (mean age 22.8 vs. 28.0 years) and less well educated (mean educational level 12.5 vs. 14.5 years) although they did not differ with respect to child rearing experience.

The results of this small scale additional study were clear. Mothers of 1-week-old infants also reported a substantial number of emotions. Interest and joy were noted by 95%, anger by 78%, distress by 65%, and surprise by 68%. Sadness and disgust were observed in their newborns by more than 40% of mothers and 35% reported fear present by 1 week of age. On the other hand, only 8% of mothers perceived shyness in their newborns and none saw guilt.[2]

The reports of guilt in infants during the last half of the first year of life is an interesting, if puzzling, result. It may be a result of some projection on the part of the mother, but it may also reflect rudimentary

---

[2]Contempt was recorded as present by 35% of mothers. But this word was clearly misunderstood by some, one of whom told us she thought it meant "content." Evidence also suggested that some mothers interpreted the word "distress" differently from others. Some interpreted it as simple discomfort while others interpreted it as a more complex emotional state. This may explain why distress was reported by only 68% of mothers of first quarter infants.

infant expressions that become better defined in the second year. Further research is needed.

We feel four possibilities need to be examined in attempting to explain the high frequency with which mothers perceive certain emotions in early infancy. The first is that mothers become attuned to the subtleties and individual features of their babies' emotional expression, aspects which are not readily apparent to experimenters whose typical experience with each individual infant is limited to a single encounter. One would then expect to see increasing maternal perception of emotion with increasing infant age. This does in fact occur, but the high maternal perception of emotion in newborn infants argues against maternal experience being the main determinant of this phenomenon.

A second possibility is that mothers are interpreting relatively undifferentiated affective behaviors in the light of contextual information and are "constructing" an emotion from these two types of input. For example, a mother encountering a crying infant may in one case say, "He's sad, because that's how I would feel were I left alone," while in another situation she might say, "He's angry, because I'd be angry if I weren't fed on time."

A third possible explanation is that the perinatal experiences of the mother lead to a special "tuning up" for empathy. In other words, the physiological and environmental changes that occur with pregnancy, childbirth and related events may produce a special emotional sensitivity which lends itself to the perception of attribution by the mother of feeling states in her young infant.

A fourth possibility is that mothers are projecting their own emotions onto their infants. Our study was designed with separate emotion frequency questionnaires for mother and infant to examine this possibility. However, the correlation data do not appear to support this explanation.

Some meaningful age trends were also evident in these data. Such trends raise questions concerning the basis for changing maternal perceptions as a function of development. Does the reliance of the mother on contextual information change as more patterned responses emerge in the older infant? Does the mother learn to "read" her infant more accurately as a function of experience in day-to-day interaction? Correspondingly, does mother's "projective" contribution become less of a factor as both infant and mother move away from the perinatal period? Clearly, these questions cannot be answered in a cross-sectional design. To further explore this, a longitudinal study of 36 infants has been undertaken. Besides asking mothers what emotions they perceive in their infants, detailed interview information is being obtained in the case of each emotion perceived. Three areas are being probed: mother's description of her infant's behavior, mother's thinking about what caused the emotion, and mother's caregiving response which she feels would typically be elicited by her infant's emotional expression.

The preliminary results of this study are quite interesting. By 3 months, mothers describe behaviors of their infants as a basis for their judgments about emotion. Early on, however, these behaviors are interpreted with the aid of contextual information; later on, the behaviors are described as more patterned with their interpretation seemingly less dependent on context. In addition, the relevant contextual variables change as a function of age. For example, in early infancy fear is judged from an infant's crying after a sudden loud noise or a loss of support. Later, fear is judged when the infant has a particular expression and an unfamiliar adult approaches. Early on, eliciting stimuli tend to be objects whether animate or inanimate; later, eliciting stimuli are predominantly human and social.

Our study emphasizes that mothers perceive a number of discrete emotions in their infants and that many report these emotions very early in their infants' lives. These reports may contain information about infant emotional development as well as information about maternal attitudes which influence caregiving. More research is needed to better understand the factors influencing these perceptions and their functions in mother-infant interactions.

REFERENCES

Campos, J. J., Goldsmith, H. H., Svejda, M. J. and Stenberg, C. R. (In press). Socioemotional development. In *Handbook of Child Psychology. Vol. II. Biology and Infancy*, M. Haith and J. Campos, eds. New York: Wiley.

Ekman, P., Friesen, W. V., and Ellsworth, P. (1972). *Emotion in the Human Face*. New York: Pergamon Press.

Emde, R. N. (1980). Levels of meaning for infant emotions: A biosocial view. In *Development of Cognition, Affect and Social Relations*, W. A. Collins, ed. Minnesota Symposia on Child Psychology, Vol. 13. Hillsdale, NJ: Lawrence Erlbaum Associates.

Emde, R. N., Gaensbauer, T. J. and Harmon, R. J. (1976). Emotional expression in infancy; A biobehavioral study. *Psychological Issues, A Monograph Series*, Inc., Vol. 10, #37. New York: International Universities Press.

Emde, R. N., Kligman, D. H., Reich, J. H. and Wade, T. D. (1978). Emotional expression in infancy: I. Initial studies of social signaling and an emergent model. In *The Development of Affect*, M. Lewis and L. Rosenblum, eds. New York: Plenum Publishing Corporation.

Fuenzalida, C., Emde, R. N., Pannabecker, B. J. and Stenberg, C. R. (1981). Validation of the differential emotion scale in 613 mothers. *Motivation and Emotion*, in press.

Hiatt, S., Campos, J. and Emde, R. N. (1979). Facial patterning and infant emotional expression: Happiness, surprise, and fear. *Child Development*, 50:4, 1020–1035.

Izard, C. E. (1971). *The Face of Emotion*. New York: Appleton-Century Crofts.

Izard, C. E. (1972). *Patterns of Emotions*. New York: Academic Press.

Izard, C. E. (1977). *Human Emotions*. New York: Plenum.

Izard, C. E., Dougherty, F., Bloxom, B. M. and Kotsch, N. E. (Unpublished manuscript). The differential emotions scale: A method of measuring the subjective experience of discrete emotions.

Izard, C. E., Heubner, R. R., Risser, D., McGinnes, G. C. and Dougherty, L. M. (1980). The young infant's ability to produce discrete emotion expressions. *Developmental Psychology*, 16:2, 132–140.

Oster, H. and Ekman, P. (1980). Facial behavior in child development. In *Development of Cognition, Affect and Social Relations*, W. A. Collins, ed. Minnesota Symposia on Child Psychology, Vol. 13. Hillsdale, NJ: Lawrence Erlbaum Associates.

Sorce, J. F. and Emde, R. N. (1981). Mother's presence is not enough: The effect of emotional availability on infant exploration. *Developmental Psychology*, in press.

Sorce, J. F., Emde, R. N. and Klinnert, M. (1981). Maternal emotional signaling: Its effect on the visual cliff behavior of one-year-olds. Paper presented at Biennial Meeting of Society for Research in Child Development, Boston, April.

Sroufe, L. A. (1979). Socioemotional development. In *Handbook of Infant Development*, J. D. Osofsky, ed. New York: John Wiley & Sons.

Tompkins, S. S. (1962). *Affect, Imagery, Consciousness. The Positive Affects*. Vol. 1. New York: Springer.

Tompkins, S. S. (1963). *Affect, Imagery, Consciousness. The Negative Affects*. Vol. 2. New York: Springer.

10

Some Origins of the "Difficult" Child: The Brazelton Scale and the Mother's View of Her New-born's Character

Russell Meares

Westmead Centre, New South Wales, Australia

Robyn Penman and Jeannette Milgrom-Friedman

Austin Hospital, Australia

Kay Baker

University of Sidney, Australia

Thirty-two mothers and their new-born babies were studied in order to consider, in a limited way, the manner in which a mother comes to attribute personality traits to her infant. The child's expected "difficulty" was rated by means of a standardized inventory. In addition, a semi-structured interview was conducted with the mother, and her baby was examined by means which have been described by Brazelton. The circumstances of birth were taken from hospital records.

Mothers who did not expect the child to be difficult showed a "general flexibility" which probably related to coping ability. Babies who were seen as unlikely to be difficult had high scores on "state control" and "physiological response to stress." These measures include ratings for habituation and seem to reflect an efficient means of dealing with

Reprinted with permission from the *British Journal of Medical Psychology*, 1982, Vol. 55, 77–86. Copyright 1982 by The British Psychological Society.

This study was supported by the National Health and Medical Research Council of Australia.

stimuli. These infantile factors did not correlate with the maternal one, suggesting that a genetic explanation of the findings was not likely. The effect of the circumstances of birth was not strong, but medication level seemed important.

The transcripts of the mothers' interviews were consistent with the view that the mother's assessment of her infant's character was not only influenced by a fine observation of the infant's behavior but also by something like "projective identification." The transcripts also suggested that mechanisms which have been seen as important in the development of identity in adolescence may be operating from the first days of life.

Soon after it is born, the mother is likely to attribute personality traits to her infant. Anecdotal evidence suggests that in pathological cases at least, these attributions may persist, influencing mother-child interaction and the subsequent personality development of the child. The Genain quadruplets provided an example of this process. One of them, Hester, was seen negatively by her mother from birth. Moreover, "she was ever after treated as the baby, called the baby and expected to behave as the baby" (Rosenthal, 1963, p. 552). These four monozygotic children all became schizophrenic in later life, but in varying degrees. Hester was the most afflicted.

Despite its presumed importance for child development, the way in which a mother comes to conclusions about the personality and nature of her infant has not been the subject of a great deal of detailed study. Broussard and Hartner (1971), however, in an investigation of the mother's perception of her infant's potential "difficulty," concluded that maternal perceptions are largely based on "fantasy." Clinical evidence, however, does not entirely favor this view. It may not have been chance, for example, that Mrs. Genain perceived Hester as weak and bad, since she was the smallest of the quads and the least healthy after birth. On the other hand, Mrs. Genain's feeling about each baby was influenced by how she felt about herself. Indeed she acted as if to parcel out pieces of herself and project them upon her infants (p. 548).

In this study we make a limited excursion into the way in which "normal" mothers perceive their infants. We chose to confine the possible infant attributes to "difficult" (which is often equated with bad) and "not difficult." Thomas et al. (1978) have identified a particular constellation of temperament traits in "the difficult child." These traits include irregularity in biological functions (e.g., sleeping, eating), slow adaptability to change, and intense and negative mood expressions.

We speculated that the mother's tendency to attribute difficulty to her new-born may depend upon two main factors:

(i) a general sense of her own competence and preparedness for motherhood;
(ii) a reasonably accurate perception of her new-born's behavioral characteristics.

In order to consider the latter possibility, we assessed the infants by means which have been developed by Brazelton. His neurophysiological and psychological assessment procedures give an index of the neonate's "competence" (Bower, 1974). For example, it tests the baby's ability to calm itself and to deal with unpleasant stimuli. A final possible factor in the mother's perception of her infant might be the circumstances surrounding the birth. These also are considered.

METHOD

Participants

Thirty-two mothers and their neonates acted as participants in this study. This sample of mothers was obtained from a local community hospital. Three sets of criteria were used in sample selection. Firstly, the women were primiparous, had English as their first language and were living in a "stable" relationship (either married or *de facto*). Secondly, they were not past term and had not had serious complications during labor. Thirdly, no woman whose infant was put under intensive care immediately post-delivery was included. The aim of these criteria was to obtain a sample of primiparae who had experienced a relatively normal birth.

The ages of the women ranged from 17 to 30, with a mean of 23.1 years. Their years of schooling ranged from nine to 15 years. Seventy percent had 10 years or less of schooling. The majority of the sample had been employed in clerical activities. The others had worked as sales, process or technical workers.

Procedures and Measures

Data for this study were obtained from four sources: (*a*) assessment of the infant using the Brazelton Neonatal Behavioural Assessment Scale

(Als et al., 1977); (*b*) hospital records; (*c*) a semi-structured interview; and (*d*) a standardized perception inventory. All data were gathered 48 to 72 hours after delivery. At this point the mothers had only a limited opportunity to judge the temperament of their infants. They had begun to feed and change their babies but had not bathed them. Nor did they see them through the night when they may have been crying. It was hospital practice to have the mothers with their babies from 5.00 a.m. to 9.00 p.m. Most women were in small dormitories but occasionally they occupied single rooms.

(i) *Infant characteristics.*—This assessment was conducted, prior to interviewing the mother, by one of us (K.B.) trained to reliability by Brazelton in the use of his scale. The scale measures four dimensions of infant behavior and has had a number of validity tests to support its use (e.g., Als et al., 1977; Sostek & Anders, 1977). The four dimensions are:
   (*a*) Interactive processes: this rates the infant's capacity for attention and its social responsiveness to cuddling and other stimuli, such as a voice or a face.
   (*b*) Motoric processes: this rates aspects of musculo-skeletal development such as muscle tone and coordination.
   (*c*) Organization processes—state control: these items indicate the infant's capacity for controlling his state of consciousness. Habituation to various stimuli is an important aspect of this test.
   (*d*) Organization processes—physiological response to stress: this indicates the infant's response to an unpleasant stimulus. The immature infant responds with a greater startle.

(ii) *Mother's perceptions.*—This was measured at the beginning of the interview with the mother, using the Neonatal Perception Inventory (Broussard & Hartner, 1971). With this inventory mothers were asked to assess how much difficulty they expected to have with their own infant's crying, bowel movements, sleeping, feeding and scheduling —irregularities in these functions being part of Thomas et al.'s (1978) constellation for the "difficult child." They were also asked to rate the typical infant for the same behaviors. The mother's perception of the typical infant is used in comparison with her perception of her own infant. Different scores on each of the five scales are summed to give the Neonatal Perception Inventory score, ranging from -25 to $+25$. Broussard and Hartner designed their scale according to clinical experience. We, however, removed the item concerning vomiting since it did not seem to reflect a common difficulty for our sample of mothers. Only 24 mothers completed this inventory fully, because of administrative difficulties not directly related to the inventory.

(iii) *Pre- and perinatal events.*—Data for the perinatal variables were obtained from hospital records. The variables measured were extent of forceps use, length of labor, induced or spontaneous labor, and level of analgesic medication. "Medication level" was scored according to the type of drug and the amount administered, as follows:

1 = none; 2 = tranquillizer; 3 = tranquillizer and single opiate, or single opiate only; 4 = two or more administrations of opiate.
Forceps use was scored 0 = 1; low = 2; mid = 3.
Induction was scored on a binary scale.

(iv) *Maternal variables.*—A semi-structured interview was conducted in the mother's hospital room. The interviews were tape-recorded and later transcribed verbatim. The typescript was used to rate the mother in terms of: (*a*) her pregnancy planning and preparation for motherhood; (*b*) aspects of her perceived temperament of relevance to mothering; and (*c*) her immediate feelings towards the birth of the infant. In all, 11 measures were specified and rated on a five-point scale. These variables are defined in the Appendix.

The reliability of these ratings was tested on the transcripts of 10 subjects. The overall reliability between two raters was 86 percent, with reliability for individual items ranging from 80 to 93 percent. One of these raters had been the interviewer. On this ground, her ratings were used in the analysis since they seemed more likely to be accurate. The "blind" rater was given instructions as shown in the Appendix.

RESULTS

(A) Smaller Sample (n = 24)

The correctional data for the 24 women and babies who completed the Neonatal Perception Scale are summarized in Fig. 1. It shows only significant correlations ($P \leqslant 0.05$). No correlations are omitted.

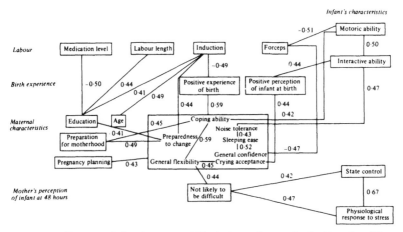

Figure 1. Significant correlations between variables in the smaller sample of subjects ($n = 24$). $P < 0.01$ where $r > 0.51$. No significant correlations are omitted. 'Not likely to be difficult' refers to the score on the Neonatal Perception Scale (NPS).

(B) Larger Sample ($n = 32$)

The correlation matrix for the larger group of 32 mothers and babies is shown in Table 1. In general, it suggests that the additional data from eight more subjects have not substantially changed the degree and direction of the relationships between the variables. In particular:

(i) they support the supposition that maternal characteristics such as "general flexibility," "crying acceptance," "sleeping ease," "general confidence," "preparedness to change" and "preparation for motherhood" are related to a general factor of "coping ability" since correlations amongst these items are increased in the larger sample;

(ii) they suggest that the correlation between maternal coping ability and the motoric ability of the infant is not a direct one, but a consequence of mothers with low coping ability being more likely to have a forceps delivery.

(C) Neonatal Perception Scale

A breakdown of the five individual items constituting the total Neonatal Perception Scale score showed seven significant correlations which are not shown in Table 1:

(i & ii) The infant who was perceived as not likely to be difficult in

Table 1. Correlation of NPS (n = 24) and maternal, prenatal, perinatal and infant variables (n = 32)

	1	2	3	4	5	6	7	8	9	10	11	12	13	14	15	16	17	18	19	20	21	22
1																						
2																						
3																						
4																						
5																						
6					-0·42																	
7		-0·47																				
8		0·47																				
9																						
10									0·39													
11																						
12										0·43												
13												0·39										
14			-0·35									0·39										
15																						
16			-0·52								0·35			0·42	0·61							
17											0·50	0·51			0·41							
18																						
19						-0·42																
20																						
21																		0·52		0·49		
22																0·44*				0·42*	0·47*	

* P < 0·05 for NPS; for the remainder P < 0·05 for r > 0·34; P < 0·01 for r > 0·44; P < 0·002 for r > 0·52.

Legend for variables

Maternal variables:
1. Age
2. Education

Planning and preparation
3. Pregnancy planning
4. Preparation for motherhood

Perinatal events:
5. Induced labour
6. Extent of forceps (1, 2, 3)
7. Medication level
8. Labour length

Postnatal reactions:
9. Positive reaction to birth
10. Positive perception of infant

Maternal temperament:
11. Crying acceptance
12. Sleeping ease
13. Noise tolerance
14. Preparedness to change
15. Coping ability
16. General flexibility
17. General confidence

Infant variables:
18. Interactive processes
19. Motoric processes
20. State control
21. Physiological response
22. NPS (Neonatal Perception Scale)

his sleeping habits scored high on state control and physiological response to stress ($r = 0.53$ and 0.49).

(iii & iv) The mother who had prepared for motherhood and who showed general flexibility did not perceive her infant as likely to be difficult in terms of crying ($r = 0.41$ and 0.44).

(v) The infant whose mother had been heavily medicated during labor was perceived as likely to be difficult with feeding ($r = -0.42$).

(vi) The child who scored poorly on motoric processes was perceived as not likely to be difficult in terms of crying ($r = -0.42$).

(vii) The mother who slept easily predicted some scheduling difficulty with her infant ($r = -0.41$).

The first five of these correlations are understandable. The final two do not admit to a simple explanation.

(D) Transcripts of Interviews

The actual remarks of the mothers were content analyzed in order to support the validity of the findings in (A) and (B) and also to illustrate them. Relevant extracts are reproduced in the discussion.

DISCUSSION

Kronstadt et al. (1979) studied mothers and infants who were older than a month. They found that not only is the mother's perception of her infant a function of the baby's behavior, it is also influenced by "subjective and variable" qualities in the mother. Our findings for neonates are similar.

The mothers in this study knew very little of their babies. Nor did they know much about other babies since this was their first. Yet within 48 hours of their birth they could make a decision about how their infant compared with others in terms of its "difficulty." This judgment came from two main sources: the mother's own characteristics and the baby's exhibited "competence" (Bower, 1974).

Those babies who were judged as not likely to be difficult scored higher for "state control," i.e., they habituated well, showing the apparent ability to block out stimuli which is a fundamental means of coping with the sensory environment. Furthermore, they showed no exaggerated responses to stimuli. In this sense they may have been fairly accurately perceived by their mothers. This supposition is consistent with the finding that mothers using a modified version of the Brazelton Neonatal Behavioral Assessment Scale were almost as objective as independent raters (Field et al., 1978).

The mother's perception of her infant also seemed to be influenced by her own temperament—in particular, her "general flexibility." This item probably reflected "coping ability," since it correlated with that variable and with "crying acceptance." In the larger series of mothers ($n = 32$), "coping ability" also correlated with "preparedness to change" and "general confidence," which in turn correlated with maternal "sleeping ease." These intercorrelations suggested that each variable may have reflected different aspects of a single maternal quality—an ability to manage her life without undue difficulty. In short, they seem to describe someone who is "competent."

"Competent" mothers saw their infants as similar to themselves. In this sense, the findings are consistent with the suggestion of Broussard & Hartner (1971) that the "fantasy" upon which the mother bases her perceptions of her new-born "may reflect her sense of self or her identification with other objects in her life." Perhaps this might be expected, since Winnicott (1958) has remarked that the mother is immersed in her baby "to the exclusion of other interests, in a way which is normal and temporary." She might, in other words, experience the baby as very much part of herself. Nevertheless, a genetic explanation offers itself. Might it be that "competent" infants are born to "competent" mothers?

At first sight, the evidence shown in Fig. 1 gives some support to a genetic hypothesis. The "interactive ability" of the infant correlates with an item which presumably reflects an aspect of the mother's coping ability (noise tolerance). Furthermore, maternal "coping ability" was related to the infant's motoric maturity. These correlations, however, were lost in the larger sample in which no maternal item correlated with any of the infant variables. This larger body of evidence suggested that the correlation concerning the infant's motoric processes was an indirect one—the mother who coped well was less likely to have a forceps delivery, which in turn was associated with poor motor abilities in the infant. Nevertheless, indirect correlations, involving the new-born's "interactive ability," suggest that genetic factors may have some part to play, and that another study may reveal it.

The events surrounding birth seem to make little direct contribution to the mother's overall perception of her infant's potential difficulty, when this is rated two days later. Nevertheless, induction appears to adversely affect the mother's view of the birth and this in turn may have an effect on her initial perception of her baby, at least in terms of the evidence of the larger sample.

The mother's initial perception of her baby also appeared to have little effect on her judgment of its personality 48 hours later. There may be several explanations for this. One is obvious, and exemplified by the mother who initially perceived her child, which had been delivered by forceps, as "ugly." A second explanation can only be offered with hesitation. It might be, as Robson & Kumar (1980) suggest, that a mother's absorption in her child is not always immediate, but takes time to develop. For example:

> I didn't go berserk (at the birth), say oh he's beautiful like some people do. But the more I see him, I get more attached, naturally, so I think more of him than when I first saw him . . .

and again:

> I was just so pleased, so happy the pain was over. Just that she'd been born. I didn't really think about her at all. I didn't really think about her till the next day 'cos I was quite detached from her really . . . I remember thinking (during pregnancy) that when the baby's born I may not want it . . . maybe I'm not ready to be a mother. But I'm starting.

The inference, however, that the mother's perception of the potential difficulty of her child is uninfluenced by perinatal events is thrown into question on more detailed examination of the Neonatal Perception Scale. This shows that a mother who had been medicated was likely to perceive her infant as difficult to feed. This is consistent with accumulated evidence which suggests that drugs given to the mother during labor affect subsequently her infant's behavior (Brackbill, 1979). There appears to be no evidence, however, which considers the effect of medication upon the mother's perception of her infant, although there have been studies in the related area of mother-child interaction (e.g., Brazelton, 1971; Richards & Bernal, 1972; Brown et al., 1975).

In this study the level of medication given during labor was inversely correlated with the level of maternal education. This is consistent with the findings of Standley et al. (1978) who concluded that such factors as maternal age, social status and education "must be considered sources of infant behavior."

These mothers' perceptions of their babies had elements which are similar to those found generally in "person perception." Studies from other fields suggest that one's perception of another is influenced by the other's behavior, and also by one's own characteristics, which include one's ideas about oneself (Secord & Backman, 1964, Back, 1977). Nevertheless, in making the above interpretations, we recognize that because of the number of significant correlations computed, some of the significant correlations could be due to chance (e.g., items (C) vi & vii in "Results"). Most of them, however, are readily interpretable and in the expected direction of association. This observation together with a content analysis of the general remarks made by the mothers during the interview tend to support the validity of the correlation data. During this interview, more than half of the mothers expressed some definite idea of their infant's personality. The adjectives used were consistent with the "difficult–not difficult" dimension. On the one hand the infants were perceived as "quiet," "placid" or "good" and on the other hand as "stubborn." In the most cases these attributions depended on the mother's observations of the infant's behavior such as sleeping and feeding, or on her view of her own character. For example one mother said,

> I think he's going to be stubborn but apart from that I don't
> know. If he doesn't want to drink, he won't. He sort of puts
> his bottom lip in. I was stubborn apparently when I was young.

These interviews also suggested that in the particular case of her newborn, the influences upon a mother's perception may be somewhat more complex than in other situations. Her inferences were often based on minute observations of their babies. For example one mother, on being asked about her infant's personality, said,

> I know he's got a little habit of mine already. I've got a habit
> of sticking my finger like that when I sleep. He's started doing
> that so he's got one of my little traits so far.

The mother, however, did not always seem to regard herself as a single entity, but rather as part of a unit which included her husband. This system, in our small sample, depended upon the marital pairs seeing themselves on one hand as having identical characteristics, or on the other hand as possessing complementary traits. An example of the former situation was:

> I think she might be a little stubborn. I had trouble feeding
> her last night. She didn't want to take the breast from me.
> She was determined not to take it so she showed a little bit
> of her nature. But her mum and dad are stubborn.

Examples of the mother's perception of complementary marital traits included:

> I think she's going to be a placid sort of person. I don't think she's going to be angry like me 'cos I've got a bit of a temper. But she hasn't I don't think. My husband is placid.

or again,

> I think she'll be like my husband—quiet, gentle. I'm more sort of nervous.

There was also evidence that mechanisms which have been associated with identity development in adolescence may be operating from the first days of life. Stierlin (1973), for example, has described the adolescent who is a "delegate" of his parents, in that he lives out parental wishes and hopes which have been largely unfulfilled. In our series, a dancing teacher with almond-shaped eyes searched her child's face when she first saw her, and found the same eyes. Two days later she said,

> My husband keeps saying she's going to be a little ballerina. I said only if she wants to be. I mean obviously she'll come to class with me.

Another mechanism associated with adolescence involves negative characteristics. The child acts out unacceptable parts of the parental personality which are usually hidden (Johnson & Szurek, 1952). The emergence of this behavior presumably depends upon parental reinforcements which are not recognized as such. An example of this process at work in infancy may be the following:

> I think she'll be pretty docile really. I hope she is, 'cos if she's like either of us, God help me. My husband's a worrier, he worries himself nearly distracted then of course that annoys me. I can be very sharp tempered. I can be very, very stubborn. That's one thing I don't like is stubborn children. I don't like to have them persist in "No I don't want"—I can't stand a disobedient child saying "no" to me. I'll probably whack her when she's older if she's going to be disobedient like that.

In conclusion, while the findings of a study of this kind must be viewed with some caution, they suggest some of the factors which may be involved in the mother's judgment of her new-born infant. Our findings raise the possibility that a process akin to "projective identification" is involved in the mother's attribution of personality traits to her infant. The content analysis of the interview data suggested that the characteristics which are "projected" come from a pool which contains traits the mother finds in herself and also those which she sees in her husband. A second factor in the mother's judgment of her infant's personality is closer to "reality" and seems to involve a fairly accurate perception of his physical capabilities. The mother's predictions of her infant's personality are important because they may become self-fulfilling, perhaps in the manner of Sameroff's (1975) transactional model of child development. In a following paper we shall report on the fate of those infants who were perceived as difficult.

REFERENCES

Als, H., Tronick, E., Lester, B. M. and Brazelton, T. B. (1977). The Brazelton Neonatal Behavioral Assessment Scale (BNBAS). *Journal of Abnormal Child Psychology*, 5:215–231.

Back, K. W. (ed.) (1977). *Social Psychology*. New York: Wiley.

Bower, T. G. R. (1974). The competent newborn. *New Scientist*, 672–675

Brackbill, Y. (1979). Obstetrical medication of infant behavior. In *The Handbook of Infant Development*, J. Osofsky, ed. New York: Wiley.

Brazelton, T. B. (1971). Influence of perinatal drugs on the behavior of the neonate. In *The Exceptional Infant*, Vol. II: *Studies in Abnormalities*, J. Helmuth, ed. New York: Brunner/Mazel.

Broussard, E. R. and Hartner, M. S. S. (1971). Further considerations regarding maternal perception of the first born. In *The Exceptional Infant*, Vol. II: *Studies in Abnormalities*, J. Helmuth, ed. New York: Brunner/Mazel.

Brown, J., Bakeman, R., Snyder, P., Frederickson, W., Morgan, S. and Hepler, R. (1975). Interaction of black inner-city mothers with their newborn infants. *Child Development*, 46:677–686.

Field, T. M., Dempsey, J. R., Hallock, N. H. and Shuman, H. H. (1978). The mother's assessment of the behavior of her infant. *Infant Behavior and Development*, 1:156–167.

Johnson, A. and Szurek, S. (1952). The genesis of anti-social acting out in children and adults. *Psychoanalytic Quarterly*, 21:323–343.

Kronstadt, D., Oberklaid, F., Ferb, T. E. and Swartz, J. P. (1979). Infant behavior and maternal adaptations in the first six months of life. *American Journal of Orthopsychiatry*, 49:454–464.

Richard, M. P. M. and Bernal, J. (1972). An observational study of mother-infant interaction. In *Ethological Studies of Child Behaviour*, N. B. Jones, ed. Cambridge: Cambridge University Press.

Robson, K. and Kumar, R. (1980). Delayed onset of maternal affection after childbirth. *British Journal of Psychiatry*, 136:347–353.

Rosenthal, D. (Ed.) (1963). *The Genain Quadruplets*. New York: Basic Books.

Sameroff, A. (1975). Early influences on development: Fact or fancy? *Merrill-Palmer Quarterly*, 21:267–294.

Secord, P. F. and Backman, C. W. (1964). *Social Psychology*. New York: McGraw-Hill.

Sostek, A. M. and Anders, T. F. (1977). Relationships among the Brazelton Neonatal Scale, Bayley Infant Scales, and early temperament. *Child Development*, 48:320–323.

Standley, K., Soule, A. B., Copans, S. A. and Klein, R. P. (1978). Multidimensional sources of infant temperament. *Genetic Psychology Monographs*, 80:203–232.

Stierlin, H. (1973). The adolescent as a delegate of his parents. *Australian and New Zealand Journal of Psychiatry*, 7:S249–S256.

Thomas, A., Chess, S. and Birch, N. (1978). *Temperament and Behavior Disorder in Children*. New York: New York University Press.

Winnicott, D. W. (1958). Primary maternal preoccupation. *Collected Papers*. London: Tavistock.

APPENDIX

Description of Maternal Variables

Pregnancy planned (planning)
1. None (no thought of pregnancy, total "mistake").
2. Not sure (i.e., "one day," "eventually").
3. Distant future (planned with partner . . . later on, few years).
4. Near future ("sometime this year," "soon").
5. Definite.

Preparation for motherhood
1. None.
2. A little.
3. Moderate.
4. A good deal.
5. A great deal.
(Coded from specific question plus overall interview—i.e., amount of reading, understanding likely problems, thoughts on upbringing, source and amount of knowledge, "matter-of-fact" attitude vs. "fanciful," etc.).

Feelings re: birth and labor ("positive experience")
1. Very − ve (*much* more painful than expected).
2. Slightly − ve (mother scared, in pain).
3. Expressed no definite feelings.
4. Slightly + ve (it was good, better than expected).
5. Very + ve (very exciting, elated feeling).

Positive feeling towards infant (at birth)
1. Very − ve (no expected rush of feeling).
2. Slightly − ve (disappointed with appearance).
3. Expressed no definite feelings (too dopey).
4. Slightly + ve (pleased with sex, glad infant healthy).
5. Very + ve (thought infant beautiful).

General flexibility in personal activities
1. None (definite about working to rule, routine, etc., unable to adapt easily).
2. A little (*prefers* routine, easily hassled if routine altered).
3. Moderate (thinks routine a good idea, but not always).
4. A good deal (*likes* to "go along with things" with some order, not easily hassled).
5. A great deal (does things when feeling like it, "happy-go-lucky," doesn't care, isn't bothered).

General confidence, decision making, taking the lead, assertiveness
1. None (reliant on others' advice, prefers being led).
2. A little (reliant on others' advice, then makes up mind).
3. Moderate (depends on circumstances . . . "a bit of both"—taking the lead sometimes).
4. A good deal (usually very independent, occasionally needing back-up).
5. A great deal (very confident, independent, assertive).

Preparedness to change for infant (re: lifestyle)
1. None (wants to make sure things don't change, negative about any change).
2. A little (acknowledges change, but not prepared for many changes).
3. Moderate (assumes present "lifestyle" already caters for arrival of infant).
4. A good deal (has thoughts and plans about change, has accepted change).
5. A great deal (definite about changing to fit in with infant's requirements).

Coping ability (with unexpected events)
1. None (worries constantly about possible "unexpecteds," easily feels and/or becomes disorganized).
2. A little (fairly emotional if unexpected things happen).
3. Moderate (upset with unexpecteds, but later adjusts).
4. A good deal (learnt to ignore hassles).
5. A great deal (not bothered at all).

Crying acceptance
1. None (won't be able to cope at all).
2. A little (doesn't think will cope very well, will be upset).

3. Moderate (upset by crying, but accepts it).
4. A good deal (not easily upset by crying, looks for reason).
5. A great deal (not upset, expects crying).

Sleeping ease (if worried)
1. None (can't sleep, keeps worrying, has difficulty settling down).
2. A little (has some trouble sleeping when worried).
3. Moderate ("light sleeper," easily disturbed, has no trouble settling down).
4. A good deal (no trouble sleeping if worried, sometimes disturbed by noise).
5. A great deal (*never* has any trouble sleeping, "sleeps like a log").

Noise tolerance
1. Poor (can't stand noise, e.g., clatter in hospital, etc.).
2. A little (can't concentrate in noisy surroundings).
3. Moderate (if in bad mood, noise is irritating).
4. Fairly good (annoyed by noise, but adjusts).
5. Very good (not bothered, "blocks it out").

II

Security of Mother- and Father-Infant Attachment and Its Relation to Sociability With Strangers in Traditional and Nontraditional Swedish Families

Michael E. Lamb

University of Utah

Carl-Philip Hwang

University of Göteborg

Ann M. Frodi

University of Rochester

Majt Frodi

University of Göteborg

Fifty-one firstborn infants were seen in the Strange Situation at 11 and 13 months—once with their mothers and once with their fathers. Seventeen of the infants come from families in which the fathers were extensively involved in child care and had spent at least a month ($\bar{X}$

Reprinted with permission from *Infant Behavior and Development*, 1982, Vol. 5, 355–367.

This research was supported by the Riksbankens Jubileumsfond of Stockholm (Sweden). We are grateful to this foundation for its financial support, to the parents and children for their generous cooperation, to Marie Bondesson, Thomas Corry, Britta Forrström, Thomas Jonsson, Agneta Lindqvist, Michael Lundgren, Christina Mattsson, and Anna Nordgren for their assistance in data collection, to William P. Gardner for assistance with data analysis, and to Dante Cicchetti for many constructive comments on an earlier version of this paper.

= 2.8 months) as primary caretakers. The infants' sociability toward unfamiliar adult strangers was also assessed prior to each Strange Situation assessment. There was no significant relationship between the security of infant-mother and infant-father attachment. Infants who were securely-attached to their fathers—especially those with B1 and B2 relationships—were most sociable with strangers, but the security of infant-mother attachment was unrelated to sociability. The significant associations with the security of the father-infant attachments did not vary depending on the fathers' relative involvement in childcare, nor the sex of the stranger. Infants were more sociable with female than with male strangers.

Since the Strange Situation procedure was described by Ainsworth and Wittig (1969), several researchers have shown that behavior in this brief procedure has remarkable predictive validity. Patterns of infant-mother attachment predict social competence with peers (Easterbrooks & Lamb, 1979; Lieberman, 1977; Pastor, 1981), sociability and cooperativeness with unfamiliar adults (Main, 1973; Thompson & Lamb, 1981), task-focused persistence in problem-solving situations (Matas, Arend, & Sroufe, 1978) and ego-resiliency in a variety of contexts (Arend, Gove, & Sroufe, 1979). However, few researchers have examined the relationship between the security of infant-*father* attachment and the infant's behavior in other contexts. The present study was designed to assess the influence of both infant-mother and infant-father attachments on the infant's sociability with unfamiliar adults. To determine whether the relative predictive importance of the two relationships varied depending upon the relative involvement of the two adults in child care, the sample included a group of families in which fathers had been highly involved in childcare.

Although it was once believed that the security of the infant-mother attachment would serve as the prototype for other (later) attachment relationships (Ainsworth, 1969; Bowlby, 1969; Freud, 1940), recent research has demonstrated that infants often form relationships of different types to their mothers and fathers (Grossman, Grossman, Huber, & Wartner, 1981; Lamb, 1978; Main & Weston, 1981). Presumably, Lamb (1981) suggests, the behavior of each parent affects the infant's expectations of the specific adult, and it is these behavioral expectations that are manifest in the Strange Situation (Ainsworth, 1977; Lamb, 1981). These findings imply that the security of both infant-parent relationships should affect the child's later behavior. In a study of which we become aware after the present research commenced, Main and

Weston (1981) demonstrated that the security of the two infant-parent attachments indeed had independent influences on the "relatedness" of 12-month-olds toward an unfamiliar clown. Highest relatedness scores were obtained by those who were securely attached to both parents, then came those who were securely attached only to their mothers, followed by those who were securely attached only to their fathers, and finally those who were insecurely attached to both parents. These data suggested that the relationships with mothers had greater predictive validity, but unfortunately, relatedness and security of infant-mother attachment were assessed at the same age, whereas the security of infant-father attachment was assessed six months later. This temporal confound, rather than the fact that the mothers were primary caretakers, may help explain the greater predictive importance of the infant-mother attachment. There was no corresponding confound in the present study. In addition, we assessed sociability with two unfamiliar adults using a previously-validated, behaviorally-based measure of sociability (Lamb, 1982; Stevenson & Lamb, 1979) rather than relying upon a somewhat ambiguous rating of "relatedness." We thus hoped to replicate Main and Weston's findings using slightly different procedures and measures. Previous studies have shown that scores on our measure of sociability are related to perceived temperament (Thompson & Lamb, 1982) and to the security of infant-mother attachment (Thompson & Lamb, 1981). Even though sociability is, as we would expect, affected by temperament, it is not simply another measure of temperament since sociability scores are affected by social experiences and changes in the security of attachment whereas temperament is unaffected by such events (Thompson & Lamb, 1982).

It would not be surprising if the mother-infant relationship had greater formative significance in traditional families. Previous studies have shown that young infants show preferences for their mothers when distressed (Lamb, 1976a, 1976b), even though most are clearly attached to both parents (Lamb, 1977), and it seems reasonable to assume that preferential relationships have greater formative significance than subsidiary attachment relationships. It is not clear, however, whether the relative formative importance of the infant-parent relationships varies depending upon the amount of interaction each adult has with the infant. To further assess whether either infant-parent relationship had greater predictive validity and (if so) whether the relative importance of the two relationships was affected by the adults' relative involvement in caretaking, we included in our sample a number of families in which fathers were extensively involved in childcare. Unfortunately, none of the fathers were as involved as they had anticipated when recruited and none were primary caretakers throughout their infants' lives. However, 17 of the fathers had spent more than a month (the average was nearly 3 months) as near-exclusive caretakers. If extent of involvement affects the predictive validity of a relationship, then the relationships to these fathers should have had greater predictive validity than the relationships to the less involved fathers. Our research was conducted in Sweden, a country in which men are legally entitled to paid paternal leave, and in which most fathers—even those who do not take an appreciable amount of paternal leave—are more involved in childcare than the average American father appears to be. This should have assured that all infants had formed attachments to both parents.

Ainsworth and her colleagues (Ainsworth, Blehar, Waters, & Wall, 1978) explain the relationship between security of attachment and sociability toward unfamiliar adults by proposing that infants generalize a style of interacting with attachment figures to initial encounters with unfamiliar persons. When an infant has different prototypes from which to generalize (e.g., different patterns of attachment to mother and father), however, the relative importance of each may be affected not only by the relative salience of each relationship, but also by similarities between the unfamiliar adult and either of the attachment figures. One important dimension of similarity may be gender. Conceivably, the security of the infant-father relationship has a greater impact on interaction with male than with female strangers, whereas the security of the infant-mother attachment affects interaction with females more than the interaction with males. By observing some infants with male and some with female strangers in the present study, we sought to investigate this hypothesis. Previous studies have shown that infants typically respond more positively to female than to male strangers (e.g., Greenberg, Hillman, & Grice, 1973; Morgan & Ricciuti, 1969) but no one has yet determined whether sociability with male and female strangers is differentially affected by the security of infant-mother and infant-father attachment.

Previous attempts to explore the predictive validity of security of attachment have typically compared securely- and insecurely-attached infants on the relevant outcome measure. In such analyses, neither the two insecure patterns (avoidant and resistant) nor the four secure subgroups are distinguished. This is unfortunate, since the two insecure patterns seem related to different patterns of antecedent infant-parent interaction (Ainsworth et al., 1978) and the B1 and B2 subgroups within the secure group are related to different antecedent maternal behaviors than the B3 subgroups (Blehar, Lieberman, & Ainsworth, 1977). Main

(1973) showed that avoidantly- and resistantly-attached infants interacted differently with strangers, while Easterbrooks and Lamb (1979) showed that securely-attached B1 and B2 infants were more sociable with peers than securely-attached B3 and B4 infants. Thompson and Lamb (1981) found that B1 and B2 infants were the most sociable with unfamiliar adults. These studies thus suggest that one needs to consider group and subgroup differences as well as differences between securely- and insecurely-attached infants. In the present study, we consider four composite groups (A1 and A2; B1 and B2; B3 and B4; C1 and C2) as well as the more global secure-insecure dimension.

In sum, then, the present study was designed to address several interrelated issues. First, we sought to confirm the lack of association between patterns of infant-mother and infant-father attachment. Second, we asked whether the security of each of the two relationships would have significant effects on infant sociability with unfamiliar adults. Our hypothesis was that the infants who were securely attached to either parent would be more sociable, with those who had two secure attachments being most sociable and those who had two insecure attachments being least sociable. Third, we determined whether the predictive validity of infant-parent attachments varied depending upon relative involvement in caretaking. We expected that the security of the infant-father attachment would be more strongly associated with sociability when the fathers were highly involved than when they were less involved. Likewise, we expected the security of the infant-mother attachment to be more strongly associated with sociability when the fathers were less involved than when the fathers were highly involved. Finally, we tested the hypothesis that the security of infant-mother attachments would have greater impact on interaction with unfamiliar female adults, whereas the security of infant-father attachment would have greatest impact on interaction with unfamiliar males.

METHOD

Subjcts

The subjects were 51 Swedish couples and their firstborn infants, who were 11- and 13-months-old ($\pm$ 2 weeks) when observed. The families were all residents of Göteborg and were recruited prenatally through childbirth preparation classes to take part in a longitudinal study. In 17 of the families (designated Nontraditional), the fathers had spent more than one month ($\bar{X}$ = 2.82 months) as primary caretakers, usually starting when the infants were around 5 months of age. In the remaining 34 families, few of the fathers took parental leave, and the mothers were primary caretakers throughout the children's lives. The average age of the mothers was 27.2 years and the fathers, 30.2 years; all of the families were middle to upper class, and there were no significant differences between the groups on the Education or Occupational scales of Hollingshead's Four Factor Index of Social Position.

Procedure

All observations took place in a gaily-decorated playroom (5m × 3.5m) furnished with two chairs and a selection of interesting toys in the middle of the room. Each infant was observed twice in this laboratory playroom, once with each parent. The two sessions were scheduled two months apart in order to eliminate sensitization or order effects (cf., Ainsworth et al., 1978). The order in which the mother-infant and father-infant relationships were assessed was counter-balanced systematically: Half the infants were tested with their mothers first.

Each laboratory session comprised two parts—the sociability assessment and the Strange Situation—both of which were videotaped for subsequent data reduction. Upon arrival at the laboratory, the infant's sociability with a strange adult was assessed using a standardized procedure developed by Stevenson and Lamb (1979). In this procedure, we focused on the infants' behavior when they were: a) first greeted by the stranger as he/she entered, b) offered a toy by the stranger, c) allowed floor freedom by the parent, d) invited by the stranger to enter into a reciprocal game, and e) picked up by the stranger. Responses in each condition were recorded using behaviorally-defined 5-point scales, on which the highest scores were assigned to friendly, accepting behaviors. The rater also indicated his/her general impression of the child's sociability on a 9-point scale. The sum of scores on all of these measures constituted the child's sociability score (possible range, 6–34).[1] Further details regarding the scoring procedure are contained in Table 1. Each child was seen with a different stranger on each occasion. Half of the infants interacted with male strangers in both assessments; half inter-

---

[1]The sociability procedure employed here was identical to that employed by Stevenson and Lamb (1979). The procedure and scoring differ somewhat from the modified procedure employed by Thompson and Lamb (1981, 1982), although scores on the two scales are very highly correlated (Lamb, 1982). The Thompson revision yields scores ranging from 9 to 49, compared with the 6 to 34 point range of the scoring system employed here.

TABLE 1
Scoring Protocol for the Assessment of
Sociability toward an Unfamiliar Adult

Baby's Reaction When First Catching the Experimenter's Sight:

1. cries, becomes quite upset
2. whimpers or fusses
3. looks at parent or looks away from the experimenter
4. looks at the experimenter without smiling
5. smiles at the experimenter

Baby's Reaction to Being Offered a Toy by the Experimenter:

1. fusses or cries
2. refuses toy by looking away or pushing the toy away
3. looks at the toy
4. tentatively touches or reaches for the toy
5. accepts the toy

Baby's Behavior When Given Floor Freedom:

1. touches parent or requests him/her to pick her/him up
2. approaches or stays near parent
3. neutral—neither moving away from or towards the experimenter
4. approaches the experimenter
5. touches the experimenter or requests her/him to pick her/him up

Baby's Reaction When the Experimenter Initiates a Reciprocal Game:

1. refuses to join in
2. initially reluctant, then participates briefly
3. initially reluctant, then joins in and persists with the game
4. immediately joins in and participates briefly
5. immediately joins in and persists with the game

Baby's Reaction When the Experimenter Attempts to Pick Her/Him Up:

1. cries, becomes quite upset
2. whimpers or tusses
3. tries to get down
4. acceptance
5. smiling acceptance

Overall Impression of Sociability:

1. quite unfriendly, fussy
2. between 1 and 3
3. generally unfriendly, serious
4. between 3 and 5
5. neutral, neither friendly nor unfriendly
6. between 5 and 7
7. friendly, positive reaction
8. between 7 and 9
9. very friendly, outgoing, smiling

acted with female strangers each time.[2] Four male and seven female strangers shared responsibility for these sessions. Sociability was rated from the videotape records by individuals who were unaware of the infant's attachment classification.

The sociability assessment occurred in the parents' presence, usually lasted less than 5 minutes, and was unintrusive and not distressful. The Strange Situation procedure then took place. The Strange Situation is a structured procedure designed to allow observation of the organization of attachment behavior in response to gradually increasing stress. For analytic purposes, the primary focus is on the infant's reaction upon reunion with the parent after a brief separation. Episode-by-episode ratings of the infant's proximity and contact seeking, contact-maintaining, avoidance, resistance, distance interaction, and search behavior are used to facilitate an overall assessment of the infant-adult attachment relationship using the 8-category classification scheme described by Ainsworth et al. (1978). Further details regarding the procedure and the scoring system can be found in the volume by Ainsworth et al. (1978). For analytic purposes, we collapsed the 8 categories into 4: avoidant (A1 and A2 subgroups); resistant (C1 and C2 subgroups); secure-low contact (B1 and B2 subgroups); and secure-high contact (B3 and B4 subgroups). The avoidant and resistant groups are traditionally deemed insecurely-attached; the B groups exemplify secure attachment.

The first author was introduced to the classification procedure by Ainsworth and he took primary responsibility for the classifications. The other raters were trained extensively by him before undertaking classifications for this study. The individuals responsible for classifying the attachment relationships were unaware of the child's behavior with the other parent and at least one (often both) of the raters did not know whether the child came from a traditional or nontraditional family. One of several unfamiliar females served as a stranger during the Strange Situation assessments. Only female strangers were employed, as we wanted to replicate Ainsworth's procedures as closely as possible. Most ratings were conducted by authors Lamb and Hwang.

Reliability.—All sociability ratings and attachment classifications were performed by at least two people, working independently. Whenever a disagreement occurred, the raters discussed it until consensus was

---

[2]Our original intention was to have each infant seen once with a male and once with a female stranger, but unfortunately this aspect of the procedure was miscommunicated in translation. By the time we became aware of the problem, it was too late to change anything. This means that our test of the fourth hypothesis was weaker than it might otherwise have been.

reached. Product-moment correlations revealed agreement in the rating of sociability exceeding $r = .93$. Pairs of raters disagreed only 5 times concerning the 102 attachment classifications, and two of these were disagreements concerning subgroup assignment.

RESULTS

The sociability of each infant was assessed twice—once in the presence of mother and once in the presence of father. To create a more robust and reliable index of sociability, the two scores were combined into a composite score for the purpose of the analyses reported here. The two individual scores for each infant were only modestly correlated ($r = .39$, $p < .0025$) but both were highly correlated with the composite scores (r's $\sim .80$) and all of the analyses yielded similar results when conducted using the individual rather than the composite scores. Composite scores ranged from 28.0 to 58.5, with a mean of 44.3 and a standard deviation of 7.8.

All significant values reported below are for one-tailed tests unless otherwise noted.

Table 2 displays the distribution of infants across the major categories or types of attachment. Inspection of the table reveals that there were fewer resistant (C-type) relationships in this Swedish sample than are typically found in American samples (Ainsworth et al., 1978). As the table also suggests, there was no significant association between the security of infant-mother and infant-father attachment revealed by analyses employing any of the following dimensions of comparison: a) a two-way division into secure (B) and insecure (A and C); b) a three-way division into the major categories (A, B, C); and c) a four-way division into the four composite groups considered here (A, B1 B2, B3 B4, C).

TABLE 2
Relationship Between Patterns of Infant-Mother and Infant-Father Attachment

		Infant-Father Attachment				
		A	B1 B2	B3 B4	C	Row Totals
Infant-Mother Attachment	A	4	4	3	0	11
	B1 B2	4	7	4	0	15
	B3 B4	5	5	12	1	23
	C	0	1	0	1	2
	Col. Totals	13	17	19	2	

Somewhat surprisingly, the security of infant-father attachment was more closely related to infant sociability than the security of infant-mother attachment. A one-way analysis of variance revealed that infants who had B1 and B2 relationships with their fathers ($\bar{X}$ = 49.5, n = 17) were significantly more sociable than those with B3 and B4 ($\bar{X}$ = 41.9, n = 19) or A1 and A2 ($\bar{X}$ = 42.0, n = 13) relationships ($F3,46$ = $p <$ .005). Another one-way analysis revealed that infants who were securely attached to their fathers ($\bar{X}$ = 45.4, n = 36) were marginally more sociable than those who were insecurely attached to their fathers ($\bar{X}$ = 42.0, n = 15:$F1,49$ = 2.009, $p <$ .08). By contrast, there was no significant relationship between sociability and the security of infant-mother attachment. Infants who had B1 and B2 relationships ($\bar{X}$ = 45.8, n = 15) and those who had A1 and A2 relationships ($\bar{X}$ = 45.7, n = 11) were somewhat more sociable than those who had B3 and B4 relationships ($\bar{X}$ = 43.3, n = 23), but these differences were not statistically significant. Likewise, infants who were securely attached to their mothers ($\bar{X}$ = 44.3, n = 38) were not significantly more sociable than those who were insecurely-attached ($\bar{X}$ = 44.7, n = 13). Unfortunately, only two infants had C-type relationships with their fathers ($\bar{X}$ = 45.0), and only two had C-type relationships with their mothers ($\bar{X}$ = 39.3) so little can be said about the sociability of these infants.

The security of infant-father attachment was related to sociability and the security of infant-mother attachment was unrelated to sociability in both the traditional and nontraditional families. Greater paternal involvement did not increase the predictive importance of the father-infant relationship, nor did lesser paternal involvement increase the relative predictive importance of the infant-mother attachment.

The security of the two relationships considered together was not significantly related to sociability. Similar degrees of sociability were manifest by infants who were securely attached to both parents ($\bar{X}$ = 45.4, n = 28), infants who were securely attached to their fathers only ($\bar{X}$ = 45.1, n = 8), and infants who were insecurely attached to both parents ($\bar{X}$ = 44.1, n = 5). Only those who are securely attached to their mothers and insecurely attached to their fathers were somewhat less sociable ($\bar{X}$ = 41.0, n = 10) than the other infants. As there was no relationship between the sex of the stranger used in the sociability assessment and the security of either the infant-mother or infant-father attachment, these results cannot be attributed to a confound between sex of stranger and the sex of the parent to whom the infant was either securely or insecurely attached.

Infants were substantially more sociable with female ($\bar{X}$ = 46.3, n = 25) than with male ($\bar{X}$ = 41.4, n = 26) strangers ($F1,49$ = 5.16, $p <$

.015). There was no significant relationship between attachment security and the differential sociability with male and female strangers: both securely- and insecurely-attached infants were more sociable with female than with male strangers. Likewise, there was no significant relationship between family type and differential sociability with male and female strangers: infants from both traditional and nontraditional families were more sociable with females. However, there was a tendency ($p = .10$) for children from nontraditional families to be more sociable ($\bar{X} = 45.6$, $n = 17$) than infants from traditional families ($\bar{X} = 43.8$, $n = 34$).

DISCUSSION

These data demonstrate once again that infants can, and frequently do, form relationships of different quality to their mother and fathers (see also Grossman et al., 1981; Lamb, 1978; Main & Weston, 1981). It thus appears that the security of attachment characterizes specific relationships between infants and their attachment figures. Presumably, the security of each relationship is independently determined by the prior pattern of interaction between the infant and the specific adult. This confirms that security of attachment is neither a personality trait nor the manifestation of a constitutional disposition or temperament (Waters & Deane, 1982). Nor is it the case, as was once believed, that the relationship with the primary caretaker serves as a prototype for all other attachment relationships (cf., Bowlby, 1969; Freud, 1940). Once infants have had sufficient interaction with adults to form attachments, they have distinctive expectations of each attachment figure. The infant's behavior in the Strange Situation thus seems to reflect its expectation of the specific adult's reliability and behavioral tendencies (Lamb, 1981).

Our results also confirm that the security of infant-adult attachment affects the infant's behavior in initial encounters with unfamiliar adults. To our surprise, however, the security of the infant-father relationship was a better predictor of sociability with unfamiliar adults than was the security of the infant-mother relationship. Previous researchers have shown that infants who are securely-attached to their *mothers* are more sociable towards strangers than infants who are insecurely-attached (Main, 1973) and that infants who have B1 or B2 (secure) relationships with their mothers are most sociable (Thompson & Lamb, 1981). No such associations were obtained in the present study, although we did find that infants who were securely-attached to their *fathers*—especially those with B1 and B2 relationships—were most sociable. There is no obvious reason why the security of the infant-mother attachment should have been unrelated to the measure of infant sociability. Although all of our fathers (especially the nontraditional men) were more involved in childcare than traditional American fathers, their wives were invariably involved as well. Thus the results do not simply reflect the complete uninvolvement or insignificance of the mothers. All of the infants appeared attached to their mothers, but the quality of these relationships apparently did not affect the infants' sociability in any significant way.

Our findings in this regard were neither predictable nor consistent with previous findings. An earlier study by Main and Weston (1981) revealed that both infant-mother and infant-father attachments had independent and additive effects on the infant's sociability (or "relatedness") toward an unfamiliar adult. In the present study, we found that when the security of the two infant-parent relationships were considered simultaneously, there was no significant relationship to sociability. Contrary to Main and Weston's findings, the infants with two secure relationships were not most sociable and the infants with two insecure attachments were not least sociable. There was not even a trend in the appropriate direction. Both theoretical considerations (Lamb, 1981) and Main and Weston's findings led us to expect that the extent of the relationship between the security of either attachment and the infants' sociability would vary depending on the relative involvement of the two parents in infant care, but no such effect was evident. Regardless of the relative involvement in child care, the security of the infant-father attachment was related to sociability, whereas the security of the infant-mother attachment was not.

Although it is not clear why we obtained these results, several possible explanations can be ruled out. First, it seems unlikely that our assessments of attachment security were rendered invalid by the inclusion of sociability assessments prior to each Strange Situation. Thompson and Lamb (1981) used the same procedure in their study, yet found clear relationships between sociability and the security of infant-mother attachments. In addition, the sociability assessment is brief, nonintrusive, pleasant, and informal; it involves little more than formalizing the interactions that may often take place when experimenters prepare parents and infants for the Strange Situation. Second, it is unlikely that the sex of the strangers employed in the sociability assessment affected our results. Main and Weston (1981) had only one male stranger, and Thompson and Lamb (1982) employed a variety of female strangers, yet both found a relationship between the security of infant-parent attachment and the infants' sociability with unfamiliar adults. Further, there was no relationship in the present study between the sex of the stranger and the security of either infant-parent attachment, indicating that our results could not be attributed to a confound between sex of the stranger and sex of the parent to whom the infant was either securely or insecurely attached. Third, the problem should not lie in the procedure we used to assess sociability, since we did find a relationship between sociability and the security of the infant-father attachment, while Thompson and Lamb (1982) found relationships between the security of infant-*mother* attachment and sociability assessed using a procedure very similar to ours. In the absence of further research, one possible explanation remains: that the Strange Situation procedure does not satisfactorily assess the quality of parent-infant attachments in at least some cultures other than our own. Unfortunately, the relationship between parent-infant interaction at home and the patterns of behavior observed in the Strange Situation have thus far only been assessed in the United States.

Most studies conducted in the United States have found that roughly 60% to 65% of their sample have secure attachments, 20% to 25% are avoidantly attached, and 10% to 15% are resistantly attached (Ainsworth et al., 1978; Main & Weston, 1981; Thompson, Lamb, & Estes, 1982; Vaughn, Egeland, Sroufe, & Waters, 1979; Waters, 1978). The distribution obtained in the present study deviated only marginally from this, with 73% of the infants securely attached, 24% avoidant, and only 4% resistant. Within the secure category, the low-contact subgroups (B1 and B2) were more common than in American samples. The distribution we obtained was thus more similar to that typically found in the U.S. than to that reported by Grossman et al. (1981) in Germany. Only 30% of their subjects were securely-attached and 60% were avoidant. Although the deviation from the American distribution was not significant, we were intrigued to find so few resistantly-attached (C-type) infants and somewhat fewer of the high-contact secure subgroups (B3 and B4), since this finding is consistent with our informal observation that Swedes are less expressive than Americans. Conceivably, these Swedish babies were constitutionally less excitable and expressive, or their patterns of emotional expressiveness had been shaped during the preceding months of interaction with their parents in the manner suggested by Thompson and Lamb (in press). There is clearly a need for more research on cultural and temperamental influences on the patterns of infant-parent interaction in the Strange Situation.

Consistent with previous studies (Greenberg, Hillman, & Grice, 1973; Morgan & Ricciuti, 1969), the infants responded more positively to female than to male strangers. This is probably due to the facts that the infants had more experience with female than with male adults and that the male strangers employed in this study were less experienced with infants than the females were. However, contrary to our expectations, infants with highly involved fathers were not more sociable with males than the infants with less-involved fathers. This may mean that experience with a variety of male or female adults affects sociability, rather than intensive experience with a single specific male or female.

In sum, these data confirm that infants frequently do form relationships of differing quality with their mothers and fathers, presumably in response to differences in prior patterns of interaction with each attachment figure. In addition, it is clear that the security of the infant-father relationship does affect at least some aspects of the infants' socioemotional behavior in other contexts. It is unclear, however, why we were unable to replicate previously-reported relationships between the security of infant-mother attachment and infant sociability. This finding, together with the finding that the relative formative importance of the infant-parent attachments did not vary depending on the adults' relative involvement in childcare, suggest that there is much we have yet to learn about the way in which infant-parent attachments affect social and personality development.

REFERENCES

Ainsworth, M. D. S. (1969). Object relations, dependency and attachment: A theoretical review of the infant-mother relationship. *Child Development*, 40:969–1025.

Ainsworth, M. D. S. (1977). Affective aspects of the attachment of infant to mother: Individual differences and their correlates in maternal behavior. Paper presented to the American Association for the Advancement of Science. Washington, February.

Ainsworth, M. D. S., Blehar, M., Waters, E. and Wall, S. (1978). *Patterns of Attachment*. Hillsdale, NJ: Lawrence Erlbaum Associates.

Ainsworth, M. D. S. and Wittig, B. A. (1969). Attachment and exploratory behavior of one-year-olds in a strange situation. In *Determinants of Infant Behavior* (Vol. IV), B. M. Foss, ed. London: Methuen.

Arend, R., Gove, F. and Sroufe, L. A. (1979). Continuity of individual adaptation from infancy to kindergarten: A predictive study of ego-resiliency and curiosity in preschoolers. *Child Development*, 50:950–959.

Blehar, M. C., Lieberman, A. F. and Ainsworth, M. D. S. (1977). Early face-to-face interaction and its relation to later infant-mother attachment. *Child Development*, 48:182–194.

Bowlby, J. (1969). *Attachment and Loss*. Vol. 1. *Attachment*. New York: Basic Books.

Easterbrooks, M. A. and Lamb, M. E. (1979). The relationship between quality of infant-mother attachment and infant competence in initial encounters with peers. *Child Development*, 50:380–387.

Freud, S. (1940). *An Outline of Psychoanalysis*. New York: Norton.

Greenberg, D. G., Hillman, D. and Grice, D. (1973). Infant and stranger variables related to stranger anxiety in the first year of life. *Developmental Psychology*, 9:207–212.

Grossman, K. E., Grossman, K., Huber, F. and Wartner, U. (1981). German children's behavior towards their mothers at 12 months and their fathers at 18 months in Ainsworth's Strange Situation. *International Journal of Behavioral Development*, 4:157–182.

Hollingshead, A. B. (1975). The four-factor index of social status. Unpublished manuscript, Department of Sociology, Yale University.

Lamb, M. E. (1976). Effects of stress and cohort on mother- and father-infant interaction. *Developmental Psychology*, 12:435–443. (a)

Lamb, M. E. (1976). Twelve-month-olds and their parents: Interaction in a laboratory playroom. *Developmental Psychology*, 12:237–244. (b)

Lamb, M. E. (1977). Father-infant and mother-infant interaction in the first year of life. *Child Development*, 48:167–181.

Lamb, M. E. (1978). Qualitative aspects of mother- and father-infant attachments. *Infant Behavior and Development*, 1:265–275.

Lamb, M. E. (1981). Developing trust and perceived effectance in infancy. In *Advances in Infancy Research*, Vol. 1, L. P. Lipsitt, ed. Norwood, NJ: Ablex.

Lamb, M. E. (1982). Individual differences in infant sociability: Their origins and implications for cognitive development. In *Advances in Child Development and Behavior*, Vol. 16, H. W. Reese and L. P. Lipsitt, eds. New York: Academic Press.

Lieberman, A. F. (1977). Preschoolers' competence with a peer: Influence of attachment and social experience. *Child Development*, 48:1277–1287.

Main, M. (1973). Exploration, play, and cognitive functioning as related to child-mother attachment. Unpublished doctoral dissertation, Johns Hopkins University.

Main, M. and Weston, D. (1981). Security of attachment to mother and father: Related to conflict behavior and the readiness to establish new relationships. *Child Development*, 52:932–940.

Matas, L., Arend, R. and Sroufe, L. A. (1978). Continuity of adaptation in the second year: The relationship between quality of attachment and later competence. *Child Development*, 49:547–556.

Morgan, G. A. and Ricciuti, H. N. (1969). Infants' responses to strangers during the first year. In *Determinants of Infant Behavior*, Vol. IV, B. M. Foss, ed. London: Methuen.

Pastor, D. L. (1981). The quality of mother-infant attachment and its relationship to toddlers' initial sociability with peers. *Developmental Psychology*, 17:326–335.

Stevenson, M. B. and Lamb, M. E. (1979). Effects of infant sociability and the caretaking environment on infant cognitive performance. *Child Development*, 50:340–349.

Thompson, R. A. and Lamb, M. E. (1981). The relationship between stranger sociability, temperament, and social experiences at 12½ and 19½ months of age. Paper presented to the Midwestern Psychological Association, Detroit, April.

Thompson, R. A. and Lamb, M. E. (1982). Strange sociability and its relationship to temperament and social experience during the school year. *Infant Behavior and Development*, 5, in press.

Thompson, R. A. and Lamb, M. E. (In press). Individual differences in dimensions of socioemotional development in infancy. In *Emotion: Theory, Research and Experience*, Vol. 2, *Emotions in Early Development*, R. Plutchik and H. Kellerman, eds. New York: Academic Press.

Thompson, R. A., Lamb, M. E. and Estes, D. (1982). Stability of infant-mother attachment and its relationship to changing life circumstances in an unselected middle class sample. *Child Development*, 53:144–148.

Vaughn, B., Egeland, B., Sroufe, L. A. and Waters, E. (1979). Individual differences in infant-mother attachment at twelve and eighteen months: Stability and change in families under stress. *Child Development*, 50:971–975.

Waters, E. (1978). The reliability and stability of individual differences in infant-mother attachment. *Child Development*, 49:483–494.

Waters, E. and Deane, K. E. (1982). Infant-mother attachment: Theories, models, recent data, and some tasks for comparative developmental analysis. In *Parenting: Its Causes and Consequences*, L. W. Hoffman and H. R. Schiffman, eds. Hillsdale, NJ: Lawrence Erlbaum Associates.

12

Stranger Sociability and Its Relationships to Temperament and Social Experience During the Second Year

Ross A. Thompson

University of Nebraska

Michael E. Lamb

University of Utah

The relationships between stranger sociability, temperament, and social experience were examined in a short-term longitudinal investigation. At 12½ and 19½ months, sociability was assessed using a brief procedure based on that of Stevenson and Lamb (1979). After each assessment, mothers completed a questionnaire concerning caregiving arrangements and family circumstances which included the

Reprinted with permission from *Infant Behavior and Development*, 1982, Vol. 5, 277–287.

This research is based on a dissertation conducted by the first author in partial fulfillment of the requirements for the degree Doctor of Philosophy in the Rackham School of Graduate Studies at the University of Michigan. It was supported by a grant from the Riksbankens Jubileumsfond of Sweden to author Lamb, and by a dissertation grant from Rackham to author Thompson. While the research was conducted, Thompson was a predoctoral fellow in the Bush Program in Child Development and Social Policy at the University of Michigan and a National Science Foundation predoctoral fellow. An earlier version of this paper was presented at the annual meetings of the Midwestern Psychological Association, Detroit, April 30 to May 2, 1981.

We are very grateful for the assistance provided by Lisa Colvin, Susan Dickstein, Melinda Feller, Leslie Fried, Margaret Madden, Susan Piconke, Jane Stein, Jamie Steinberg, Susan Strzelecki, and Michele Tukel. David Estes and Catherine Malkin provided special help with testing and scoring. We are also appreciative of technical assistance provided by Lee Davis. George A. Morgan and Mary K. Rothbart provided helpful comments on an earlier version of this manuscript. Finally, we wish to express a special debt to the families who participated in this study.

*Infant Behavior Questionnaire (Rothbart, 1981), which is a measure
of infant temperament. At 19½ months, temperament measures for
fearfulness, distress to limitations, smiling and laughter, and activity
level were related to stranger sociability. There were fewer significant
correlations between sociability and temperament at 12½ months, and
few relationships between sociability and social experience variables
at either age. However, changes in family circumstances, especially
those changes in parental employment status, were associated with
lower sociability scores at 19½ months. At each age, sociability scores
correlated negatively with the temperament dimension of fearfulness.
Measures of both sociability and temperament showed significant stability over the 7-month period.*

The nature of an infant's reactions to unfamiliar adults has long been
of interest to developmentalists. Although early work in this area was
concerned with "stranger anxiety" or fear (e.g., Decarie, 1974; Rheingold
& Eckerman, 1973; Scarr & Salapatek, 1970; Schaffer, 1966), researchers
now tend to focus on affiliative as well as wary tendencies, usually with
the goal of relating individual differences in stranger sociability to other
aspects of socioemotional development (Beckwith, 1972; Bretherton,
1978; Clarke-Stewart, Umeh, Snow, & Pederson, 1980; Stevenson &
Lamb, 1979; Thompson & Lamb, in press). Individual differences in
stranger sociability—assessed in terms of the quality of the infant's social
initiatives and socioemotional responses to the overtures of an unfamiliar
adult—are significantly related to cognitive performance (see review by
Lamb, 1982), the quality of the caregiving environment (Clarke-Stewart
et al., 1980; Lamb, 1982; Stevenson & Lamb, 1979) and the security of
the infant-mother attachment relationship (Main, 1973; Owen, Chase-
Lansdale, & Lamb, in preparation; Thompson & Lamb, in press).
    The origins of individual differences in stranger sociability have re-
ceived little attention, however. Although it is reasonable to expect that
sociability is affected by the infant's prior experience with other people
(such as the number of regular caregivers, experience with other children, and the number of siblings), the evidence for this proposition is
mixed. Clarke-Stewart and her colleagues (1980) found that infants who
experienced greater amounts of nonparental care behaved more negatively with strangers than did other infants, but they found no other
consistent relationships. Stevenson and Leavitt (1980), Beckwith (1972),
Morgan and Ricciuti (1969) and Harmon, Morgan, and Klein (1977)
have all reported nonsignificant associations between stranger sociability
and the baby's range of social experiences.
    Meanwhile, several researchers have explored an alternative propo-

sition: that stranger sociability is related to constitutionally-based aspects of temperament. Scarr and Salapatek (1970) reported that babies who were more active, adaptable, positive of mood, more likely to approach novel stimuli and had a higher response threshold (all assessed using a variant of Thomas, Chess, Birch, Hertzig, & Korn's [1963] parent interview) were less fearful of strangers. Other researchers, however, have reported more modest results. Morgan, Levin, and Harmon (1975) found no associations between stranger responsiveness and parent report measures of the baby's adaptability, sensitivity to stimuli, and physiological sensitivity, although Harmon and colleagues (1977) found that babies who were generally fussy also tended to avoid a stranger. Paradise and Curcio (1974) found relationships only between approach and stranger fearfulness. Finally, employing Carey and McDevitt's (1978) Infant Temperament Questionnaire, Stevenson and Leavitt (1980) found that high sociability scores at 12 months were related to low activity level, a greater tendency to approach new stimuli, and greater distractability, but not to the other six subscales. In view of these inconsistent findings, one goal of the present study was to further investigate and compare the contributions of social experience and temperament to individual variations in sociability during the second year.

Most of these studies have assessed stranger sociability on only one occasion, and thus it is unclear whether individual differences in sociability reflect relatively enduring response tendencies, or are more transient. Consequently, a second goal of the study was to examine the relationships between sociability, temperament and social experience at two points in time: 12½ and 19½ months of age. The test-retest design permitted us to examine not only the temporal stability of sociability scores over a 7-month period, but also to study the effects of social experiences occurring between the two assessments on changes in sociability. We were particularly interested in the effects of critical intervening experiences, such as a major separation from the mother or changes in family circumstances which might influence the infant's social experiences.

We studied stranger sociability during the infant's second year because this is a period of rapidly developing social responsiveness, during which infants become more sophisticated social partners due to their expanding communicative repertoire and their growing autonomy. Thus sociability scores in the second year reflect individual differences in the development of more sophisticated and complex social skills than during the first year, and we expected that the correlates of these differences would yield important information concerning the early development of social responsiveness.

Since no temperament questionnaire has been standardized for infants older than 12 months, the measurement of temperament was potentially problematic. We selected the Infant Behavior Questionnaire (IBQ), developed by Rothbart (1981), for several reasons. First, it involves behaviorally-based and situationally-specific appraisals of the infant's behavior over limited periods of time (i.e., one-week or, in certain cases, two-week periods), and thus the effects of biased parental reporting are minimized. Second, the situations assessed in the questionnaire—feeding, sleeping, bathing, dressing, play, soothing, and "daily activities"—seem relevant to 19½-month-olds as well as to younger infants, even though the IBQ was standardized on 3- to 12-month-olds. Third, the six IBQ subscales (activity level, distress to limitations, fear, duration of orienting, smiling and laughter, soothability) comprise affectively-based temperamental dimensions which are likely to be related to stranger sociability. Finally, the IBQ permits the respondent to indicate that a particular question seems inapplicable or irrelevant. This provided one way of appraising the usefulness of the IBQ for assessing infants older than 12 months.

METHOD

Subjects

The subjects for this study were 43 infants (21 males, 22 females), 15 of whom were firstborns. They were tested at 12½ months (± 2 weeks), and again at 19½ months (± 2 weeks).[1] Approximately half the families were contacted through a subject pool administered by the developmental psychology program at the university; the other half were recruited through birth announcements published in a local newspaper. All families were contacted by phone; roughly 78% of the families we called agreed to participate.

The families in this study ranged from upper-middle-class professionals to lower-middle-class blue-collar workers. Educational level ranged from graduate degrees to high-school training. All families except one were intact, two-parent families. Taken together, the heterogeneity of this middle-class sample is reflected in scores on Hollingshead's Four-Factor Index of Social Position (Hollingshead, 1975). Fourteen families were in Hollingshead's Class I (major professional and business),

---

[1] There were two exceptions. One infant was initially tested three weeks before his first birthday; another was seen for the second time one week following her 20-month anniversary. Inspection of the data revealed that these infants did not differ from others in relevant behaviors, so their data were included.

12 in Class II (minor professional and technical), 13 in Class III (skilled craftsmen, clerical, sales workers), and four in Class IV (machine operators and semiskilled workers). All families were white except one, which was Puerto Rican.

Procedure

Stranger sociability in infants was assessed using a modified version of a semistandardized procedure developed by Stevenson and Lamb (1979), which was designed to measure an infant's responses to initial encounters with an unfamiliar adult. The procedure involves a series of social overtures of gradually increasing intrusiveness conducted by a female stranger in mother's presence. The initial social bids occur while the infant is seated on mother's lap: first an interesting toy is offered the baby, and then the stranger attempts to initiate a give-and-take exchange. Following this, the infant is placed on the floor, and the baby's initial response to floor freedom is observed. The stranger then moves to the floor, again offers the baby a toy, and initiates a turn-taking exchange. After a few moments of play, the stranger attempts to pick up the baby, before finally leaving the room. The total session typically lasts about five or six minutes (see Table 1).

The sociability assessment was conducted in a large, carpeted playroom (5.75 m. × 4.5 m) containing two chairs (for mother and stranger), a table, and an assortment of age-appropriate toys for the baby in the middle of the room. Eight highly-trained female college students served as strangers; a different group of four students was employed for the assessments at each age. Sessions at both ages were videotaped from behind one-way windows; ceiling microphones were used to record sound.

From videotape records, the infant's initial response to each successive initiative was scored on a 1 (withdrawal, distress) to 5 (outgoing, friendly) point scale. The baby's responses to the stranger's entrance and departure were similarly appraised. Finally, the rater made a summary assessment of the baby's responsiveness to the stranger on a 9-point scale. The sum of these ratings constituted the infant's score for stranger sociability (see Table 1).

Scoring was conducted by two highly-trained research assistants with whom a high level of inter-rater reliability had been achieved. Scoring of the 19½-month assessments was conducted blind to the 12½-month ratings. Periodic reliability checks performed on a total of eight assessments at each age yielded coefficients of exact agreement on subscales exceeding 87% each time. Although different assistants rated the 12½-month and 19½-month assessments, consistency was assured by having a single researcher (the first author) conduct the training and reliability checks at each age. In addition, the rater of the 19½-month assessments rescored five 12½-month assessments, and achieved 95% exact agreement with the original rater.

Questionnaires

Following each laboratory assessment, mothers were given questionnaires to complete at home and return by mail. Each questionnaire included inquiries concerning the parents' occupations, the identities of other major caregivers (if any), the amount of time weekly that each spent with the baby, and the composition of the family group. In addition, the 19½-month questionnaire included inquiries concerning the incidence of major separations (i.e., 24 hours or longer) experienced by the baby since birth, important changes in family circumstances (e.g., moving to a new home, change in employment status for either parent,

TABLE 1
Procedure for Assessing Stranger Sociability

A. *Baby's Initial Reaction to the Stranger*
   1. Cries, becomes quite upset
   2. Whimpers or fusses
   3. Turns to mother or away from the stranger, sometimes with a shy smile
   4. Looks at the stranger intently without smiling
   5. Smiles at the stranger

B. *Baby's Initial Reaction to Being Offered a Toy by Stranger on Mother's Lap (Score First 10 Seconds Following Initiation of Bid)*
   1. Fusses, cries or turns toward mother
   2. Refuses toy by looking away, pushing it away, turning toward another toy, or using words (e.g., "no")
   3. Looks at toy without reaching for it
   4. Tentatively reaches for or touches toy
   5. Accepts toy from stranger with little hesitation

C. *Baby's Reaction to the Stranger's Initiation of a Give-and-Take Exchange on Mother's Lap (Score First 30 Seconds Following Initiation of Bid, or Two Attempts to Get a Game Started)*
   1. Crying, fussing or other indications of distress
   2. Refusal to join in by turning toward mother or another toy, turning away from stranger, just looking at stranger, or using words (e.g., "no")
   3. Initially reluctant, then participates
   4. Immediately joins in and participates with stranger
   5. Actively participates in game with stranger by smiling, initiating exchanges, anticipating give-and-take, changing the game, acting playfully or teasing the stranger, etc.

TABLE 1
(Continued)

D. *Baby's Behavior When Given Floor Freedom*
1. Touches mother or requests to return to lap
2. Approaches or turns toward mother
3. Stays where s/he is or moves away from mother to play with toys
4. Approaches stranger
5. Touches stranger or requests to be picked up

E. *Baby's Initial Reaction to Being Offered a Toy by Stranger on Floor (Score First 10 Seconds Following Initiation of Bid)*
1. Fusses, cries or turns toward mother
2. Refuses toy by looking away, pushing it away, turning toward a different toy, or using words (e.g. "no")
3. Looks at toy without reaching for it
4. Tentatively reaches for or touches toy
5. Accepts toy from stranger with little hesitation

F. *Baby's Reaction to the Stranger's Initiation of a Give-and-Take Exchange on the Floor (Score First 30 Seconds Following Initiation of Bid, or Two Attempts to Get a Game Started)*
1. Crying, fussing or other indications of distress
2. Refusal to join in by turning toward mother or another toy, turning away from stranger, just looking at stranger, or using words (e.g., "no")
3. Initially reluctant, then participates
4. Immediately joins in and participates with stranger
5. Actively participates in game with stranger by smiling, initiating exchanges, anticipating give-and-take, changing the game, acting playfully or teasing the stranger, etc.

G. *Baby's Reaction When the Stranger Attempts a Pick-Up*
1. Immediately cries, becomes quite upset
2. Whimpers or fusses; milder distress reaction
3. Tries to get down, wiggles in stranger's arms, or turns and reaches toward mother
4. Minimal acceptance of pick-up, but baby turns away from stranger, avoids eye-contact, and/or doesn't mold to her
5. Positive acceptance of pick-up, with molding, sometimes smiling, etc.

H. *Baby's Reaction to the Stranger's Departure*
1. Returns to mother as stranger walks out of room, or clings to her
2. Ignores stranger's departure entirely
3. Looks up fleetingly as stranger leaves the room
4. Sustained visual regard of the stranger as she leaves
5. Smiles at the stranger, waves or says "bye-bye," follows stranger to the door, etc.

I. *Overall Impression of Sociability*
1. Quite unfriendly, fussy, fearful
2. Between 1 and 3
3. Generally unfriendly, serious, wary
4. Between 3 and 5
5. Neutral, neither friendly nor unfriendly
6. Between 5 and 7
7. Friendly, positive reaction
8. Between 7 and 9
9. Very friendly, outgoing, smiling

birth of a new baby, etc.) since the baby's birth, and the infant's peer experiences.

The Infant Behavior Questionnaire was also completed and returned by mail. In completing the IBQ, the mother was asked to consider a variety of situations and indicate how her baby typically behaved in those situations. The mother was asked to consider only events occurring during the preceding week (or, in some instances, two weeks). A special rating ("X") was used when questions referred to situations which did not occur during the specified time period, or were otherwise inapplicable. Scoring the 92-item questionnaire involves computing mean values for each of the six subscales; activity level, distress to limitations, fear, duration of orienting, smiling and laughter, and soothability (see Rothbart, 1981, for further details).

RESULTS

Mean stranger sociability scores were very similar at each age (12½ months: 34.53; 19½ months: 34.95), and the scores were significantly correlated over time ($r = .40$, $p < .01$).[2] Scores for each IBQ subscale were also highly correlated over time (activity level: $r = .53$; distress to limitations: $r = .61$; fear: $r = .65$; duration of orienting: $r = .67$; smiling and laughter: r .76; soothability: $r = .46$; all $p < .005$). There were some age-related changes in temperament: at 19½ months, infants exhibited more smiling and laughter ($t = 2.06$, $df = 41$, $p < .05$), longer orienting duration ($t = 3.47$, $df = 41$, $p < .0015$), and diminished activity level ($t = 2.39$, $df = 41$, $p < .025$) than at 12½ months. Developmental differences on other IBQ subscales were nonsignificant.

At 12½ months, stranger sociability scores were significantly, and negatively, correlated only with the infant's reported fearfulness. At 19½ months, by contrast, sociability scores were negatively associated with IBQ scales for activity level, distress to limitations, and fear, and positively related to smiling and laughter (see Table 2). Other correlations were small and nonsignificant. At each age, the temperament scale assessing fearful reactions was most strongly associated with sociability. In general, relationships between sociability and temperament were stronger at 19½ months than at 12½ months.

The t-tests revealed fewer significant relationships between stranger sociability scores and prior social experience than with temperament. The following variables were not significantly related either to 12½ or

---

[2]All reported p-values are for two-tailed tests, even though one-tailed tests were justified in many cases.

TABLE 2
Correlations Between IBQ Temperament Subscales
and Stranger Sociability Scores

Temperament Subscale	12½ Months	19½ Months
Activity Level	− 14	−.45**
Distress to Limitations	−.19	−.34*
Fear	−.38*	−.47**
Duration of Orienting	.08	.11
Smiling and Laughter	.18	.36*
Soothability	.07	.14

*p<.05
**p<.005

19½-month sociability scores or to changes in sociability over the 7-month period: the number of siblings, whether the child had regular experiences with peers, and whether the infant had experienced a major separation (≥ 24 hours) from the mother during the first year, or between the two assessments. There were also no significant associations between 12½-month sociability scores and: changes in family circumstances during the baby's first year, maternal employment during the first year, the father's assumption of regular caregiving responsibilities, and the regular involvement of extra-familial caregivers (e.g., babysitter, child care agency).

One set of relationships was informative, however. Those infants who experienced one or more important changes in family circumstances (e.g., employment change for either parent, moving to a new home, birth of a new baby) between the two assessments had lower sociability scores at 19½ months ($\bar{X}$ = 32.06, N = 16) than did other babies ($\bar{X}$ = 36.67) (t = 2.21, df = 41, p < .035). In particular, changes in the employment status of either father or mother had the greatest impact upon stranger sociability (19½-month mean sociability score for these babies was 29.44 (N = 9); for all others, $\bar{X}$ = 36.41; t = 2.92, df = 41, p < .006). These employment changes, in turn, typically influenced the nature of caregiving arrangements for the child. Sociability scores at 19½ months were lower when the father assumed a major caregiving role ($\bar{X}$ = 29.87, N = 8) than when he did not ($\bar{X}$ = 36.11) (t = 2.43, df = 41, p < .02). Greater paternal involvement in caregiving was, in fact, associated with a decrease in sociability scores over the two assessments ($\bar{X}_{change}$ = − 5.00) compared to an increase when he was minimally involved ($\bar{X}_{change}$ = 1.66) (t = 2.38, df = 41, p < .025). On the other hand, sociability scores tended to increase when the child experienced regular extrafamilial care (e.g., babysitter, child care agency) ($\bar{X}_{change} = 5.67$, $N = 6$) and to remain the same ($\bar{X}_{change} = -0.43$) when there was not ($t = 1.90$, $df = 41$, $p < .065$).

The temporal association between stranger sociability and temperament was examined using cross-lagged correlations. The analysis of 12½-month temperament and 19½-month sociability scores yielded significant negative associations between sociability and activity level ($r = -.35$, $p < .05$), distress to limitations ($r = -.42$, $p < .01$) and fear ($r = -.30$, $p < .05$). Sociability scores at 12½ months were significantly associated with only one 19½-month IBQ subscale: fear ($r = -.38$, $p < .05$).

The number of significant relationships between social experience variables and temperament scores at 12½ and 19½ months were fewer than would be expected by chance, and were nonsystematic. There were modest sex differences in sociability: at 19½ months, girls scored higher than boys ($t = 2.59$, $df = 41$, $p < .015$). There was a similar tendency at 12½ months, but the difference was not significant. On the temperament subscales, boys received higher scores than girls for smiling and laughter at 12½ months ($t = 1.91$, $df = 41$, $p < .065$); there were no other differences by sex.

Finally, we compared the number of items receiving an "X—Does not apply" rating at 19½ and 12½ months on the IBQ. The difference was minimal: out of 84 questions relevant to the IBQ subscales, an average of 78.70 received scorable ratings at 12½ months, compared with 76.95 at 19½ months. The proportions of questions omitted were relatively equal across subscales, and were similar at each age.

DISCUSSION

These findings suggest that both temperament and prior social experiences affect the development of stranger sociability, but in importantly different ways.

First, scores on the IBQ subscales were clearly and meaningfully related to sociability scores at 19½ months; trends in the same direction were evident at 12½ months. At both ages, sociability was most strongly, and negatively, correlated with the scale assessing fearful reactions. This finding, which is similar to those reported by other researchers, implies that affiliative/sociable and fear/wariness response systems are inversely related in infancy. More important, it suggests that sociability during the first two years is related to a more general, situationally-nonspecific response tendency. In other words, infants who tend to approach and engage novel stimulus events also do so in their initial encounters with unfamiliar adults.

Sociability scores were also negatively correlated with the IBQ subscales assessing activity level and distress to limitations, and positively associated with the index of smiling and laughter. While the relationships with distress to limitations and smiling and laughter are intuitively reasonable, the negative association with activity level, which was also reported by Stevenson and Leavitt (1980), deserves further consideration. It may well be that the ability to engage in friendly, well-modulated interaction with an unfamiliar adult requires the capacity to inhibit ongoing activity in order to attend and respond to the partner's initiatives.

In general, there were more significant relationships between stranger sociability and temperament than between sociability and the breadth of prior social experiences. There was little evidence that infants who had had a wider range of social experiences—through regular interaction with non-maternal caregivers (including the father), or frequent contact with peers or siblings—were more sociable than infants with a more limited range of social experiences. Indeed, the only significant associations were somewhat inconsistent: while regular extra-familial caregiving was associated with an *increase* in sociability between the two assessments, those infants whose fathers assumed a major caregiving role *declined* in sociability. Nor were critical experiences—such as a major separation from the mother—related to sociability scores or to their change over time. On the other hand, changes in family circumstances did seem to affect the development of stranger sociability. In particular, changes in the employment status of either parent were associated with lower sociability scores at 19½ months, perhaps because they affected the nature of interactions within the home which, in turn, influenced responsiveness to nonfamilial persons.

In light of this finding, and in view of repeated failures to find systematic, meaningful and replicable associations between the infant's prior experience with other people and responsiveness to strangers (e.g., Beckwith, 1972; Clarke-Stewart et al., 1980; Harmon et al., 1977; Morgan & Ricciuti, 1969, Morgan et al., 1975; Paradise & Curcio, 1974; Stevenson & Leavitt, 1980; this study), we suggest that further research on the origins of stranger sociability in infancy should focus on the quality of mother-infant interaction as well as the baby's range of experience with other social partners. Several researchers have shown that responsiveness to strangers is influenced by the quality of infant-mother interaction. Main (1973), for example, found that infants who were securely attached to their mothers at 12 months exhibited greater friendliness and cooperation toward unfamiliar adults at 20 months than did insecurely-attached infants. In a previous analysis of these data, Thompson (1981) likewise found a strong association between stranger sociability and the security of infant-mother attachment: when attachment classification was the same at 12½ and 19½ months, sociability scores were highly stable over time ($r = .74$, $p < .0001$, $N = 23$); when attachment status was temporally unstable, so too was stranger sociability ($r = -.18$, $N = 20$). In the absence of changes in the security of infant-mother attachment, therefore, stranger sociability appears to be highly stable over time. We also found that individual differences in sociability scores were related to the security of infant-mother attachment, although only sociability scores (not attachment status) were related to temperamental characteristics. Clarke-Stewart and colleagues (1980) and Stevenson and Lamb (1979) also reported relationships between sociability and the mother's interactive style. Stranger sociability may thus reflect, in part, the generalization of interactive capacities which the infant has learned in exchanges with the mother. Clearly, this is an area meriting further investigation.

In sum, individual differences in stranger sociability appear to be more strongly related to variation in temperament—especially fearfulness—than to the dimensions of prior social experience assessed in this study, Moreover, cross-lagged correlations suggested a stronger relationship between 19½-month sociability scores and earlier ratings of distress to limitations and activity level than the reverse. Thus temperamental traits appear to be importantly implicated in the development of stranger sociability, and were themselves weakly related to the social experience variables.

The validity of our results is buttressed by evidence concerning the usefulness of the Infant Behavior Questionnaire for assessing stable dimensions of infant temperament during the second year of life. Ratings on all six IBQ subscales were remarkably stable over time; indeed, they were more strongly correlated over the 7-month period than they were over comparable periods during the first year in Rothbart's larger sample (Rothbart, 1981). Moreover, the mothers in our sample evidently felt comfortable using the questionnaire to describe their 19½-month-olds: there was no appreciable increase over time in "Does not apply" ratings, and item omissions were evenly distributed over IBQ subscales at each age. While there remains a need, of course, to assess the validity and reliability of the IBQ when used with older infants, our findings are certainly promising, and suggest also that the measure has external validity when used with 19½-month-old infants.

Indeed, since we consistently found stronger relationships among the variables at 19½ months than at 12½ months, there is evidently a real need for further study of sociability and its correlates during the second year of life. Since this is a time of rapidly developing social skills, individual differences in stranger sociability during the second year may also yield important relationships with other dimensions of socioemotional development. Moreover, in contrast to the short-term variability of measures of stranger responsiveness during the first year (e.g., Emde, Gaensbauer, & Harmon, 1976; Schaffer, 1966), we found that sociability scores were significantly correlated between 12½ and 19½ months, and mean scores were similar at each age. In short, individual differences in stranger sociability appear to be more stable during the second year, and may also be more informative concerning important dimensions of early social responsiveness.

REFERENCES

Beckwith, L. (1972). Relationships between infants' social behavior and their mothers' behavior. *Child Development*, 43:397–411.

Bretherton, I. (1978). Making friends with one-year olds: An experimental study of infant-stranger interaction. *Merrill-Palmer Quarterly*, 24:29–51.

Carey, W. B. and McDevitt, S. C. (1978). Revision of the Infant Temperament Questionnaire. *Pediatrics*, 61:735–739.

Clarke-Stewart, K. A., Umeh, B. J., Snow, M. E. and Pederson, J. A. (1980). Development and prediction of children's sociability from 1 to 2½ years. *Developmental Psychology*, 16:290–302.

Decarie, T. G. (1974). *The Infant's Reaction to Strangers*. New York: International Universities Press.

Emde, R. N., Gaensbauer, T. J. and Harmon, R. J. (1976). Emotional expression in infancy: A biobehavioral study. *Psychological Issues*, 10, Monograph 37. New York: International Universities Press.

Harmon, R. J., Morgan, G. A. and Klein, R. P. (1977). Determinants of normal variation in infants' negative reactions to unfamiliar adults. *Journal of the American Academy of Child Psychiatry*, 16:670–683.

Hollingshead, A. B. (1975). Four factor index of social status. Unpublished manuscript, Yale University.

Lamb, M. E. (1982). The origins of individual differences in infant sociability and their implications for cognitive development. In *Advances in Child Development and Behavior*, Vol. 16, H. W. Reese and L. P. Lipsitt, eds. New York: Academic Press.

Main, M. (1973). Exploration, play, and cognitive functioning as related to child-mother attachment. Unpublished doctoral dissertation, Johns Hopkins University.

Morgan, G. A., Levin, B. and Harmon, R. J. (1975). Determinants of individual differences in infants' reactions to unfamiliar adults. *JSAS Catalog of Selected Documents in Psychology*, 5:277 (Ms. No. 1006).

Morgan, G. A. and Ricciuti, H. N. (1969). Infants' responses to strangers during the first year. In *Determinants of Infant Behavior*, Vol. IV, B. M. Foss, ed. London: Methuen.

Owen, M. T., Chase-Lansdale, L. and Lamb, M. E. (1981). Mothers' and fathers' attitudes, maternal employment, and the security of infant-parent attachment. Manuscript in preparation, University of Michigan.

Paradise, E. B. and Curcio, F. (1974). Relationship of cognitive and affective behaviors to fear of strangers in male infants. *Developmental Psychology*, 10:476–483.

Rheingold, H. and Eckerman, C. (1973). Fear of the stranger: A critical examination. In *Advances in Child Development and Behavior*, Vol. 8, H. W. Reese and L. P. Lipsitt, eds. New York: Academic Press.

Rothbart, M. K. (1981). Measurement of temperament in infancy. *Child Development*, 52:569–578.

Scarr, S. and Salapatek, P. (1970). Patterns of fear development during infancy. *Merrill-Palmer Quarterly*, 16:53–90.

Schaffer, H. R. (1966). The onset of fear of strangers and the incongruity hypothesis. *Journal of Child Psychology and Psychiatry*, 7:95–106.

Stevenson, M. B. and Lamb, M. E. (1979). Effects of infant sociability and the caretaking environment on infant cognitive performance. *Child Development*, 50:340–349.

Stevenson, M. B. and Leavitt, L. A. (1980). Associations among temperament, sociability and social experiences in one-year-olds. Paper presented to the biennial meetings of the International Conference for Infant Studies, New Haven, April.

Thomas, A., Chess, S., Birch, H. G., Hertzig, M. E. and Korn, S. (1963). *Behavioral Individuality in Early Childhood*. New York: New York University Press.

Thompson, R. A. (1981). Continuity and change in socioemotional development during the second year. Unpublished doctoral dissertation, University of Michigan.

Thompson, R. A. and Lamb, M. E. (1981). Security of attachment and stranger sociability in infancy. *Developmental Psychology*, 18, University of Michigan. (In press.)

Part III

LANGUAGE, COGNITION, AND LEARNING

Language, cognition, and learning are closely interrelated, and at the same time encompass a wide variety of phenomena and issues. This is clear throughout the papers in the third section.

Baker and Cantwell consider the developmental, social, and behavioral concomitants and consequences of speech and language disordered children. Both groups in their study tended to have a high rate of behavior problems which could not be explained by adverse social or family factors. The children with language problems, or dysphasias, were at higher risk for behavioral, social, and developmental problems than were the youngsters with speech difficulties. The authors emphasize the implications of their findings for psychiatric screening and intervention.

Yarrow and his co-workers report a relationship of persistence at tasks with levels of cognitive functioning and competence in infancy. They consider the relationship to be reciprocal, with persistent infants becoming more competent and competent infants becoming more persistent. The authors consider task persistence as one aspect of infants' motivation to master the environment. Whether the persistence is motivational or temperamental in origin, or a combination of both, is not clear from the authors' data.

Clarke's paper provides a useful review of a number of issues in psychology and education, such as cognitive views of learning, learning time, teacher-pupil interactions, and the relative importance of school and home influences on school achievement. The author emphasizes the complex interrelationships of biological and social factors, and points out the value of naturalistic as contrasted to laboratory studies.

13

Developmental, Social and Behavioral Characteristics of Speech and Language Disordered Children

Lorian Baker and Dennis P. Cantwell

University of California at Los Angeles

This paper reports on an epidemiological study of psychiatric disorder in children with speech and language disorders. Earlier preliminary analyses of data on the children presenting to a speech clinic suggested that these children are at risk for the development of psychiatric disorder. Data on a larger number of children are analyzed in the present paper, and particular attention is given to the developmental, demographic and linguistic factors which may play a role in the etiology of psychiatric disorder or communication disorder. The data confirm that communication disordered children are at risk for the development of psychiatric disorder, and indicate that adverse environmental conditions do not seem to be responsible for this risk. A subgroup of children who are at greatest risk is identified and described.

There is now a growing body of data suggesting that children with speech or language problems are "different" developmentally, socially, and/or behaviorally from children in the general population who do not have speech or language problems. A review by the present authors[1] of

Reprinted with permission from *Child Psychiatry and Human Development*, 1982, Vol. 12, No. 4, 195–206.

Dr. Baker is a Research Associate specializing in psycholinguistics at the Neuropsychiatric Institute, University of California at Los Angeles. Dr. Cantwell is Joseph Campbell Professor of Child Psychiatry at the Neuropsychiatric Institute.

the literature on speech and language disordered children has revealed a number of case reports written by speech/language pathologists, school teachers, guidance counselors, and other professionals which indicate that speech or language disordered children tend to have numerous social and behavioral difficulties. Studies of psychiatric practices or child guidance clinics[2,3,4] have shown that there is a high prevalence of speech and language problems among the emotionally disturbed children attending these facilities.

Epidemiological studies from the general population have provided further evidence of the "abnormality" of children with speech and language problems. The most comprehensive such epidemiological study to date has been done in England by Richman and Stevenson.[5-9] They found that in a random sample of three-year-old children living in one outer-London borough, 22 children had a delay in expressive language, 16 children had a severe delay in expressive language, and 10 had a specific expressive language delay. Comparisons of the language delayed children to the remaining children in the sample revealed that the language delayed children were different in several ways. First, the children with language problems had significantly more behavior problems than the children with normal language development: 58 percent of the language delayed had behavior problems compared to only 14 percent of the non-language delayed children. In addition, in this sample the presence of language delay was associated with the presence of family discord, maternal depression, large family size, and the presence of psychosocial stress.

The present authors have conducted an epidemiological study of psychiatric disorder in children presenting to a community speech clinic. Data from the first 100 children seen in this study were reported earlier in this journal.[10] It was found that the parents of these children noted an average of 18 behavioral symptoms per child, and the teachers of the children noted an average of 17 symptoms per child. Commonly reported symptoms included: having a short attention span, being easily frustrated, fidgeting, having poor coordination, being shy, being overly sensitive, and having frequent temper tantrums. Psychiatric diagnosis of the first 100 children seen in this study revealed the presence of a diagnosable psychiatric disorder, according to DSM-III criteria,[11] in approximately one-half of the group of children.[12] Developmental disorders (reading, math, etc.) were found in approximately one quarter of the first 100 children. Thus, speech and language disordered children as a group seem to be at risk for both psychiatric disorder and developmental disorders.

More detailed analysis of the data on the first 100 children revealed the very interesting finding that the children presenting to a typical speech clinic are not a homogeneous group. Rather, the children fall into two major subgroups according to linguistic diagnosis. These two groups are *"pure speech disordered children"* who have disorders of the production of the phonetic speech string (including articulation disorders, fluency disorders or voice disorders), but whose language (grammar and vocabulary) is normal; and *"speech and language disordered children"* who have disorders involving both speech (articulation, fluency or voice) and language (grammar or vocabulary). The data from the first 100 cases seen indicated that the children with disorders involving language seem to be more at risk for psychiatric problems than the children whose problems were confined to speech production.[13] Of those children who were psychiatrically ill, the majority (87 percent) were found to have disorders involving language, whereas of the psychiatrically well children, only a minority (36 percent) had disorders involving language. In addition to having different rates of psychiatric illness, it appears that language disordered children are different from purely speech disordered children in the types of problems they have. Analysis of parent and teacher reports[14] indicated a greater frequency of complaints about hyperactivity and developmental problems in the language disordered group and a greater frequency of somatic complaints in the purely speech disordered group. The frequency of complaints by parents and teachers about conduct, emotional problems and peer relationships did not distinguish the two types of communication impaired children.

The aim of the present paper is to further describe a typical speech clinic population of children. Data from a larger sample will be reported with special regard to such factors as developmental milestones, biological and medical history, demographics, family structure, behavioral symptoms, and psychiatric diagnosis. Despite the previous studies done by various authors on special subgroups of speech or language impaired children,[1] there is still no comprehensive report known to the present authors on the social, behavioral, and other problems of a "typical" group of children presenting to a "typical" speech clinic. The present paper will attempt to: confirm whether such children are at risk for psychiatric disorder, determine if they are at risk for particular types of psychiatric disorder, determine if they are at risk for other problems, determine if there are certain demographic or developmental features by which such children may be identified, confirm that children with pure speech disorders are less at risk for psychiatric problems than children with disorders involving language, and determine whether there are any develop.mental or demographic features which differentiate between purely speech disordered children and language disordered children who present to a speech clinic.

METHOD

Subjects for the study were patients of the Community Speech and Hearing Clinic, a large speech clinic in the greater Los Angeles area which serves a broad social spectrum of cases. The clinic did not offer psychiatric evaluation or services of any type. All children coming to the clinic for a speech or language evaluation who were between the ages of two and sixteen years and who had been found by screening or testing to have hearing within normal limits, were asked to take part in the study. The refusal rate was quite low (less than two percent), and hence the patients taking part in the study are believed to be representative of children with speech and language disorders, coming to a general speech clinic.

The study consisted of a comprehensive clinical, social, and linguistic evaluation of each child. Standard language, intelligence, and achievement tests were done (including, as appropriate for the child's age and abilities, the Peabody Picture Vocabulary Tests, the Wechsler Primary and Preschool Scale of Intelligence or the Wechsler Intelligence Scale for Children, the Receptive-Expressive-Emerging Language Scale, the Goldman-Fristoe Test of Articulation, the Carrow Test of Auditory Comprehension of Language, the Illinois Test of Psycholinguistic Abilities, the Wide Range Achievement Test, and the Gray Oral Reading Test). The child was given a developmental neurological examination for "soft signs" and was interviewed by a child psychiatrist. The child's parents were interviewed regarding family history, medical history, developmental history, child's history of behavioral problems and social environment. In addition, questionnaires designed by Rutter[15] and Conners[16] were given to both the child's parents and his teacher (if he had one). These questionnaires enumerated certain behaviors and asked for additional comments about the child. More detailed descriptions of the evaluation instruments used in this study are provided in previous publications.[10,12-14]

The present paper reports on the results of these comprehensive evaluations for 180 children. Seventy-six of these children had pure speech disorders, and 104 had disorders involving language development.

Of the 76 children with a "pure" speech disorder, 81 percent had an articulation problem, 17 percent were dysfluent, and two percent had a voice disorder or spoke too fast. Of the articulation impaired children, 61 percent were diagnosed as having a developmental articulation disorder, eight percent as having a speech disorder resulting from structural abnormality of the speech mechanism, and five percent as having a speech disorder due to neurological abnormality. Seven percent of the articulation impaired children had a simple lisp.

Of the 104 language impaired children, 27 percent were found to have an expressive language disorder, with comprehension within normal limits, whereas 73 percent of the children had a disorder affecting both expressive and receptive language.

The speech disordered children ranged in age from 2.3 to 11.7 years of age, and had a mean age of 5.6 years. The language disordered children ranged in age from 1.9 to 12.1 years of age and had a mean age of 4.8 years. Both the speech disordered group and the language disordered group were 72 percent male and 38 percent female.

RESULTS

Demographic Characteristics of Speech and Language Disordered Children

The "typical" child presenting to the speech clinic for evaluation was a male Caucasian early-born child from a small family. This characterization is true for both the purely speech disordered children and for the language disordered children. Seventy-two percent of the children in both the pure speech group and the language group were males. The speech impaired children and the language impaired children were also similar in family size, birth order, and ethnic background. Large families were not common among the group of children studied, with only nine percent of the language disordered children and seven percent of the speech disordered children coming from families of four or more children. In fact, 69 percent of the language impaired children and 67 percent of the speech impaired children came from either one or two child families. The distribution of birth orders was not significantly different for the speech and language disturbed groups of children. In both groups, children tended to be early-, rather than later-borns. In the language disordered group of children, 44 percent of the children were first borns, 35 percent were second borns, 11 percent were third borns, two percent were fourth borns, and four percent were fifth or sixth borns. In the speech impaired group, 45 percent of the children were first borns, 41 percent were second borns, 11 percent were third borns, and 3 percent were fourth borns. The vast majority of the children studied were of Caucasian origin. In both the speech disordered group and the language disordered group, approximately five percent of the children had non-white parents.

The speech disordered children differed from the language disordered children in severai social class indicators. Fathers of the language impaired children tended to have lower status occupations than fathers of the speech impaired children. Nineteen percent of the fathers of the language impaired children were employed in unskilled labor jobs, whereas only three percent of the fathers in the speech impaired group held such jobs. Thirty-four percent of the fathers of the language impaired children had professional jobs, whereas forty-seven percent of the fathers of the speech impaired children held professional positions. These differences were significant to the 0.01 level. The fathers of the speech disordered children also tended to be better educated than the fathers of the language disordered children, although this difference did not reach statistical significance. Forty-six percent of the language disordered children had fathers with a college degree, whereas sixty-eight percent of the speech disordered children had fathers with college degrees. There was a significant difference (.001) between the two groups of children in terms of mothers' education. Twenty-three percent of the language disordered children had mothers with college degrees, whereas 51 percent of the speech disordered children had mothers with college degrees. There was a trend, but it was not statistically significant, for the mothers of the language disordered group to hold lower status jobs. Only nine percent of the mothers in the language disordered group had such jobs. The average age of fathers in the language disordered group was 34 years, and in the speech disordered group it was 35 years. Mothers of the language disordered children averaged 30 years, whereas mothers of the speech disordered children averaged 32.5 years. Although the ages of the mothers in the language disordered group is significantly younger than the ages of mothers in the speech disordered group, it must be remembered that the language disordered children were significantly younger than the speech disordered children, so that the ages of mothers at the time of the children's births were not significantly different.

Developmental Characteristics of Speech and Language Disordered Children

In general, children in the language disordered group were significantly later in reaching developmental milestones than children in the speech disordered group. However, mean ages for reaching motor milestones were still within the normal range for the language impaired group. The mean age for sitting was 7.8 months in the language disordered group (versus six months in the speech impaired group). The mean age for crawling was 9.3 months in the language impaired group (versus 7.2 months in the speech impaired group). The mean age for standing alone was 13.1 months for the language impaired group (versus 9.7 months for the speech impaired group). The mean age for unaided walking was 16.2 months in the language impaired group (versus 13.4 months in the speech impaired group).

Performance I.Q.'s were significantly higher in the speech impaired group than in the language impaired group, although mean I.Q.'s were in the normal range for both groups. The mean performance I.Q. (based on WISC or WPPSI) was 94 for the language delayed group and 116 for the speech impaired group.

Although developmental milestones and performance intelligence scores were significantly lower in the language delayed group than in the speech delayed group, these data could not be explained by medical or neurological factors. The birth weights of the two groups of children were not significantly different. The frequency of past or current medical disorders (including known brain damage, seizures, hearing impairment, or tonsillectomies) was essentially the same for the two groups of children, with 40 percent of the speech disordered group having had or having some medical complications and 47 percent of the language disordered group being so affected. Performance of the two groups of children in a neurological examination (including skipping, hopping, and finger tapping) was essentially the same.

Frequency and Types of Behavior Problems Occurring in Speech and Language Disordered Children

Parents' and teachers' questionnaires revealed a variety of behavioral problems among the children studied. The most frequent complaint of parents of the speech impaired children was that their children's feelings were too easily hurt. This problem was reported in 30 percent of the children. The second most commonly occurring problem was being too easily frustrated. This was reported by parents of 21 percent of the children. Other frequently reported symptoms were: thumb-sucking, shyness, being a picky eater, being frightened of new situations (all occurring in 15 percent of the speech impaired children).

Having feelings that were too easily hurt and being frustrated too easily were also the most common problems of the language impaired children. However, the parents of these children cited these problems much more frequently, claiming that 40 percent of the language delayed children had feelings easily hurt and that 38 percent were easily frustrated. Other complaints were also much more common among parents of the speech and language disordered children. Thirty-six percent of the children were classified as being too excitable, 30 percent of the children were said to have a short attention span and 28 percent were considered worriers and immature for their age. Twenty-seven percent of the children wet their pants or beds, 22 percent were reported unhappy and 21 percent were solitary.

School teachers made fewer complaints about the speech disordered children than parents did, although the teachers' complaints about the language impaired children occurred at the same frequency as the parental complaints about these children. The most frequent complaints made by teachers about the speech disordered children were of submissiveness, restlessness, short attention span, solitary behavior and poor coordination. These symptoms occurred in from 12 percent to 14 percent of the speech disordered children.

The most frequently cited behavior of the language disordered children cited by the teachers was short attention span, occurring in 52 percent of the language disturbed children. Lack of leadership quality occurred in 36 percent of these children. Fidgeting and solitary behavior were, according to the school teachers, problems for 30 percent of the language impaired children. Restlessness was a problem for 28 percent of the children, and stubbornness was a problem for 26 percent. Excitability and excessive demands for attention were also common problems in the language impaired children, affecting 23 percent of the group according to teachers' reports.

A number of problems occurred significantly more frequently in the speech and language impaired group of children than in the purely speech impaired group of children. Parents and teachers both found short attention spans and excitability were more common in the language impaired group of children. According to parental ratings, wetting, soiling, unhappiness, clinging, worries, immaturity, squirminess and constant climbing were also more common in the children whose language was affected. According to the school teachers' reports, fidgeting, quick mood changes, solitary behavior, lack of leadership, resentfulness, defiance, excessive demands for attention and stubbornness were significantly more common in the language impaired children than in the speech impaired children.

Factor analysis of the parents' and teachers' reports using the Rutter and Conners factors revealed a significantly greater hyperactivity factor (according to both the parents' and teachers' questionnaires) in the language disordered group than in the speech disordered group. In addition, significantly greater conduct disorder and passivity disorder factors were found in the language disordered group. In addition, significantly greater conduct disorder and passivity disorder factors were found in the language disordered children according to the teachers' reports.

Prevalence and Types of Psychiatric Illness Found in Speech and Language Disordered Children

Psychiatric diagnoses of the children were made by child psychiatrists, using the operational diagnostic criteria of DSM-III. Over half (53 percent) of the children studied had some psychiatric disorder, according to DSM-III criteria. The most frequently occurring disorder was attention deficit disorder which affected 16 percent of the children studied. Oppositional disorder and avoidant disorder were the next most common disorders, with both of these disorders occurring in six percent of the children studied. A variety of other psychiatric disorders were found, with each occurring in less than five percent of the total sample. The diagnoses found and their frequencies of occurrence are listed in Table 1.

The prevalence rates for psychiatric illness were not the same in the purely speech disordered children as in the language disordered children. Psychiatric illness was significantly more common in the language impaired children than in the purely speech impaired children. Sixty-three percent of the language impaired children were found to have a psychiatric disorder, whereas only 25 percent of the speech impaired children were found to have psychiatric illness. Attention deficit disorder was the more frequently occurring diagnosis in both groups, but the frequency of occurrence for other psychiatric diagnoses differed somewhat between the two groups. Oppositional disorder was notably more common in the language disordered children than in the speech disordered children.

DISCUSSION

The data presented indicate that children with either speech or language difficulties tend to have a high rate of emotional and behavioral problems. Thirty-three percent of the children studied were described

TABLE 1

PREVALENCE AND TYPES OF PSYCHIATRIC DISORDER IN CHILDREN
WITH SPEECH AND LANGUAGE DISORDERS

	Whole Sample N = 180		Pure Speech Disorders Group N = 76		Language Disordered Group N = 104	
	N	%	N	%	N	%
Any psychiatric disorder	95	53%	19	25%	66	63%
Attention deficit disorder	28	16%	3	4%	25	24%
Oppositional disorder	11	6%	1	1%	10	10%
Avoidant disorder	11	6%	3	4%	8	8%
Unspecified illness	8	4%	3	4%	5	5%
Adjustment disorders	6	3%	2	3%	4	4%
Conduct disorder	5	3%	1	1%	4	4%
Separation anxiety disorder	4	2%	1	1%	3	3%
Overanxious disorder	3	2%	1	1%	2	2%
Chronic hypomanic disorder	3	2%	1	1%	2	2%
Infantile autism	2	1%	0	0	2	2%
Parent-child problem	2	1%	1	1%	1	1%
Other interpersonal problem	1	1%	1	1%	0	0
Schizoid disorder	1	1%	1	1%	0	0

(Percentages have been rounded off to whole numbers. Hence, totals do not equal 100.)

by their parents as having their feelings too easily hurt, 28 percent were described as having low tolerance for frustration, 19 percent were considered to have an abnormally short attention span, and 16 percent were having problems with wetting their pants. Although there is no control group of non-speech or language disordered available for direct comparison with the children studied, it appears from epidemiological studies of behavior problems in children that these figures are considerably higher than would occur in the general population of children.[5,12,15]

The behavioral, emotional and developmental problems found in this group of children cannot be explained entirely by adverse social or family factors. Indeed, the children in the study were generally early borns from small-sized families cf middle class backgrounds. Neurological examination results were normal for the vast majority of the children, and both developmental milestones and non-verbal intelligence scores were within the normal range for the children studied.

Richman and Stevenson[7] predicted that children attending speech programs would be different from the language delayed children that they identified in the general population in that specific language delays would be more prevalent and adverse environmental and social factors less common. It is true that the speech clinic sample of children in the present study had fewer adverse social and environmental factors than the children from the general sample studied by Richman and Stevenson. However, it is significant to note that behavioral problems are almost as prevalent in the present sample as in the sample studied by Richman and Stevenson.

Clearly, speech or language disordered children are "at risk" for emotional and social problems, and this fact must be taken into account in planning treatment and education for such children. Speech and language clinicians in particular need to be made aware that a significant number of the children seen in their practices are likely to have a significant behavioral-emotional problem that may require intervention beyond the competence of the speech and language therapist.

The comparisons made of children with speech problems versus children with language problems indicate that it is the children with *language* disorders that are most seriously at risk for behavioral, social, and developmental problems. Although still within normal limits, the developmental milestone ages and non-verbal intelligence scores are significantly lower in the language impaired children than in the speech impaired children. Most of the behavioral problems found occur with twice the frequency in the language disordered children as in the speech disordered children. Diagnosable psychiatric illness is more than twice as prevalent in the language disordered group as in the purely speech disordered group.

These facts suggest that psychiatric screening and intervention programs for communication disordered children should concentrate on those children who show deficits in language rather than on those children who have deficits in speech only. There is a high likelihood that such children will suffer from psychiatric disorders (in particular attention deficit disorder or oppositional disorder) and other (non-language) developmental disorders. Since there do not appear to be any demographic variables by which these high risk children can be identified, early language screening programs may be the most effective way of identifying these children.

REFERENCES

1. Cantwell, D. P..and Baker, L. (1977). Psychiatric disorder in children with speech and language retardation. A critical review. *Archives of General Psychiatry,* 34:583–591.
2. Weber, J. L. (1965). The speech and language abilities of emotionally disturbed children. *Canadian Psychiatric Association Journal,* 10:417–420.
3. Chess, S. and Rosenberg, M. (1974). Clinical differentiation among children with initial language complaints. *Journal of Autism and Childhood Schizophrenia,* 4:99–109.
4. Friedlander, B. Z., Wetstone, M. S., and McPeek D. L. (1974). Systematic assessment of selective language listening deficit in emotionally disturbed children. *Journal of Child Psychology and Psychiatry,* 15:1–12.
5. Richman, N. (1977). Behaviour problems in pre-school children: Family and social factors. *British Journal of Psychiatry,* 131:532–527.
6. Richman, N., Stevenson, J. and Grapham, P. (1975). Prevalence of behaviour problems in 3-year-old children: An epidemiological study in a London Borough. *Journal of Child Psychology and Psychiatry,* 16:277–288.
7. Richman, N. and Stevenson, J. (1977). Language delay in 3-year-old children: Family and social factors. *Acta Paediatr. Belg.,* 30:213–219.
8. Stevenson, J. E. and Richman N. (1976). The prevalence of language delay in a population of three-year-old children and its association with general retardation. *Developmental Medicine and Child Neurology,* 18:431–441.
9. Stevenson, J. and Richman N. (1978). Behavior, language, and development in three-year-old children. *Journal of Autism and Childhood Schizophrenia,* 8:299–313.
10. Mattison, R., Cantwell, D. P. and Baker, L. (1980). Behavior problems in children with speech and language retardation. *Child Psychiatry and Human Development,* 10:246–257.
11. American Psychiatric Association, Task Force on Nomenclature and Statistics. (1980). *Diagnostic and Statistical Manual of Mental Disorders,* 3rd edition. Washington, D.C.: APA.
12. Cantwell, D. P., Baker, L. and Mattison, R. E. (1979). The prevalence of psychiatric disorders in children with speech and language disorder: An epidemiologic study. *Journal of the American Academy of Child Psychiatry,* 18:450–461.
13. Cantwell, D. P., Baker, L. and Mattison, R. E. (1980). Factors associated with the development of psychiatric disorder in speech and language retardation. *Archives of General Psychiatry,* 37:423–426.
14. Baker, L., Cantwell, D. P. and Mattison, R. (1980). Behavior problems in children with pure speech disorders and in children with combined speech and language disorders. *Journal of Abnormal Psychology,* 8:245–256.
15. Rutter, M., Graham, P. and Yule, W. (1970). *A Neuropsychiatric Study in Children.* Clinics in Developmental Medicine, No. 35/36. London: Heinemann.
16. Conners, D. K. (1973). Rating scales for use in drug studies with children. *Psychopharmacological Bulletin* (Special Issue), 24–59.

14

Infants' Persistence at Tasks: Relationships to Cognitive Functioning and Early Experience

Leon J. Yarrow

National Institute of Child Health and Human Development
National Institutes of Health
Bethesda, Maryland

George A. Morgan

Colorado State University

Kay D. Jennings

University of Pittsburgh

Robert J. Harmon

University of Colorado School of Medicine

Juarlyn L. Gaiter

Children's Hospital National Medical Center

A technique for measuring one aspect of infants' motivation to master the environment—persistence at tasks—is described. Forty-four 13-

Reprinted with permission from *Infant Behavior and Development*, 1982, Vol. 5, 131–141.
The Developmental Psychobiology Research Group Endowment Fund, Department of Psychiatry at the University of Colorado School of Medicine, provided assistance in the preparation of the manuscript. The data were collected while the authors were at the National Institute of Child Health and Human Development. We wish to acknowledge the assistance of Joan Suwalsky, Myrna Fivel and Claire Bennett Freeland. Robert Klein, Peter Vietze, Frank Pedersen, Rex Culp and several reviewers made helpful comments on earlier drafts.
Robert Harmon is currently supported by Research Scientist Development Award #1 K01-MH34005-02.

month-old infants engaged in persistent, task-directed behaviors about 60% of the time during 11 mastery tasks. As a measure of concurrent validity, persistence during a Bayley examination was rated by another examiner; a moderately high correlation (r = .48) was found. Significant relationships were also found between persistence at the mastery tasks and Bayley MDI, suggesting considerable intertwining of cognition and motivation in infancy. In a subsample of 25 infants tested at 6 months, significant relationships were found between goal-directedness, an index of directed persistent behavior, and both cognitive functioning and infant competence on the mastery tasks at 13 months. Several aspects of the 6-month environments of these 25 infants, especially maternal kinesthetic and auditory stimulation, maternal responsiveness, and responsiveness of toys were related to persistence and competence at 13 months.

Conceptions of the young infant have changed dramatically in recent years. We now know that the infant is neither passive nor a completely helpless organism; the infant is an active, striving being who attempts to master the environment and to produce effects. We are beginning to acquire some understanding of the young child's influence on caregivers, but we have little knowledge, even on a descriptive level, about how the infant begins to master the inanimate environment. This paper describes a technique for assessing one aspect of mastery motivation—persistence at tasks.

Many theoretical threads have been woven into our thinking about mastery: Piaget's (1952) theory of cognitive development, Hunt's (1965) theoretical thinking about intrinsic motivation, and especially Robert White's (1959) conceptualization of effectance motivation. Integrating psychoanalytic theory, Eriksonian hypotheses and Piaget's insights, White (1959) articulated a theory of effectance motivation or motivation for competence. Rejecting traditional drive reduction theories, White proposed that motivation to be competent is intrinsic and independent of gratification of physiological drives. Morever, he maintained that activities in the service of competence are adaptive; they help the child acquire knowledge and skills. Hunt (1965) emphasized that competent behaviors are self-reinforcing and lead to an intrinsic motivation to act effectively.

Most research generated by this theorizing has focused either on effectance motivation in school-age children (Harter, 1978) or, in infants, on the development of competent functioning as distinguished from the motivation to become competent (W. Bronson, 1974; Wenar, 1976; B.

White, 1975). In a recent review of the literature, Ulvund (1980) concluded that cognition and motivation cannot be clearly distinguished in infancy, and that there is a continuous interaction between them.

Despite recognition of the importance of mastery motivation, there are currently no instruments, similar to those for measuring cognitive development, to assess individual differences in infants' attempts to control or master the environment. As part of this research, we have developed a set of tasks to assess mastery motivation in 1-year-old infants. In this paper, we shall focus on one aspect of mastery motivation—the infant's persistence in attempts to master the inanimate environment.

There are several basic questions with which we are concerned:

1. To what extent do 1-year-olds persist at tasks, and how is such persistence related to success at the tasks?
2. Is there cross-situational consistency in persistence? Is persistence at mastery tasks related to persistence in other settings?
3. Are the measures of persistence related to contemporaneous cognitive development?
4. Are there precursors at 6 months of persistence and competence at 1 year?
5. What aspects of early experience influence the child's persistence and cognitive functioning at one year?

METHOD

Sample

The sample consisted of 44 infants, 13 months of age: 23 boys and 21 girls; 21 were firstborns and 23 had older siblings. All were from upper-middle socioeconomic backgrounds. On the Duncan Occupational Scale, 42 of the 44 fathers were in professional or managerial occupations; 80% of the fathers and 70% of the mothers were college graduates. The mean age of the mothers and fathers was 29 and 32, respectively. All infants were normal at birth, and there were no unusual medical problems during pregnancy, delivery, or during the first 12 months of life.

Procedures

The data were obtained during two sessions. In the first session, the mastery motivation tasks were presented in a laboratory testing room.

Approximately one week later, the Bayley Scales of Infant Development were administered in the infants' homes. Each session was conducted independently, i.e., neither the tester nor the observer had knowledge of the child's performance on the other session.

As part of another study, 25 of these infants, 12 boys and 13 girls had been tested with the Bayley Scales of Infant Development when they were 6 months old. The home environment of these infants was also assessed at 6 months.

Mastery Session

We drew on several sources in the development of the "tasks" (the test items) and the "measures" (the dimensions of behavior coded). The general procedure and our thinking about specific tasks was influenced by a study concerned with developing techniques to assess the effects of intervention programs (Gordon, Moreno, Rand, Beller, Lally, Freiberg, & Yarrow, 1974). Three mastery tasks were adapted from techniques used to study detour behavior in infancy (Gaiter, 1973). The major considerations governing choice of tasks were that they be interesting to 1 year olds and that they provide an opportunity to observe individual variability in task-directed behaviors.

The 11 tasks used in this study were of three types. Five tasks gave the infant opportunities to secure feedback or produce auditory effects by using a manipulandum, such as a button, lever, or dial. A second type of task offered infants the opportunity to combine objects in appropriate ways, such as placing blocks in a bottle and pegs in holes. These tasks involved practicing skills which are just developing at 1 year of age. Four tasks required the infant to circumvent a barrier or obstacle in order to obtain a goal object. The tasks chosen were considered age-appropriate, but were sufficiently difficult to require some persistence in order to solve them.

The infants were tested by a female examiner in a large (4 × 5 meters), comfortably furnished laboratory playroom. On the first six tasks, infants sat on their mothers' laps at a table across from the examiner. The remaining tasks were administered to the baby on the floor. Mothers were asked not to talk during presentation of the tasks. The items were presented in a standardized manner with limited interaction between the infant and the female experimenter. A general instruction such as "make it work" or "get the toy" was given as each object was presented. After the infant had the opportunity to attempt the task, the items which involved producing effects and combining objects were demonstrated by the tester. After pretesting, it was decided that some variation in the length and timing of the task was desirable. The first task was presented for three minutes to allow for warm-up. Eight tasks had two one-minute trials and the other two had one two-minute trial.

Initially we had a number of measures of mastery: Latency to Task Involvement, Persistence, Exploration of the Materials, Variety of Approaches, Frequency of Solution, Variety of Effects Produced, Latency to First Solution, Affect, and Competence. All but three of the measures were eliminated because of limited variance or because they were highly intercorrelated with other measures; on a few, it was not possible to obtain adequate interobserver reliability. The analyses reported are based on the following measures: (a) Persistence at Tasks, (b) Competence, and (c) Affect. The first measure, Persistence, was the percentage of time during each task in which the child was engaged in task-directed behaviors. These behaviors included all attempts, even if not fully successful, to produce the effect, combine the objects, or secure the goal object. Looking at, touching, generalized exploration, or mouthing the toy were not scored as task directed. An overall Persistence score on the 11 tasks was obtained by standardizing the scores and then averaging them for each task.

Second, to measure Competence or skill on the tasks, we counted the number of trials on which the infant correctly produced the effect, combined the objects, or secured the goal object.

Third, an overall Affect score was obtained, based on the observer's rating on a 1 to 5 scale of the child's affective behavior during each task, e.g., crying, fussing, smiling, laughing. Most infants were rated at the midpoint on most tasks; scores of 1, predominantly unhappy, were very rare, partly because the session was interrupted and the infants were given a break between trials if they became too restless.

Interobserver reliability was obtained by having two independent observers code the behavior of 10 infants on the mastery tasks. The reliability coefficient for the overall Persistence score was .99. Overall reliability for Affect was .98. There was perfect agreement between observers on number of trials with solution. (See Morgan, Harmon, Gaiter, Jennings, Gist, & Yarrow, 1977, for a more complete description of the tasks, procedure, and scoring.)

Developmental Testing Session

About a week after the infants were given the mastery tasks, the Bayley Scales of Infant Development were administered in the infants' homes.

In addition to the Mental Development Index (MDI) and the Psycho-motor Development Index (PDI), four measures of more differentiated aspects of infant functioning were derived. All mental development items between 11 and 19 months were grouped conceptually according to the predominant skills they measured, using a procedure similar to one employed by Yarrow, Rubenstein, and Pedersen (1975). Three of these clusters—Spatial Relations, Perceptual Discrimination, and Problem Solving—were similar in content to the mastery tasks.

The Spatial Relations clusters consisted of four items requiring rep-etition of an activity involving newly emerging relational skills, such as placing cubes in a cup, beads in a box, or pegs in a board (Bayley Items 100, 107, 114, 118). The Perceptual Discrimination cluster consisted of five items involving simple form discrimination, such as placing round and square blocks in appropriate holes (Bayley Items 110, 120, 121, 129, 108). The Problem Solving cluster contained only two items: item 109 which required the infant to remove a barrier to obtain a goal object and item 122 which involved means-ends behavior. The Language clus-ter included four receptive items, such as shows shoe, and four expressive items, such as names objects (Bayley Items 101, 106, 113, 117, 124, 126, 127, 128).

Measures at Six Months

As part of another study, 25 infants from the present sample had been tested with the Bayley Scales of Infant Development when they were 6 months old. Several clusters were derived from the 6-month Bayley items using the categories developed by Yarrow, Rubenstein, and Pedersen (1975). The cluster most similar to the 13-month persistence measure was labeled Goal Directedness. This cluster consisted of five items from the Bayley Mental Scales (Items 60, 71, 80, 82, 96) which measured the infant's persistent, directed attempts to obtain objects under a variety of conditions.

At 6 months, the home environments of these infants were observed twice, using a time-sampling procedure. Two measures of the inanimate environment were derived by recording all the toys and other objects which were within reach of the infant during the observations. Respon-siveness of toys was an index of the feedback potential of the objects. Variety was the number of different objects that were within reach of the infant. Nine measures of the social environment were also obtained: the frequency of kinesthetic, tactile, auditory, and visual stimulation; social mediation of interactions with smiles and vocalizations; the mother's contingent responsiveness to the infant's positive vocalizations and to the infant's distress; and the overall level and variety of social stimulation. A detailed description of the procedure and measures is provided in Yarrow, Rubenstein, and Pedersen (1975).

RESULTS AND DISCUSSION

All analyses are reported for the total group, since there were few significant sex differences in mean scores or in relationships among the variables.

Infant's Behavior During the Mastery Session

Considerable persistence was shown on all the mastery tasks; there was, however, a great deal of individual variability. On the average, 60% of each trial was spent working on the task.

The tasks were moderately difficult; the infants were successful in 63% of the trials. The effect production tasks were intended to be easily solvable, and on the average, 86% of the infants produced the effect at least once on each trial. More than two thirds (69%) of the infants were able to combine objects appropriately, and most of them tried to do so. Although we anticipated that the detour problems would be quite difficult, they were easier than they appeared to be during pilot testing. The infants were able to circumvent the barrier to obtain the goal object on 51% of the trials.

We assumed that the infants' affect while working on or after completing challenging tasks might be a meaningful index of their feelings about mastery. Although some investigators (e.g., Bronson, 1974; Watson, 1966) have reported that infants smile when they become aware that their behavior has produced an effect, expressions of positive or negative affect during or after completion of the mastery tasks were not common. On 8 of the 11 tasks, the predominant expression was neutral. On only 1 of the 11 tasks, an effect production task, did more than 25% of the infants express positive affect. On the two other tasks, both barrier problems, more than 25% of the infants expressed some mild negative affect. These two tasks proved frustrating for infants who were unable to circumvent the detour and obtain the goal object. Perhaps more meaningful data on affect would have been obtained if we had recorded instances of positive affect immediately following solution of a task.

The interrelations of the three measures from the mastery motivation session were examined. Consistent with assumptions about the interdependence of motivation and cognition, Persistence was significantly related to the measure of Competence, Number of Trials with Solution, ($r = .69$, $p < .01$). To some extent, Persistence and Competence were necessarily related, however it was possible, and not uncommon, for an infant to put forth much effort, but not succeed. It was less common for an infant to do well with little effort or persistence. Affect was less highly related to Persistence ($r = .39$, $p < .05$), and it was not related to Competence. Thus, functioning during the session was not dependent on or highly related to the infant's general affect.

Concurrent Validity of Measures of Persistence Across Sessions

To examine the concurrent validity of the mastery motivation measure, the relation between persistence on the mastery tasks and a similar measure obtained during the Bayley testing was analyzed. Persistence in the mastery session and an independent rating of the infant's persistence on the Bayley Scales were significantly related ($r = .48$, $p < .01$), indicating some consistency on these measures.

Relations Between Persistence and Cognitive Development

We have previously reported significant relationships between qualitative aspects of infants' exploratory play used as an index of mastery motivation and cognitive functioning (Jennings, Harmon, Morgan, Gaiter, & Yarrow, 1979). Further confirmation of the interrelatedness between cognition and motivation is provided by data on the relations between the Bayley MDI and Persistence on the mastery tasks.

Persistence on the mastery tasks was significantly related to the Bayley MDI and to each of the clusters derived from the Bayley Scale (Table 1). This finding is similar to one mentioned earlier, i.e., persistence and competence within the mastery session were significantly related. These findings cannot be explained solely in terms of a general responsiveness to tests or to the experimenter, because the correlation of Persistence with the Bayley PDI was negligible.

Especially interesting are the relationships between Persistence and Competence on the mastery tasks and the Bayley clusters. Both Competence and Persistence on the mastery tasks are significantly related to three Bayley clusters: Spatial Relations, Perceptual Discrimination, and Problem Solving (Table 1). In each of these instances, the correlation with Competence on the mastery tasks is somewhat higher than the correlation with Persistence. Inasmuch as the Bayley Mental Develop-

TABLE 1
Correlations of Mastery Session Measures
with Scores from the Bayley Session at 13 Months of Age
(N = 44)

Bayley Session Measures	Mastery Session	
	Persistence	Competence
Rating of Persistence	.48**	.45**
Mental Development Index (MDI)	.60**	.72**
Spatial Relations Skills Cluster	.37*	.58**
Perceptual Discrimination Cluster	.53**	.74**
Problem Solving Cluster	.35*	.45**
Language Cluster	.42**	.16
Psychomotor Development Index (PDI)	.17	.31*

*p < .05
**p < .01

ment Index is primarily a measure of cognitive competence, these findings give some external support to our measure of Competence on the mastery tasks. A provocative finding, which is more difficult to understand, is that the Bayley Language cluster is significantly related to Persistence but is not related to the competence scores on the mastery items. This relationship suggests a link between the motivation to master the inanimate environment and early indices of language functioning, but little or no link between early language and the ability to master these problems. The language cluster at this age is primarily an index of comprehension of language. Infants who are more advanced in receptive language may be more capable in understanding the instructions to work at the task, but they may not have the fine motor or cognitive skills to complete it successfully.

Behavioral Precursors of Persistence and Competence

Since we had 25 infants in this study who had been given the Bayley at 6 months of age as part of another investigation, we were able to look at the behavioral precursors of mastery and cognitive development at 13 months. Consistent with previous findings, there were no predictive relationships between the Bayley MDI at 6 and 13 months. Nor were there any predictors of the measure of mastery motivation at 13 months, although one correlation approached significance—that between the cognitive-motivational cluster, Goal Directedness, at 6 months and the overall measure of Persistence on the mastery tasks at 13 months ($r =$

.36, $p < .08$). Goal Directedness was a measure of the infant's persistent, directed attempts to secure objects under a variety of conditions (Yarrow, Rubenstein, & Pedersen, 1975). We found several predictive relationships between Goal Directedness at 6 months and cognitive measures at 13 months. Goal Directedness was significantly related to the 13-month Bayley Problem Solving cluster ($r = .42$, $p < .05$), and to a measure of competence on the mastery tasks—the number of detour problems solved ($r = .45$, $p < .05$). These findings of a relationship between early cognitive-motivational functioning and relevant aspects of later competence suggest that early attempts to master the environment may be one antecedent of the development of competence.

Environmental Antecedents of Persistence and Competence

These 25 infants were also observed twice at home with their mothers when they were 6 months old. A significant relationship was found between the responsiveness of the infant's playthings and persistence on the mastery tasks at 13 months ($r = .40$, $p < .05$). Consistent with what one might expect, a somewhat higher correlation ($r = .54$, $p < .01$) was found between responsiveness of toys at 6 months and persistence on the effect producing mastery tasks at 13 months. Thus, those children who had responsive objects available to play with during infancy were more likely to be engaged in producing effects in the mastery situation seven months later. The Variety of Toys at 6 months was not related to persistence on the mastery tasks. Neither aspect of the 6-month inanimate environment (responsiveness or variety) was significantly related to cognitive functioning or competence on the mastery tasks of 13 months (see Table 2).

Significant relationships were found between persistence at 1 year and three aspects of maternal care when the infant was 6 months (Table 2): the amount of maternal kinesthetic stimulation, auditory stimulation, and social mediation of play. These correlations suggest a link between a stimulating, responsive early environment and later persistence at tasks.

The relationships between these 6-month maternal variables and 1-year Competence on the mastery tasks and the Bayley MDI suggest a similar linkage. Kinesthetic and Auditory Stimulation were significantly related to both measures of Competence, while maternal Contingent Responsiveness and Variety of Social Stimulation were significantly related to one measure of Competence.

The Bayley Psychomotor Index had a generally lower average correlation ($r = .23$) and a somewhat different pattern of relationships with the maternal social environment. Proximal stimulation (tactile and kin-

TABLE 2
Relationships Between 6-Month Environment
and 13-Month Infant Functioning
(N = 25)

6-Month Measures	13-Month Measures			
	Persistence at Mastery Tasks	Competence at Mastery Tasks	Bayley MDI	Bayley PDI
Inanimate Environment				
Responsiveness of Toys	.40*	.26	.13	.13
Variety of Toys	.13	.09	.27	.11
Maternal Environment				
Kinesthetic Simulation	.49*	.48*	.52*	.46*
Tactile Stimulation	.22	.18	.11	.43*
Auditory Stimulation	.46*	.43*	.44*	.13
Visual Stimulation	.02	.06	.09	−.19
Contingent Responsiveness to Distress	.28	.45*	.34	.16
Contingent Responsiveness to Positive Vocalization	.37	.36	.40*	.43*
Social Mediation of Play	.40*	.23	.36	.15
Level of Social Stimulation	.35	.31	.36	.24
Variety of Social Stimulation	.38	.30	.42*	.27

*$p < .05$

esthetic), as would be predicted, seems to be much more important than distal stimulation for motor development.

The relatively strong relationships between kinesthetic stimulation in early infancy in both cognitive and motivational functioning at one year are striking. Other studies have found relationships between kinesthetic stimulation and early cognitive development (Yarrow et al., 1975), as well as with visual alertness in young infants (Gregg, Haffner, & Korner, 1976; Korner & Thoman, 1970). One can only speculate about why this type of stimulation is so influential during the first 6 months. Korner and Thoman (1970) have suggested that since the kinesthetic-vestibular system is one of the earliest to be myelinated, it may be an especially sensitive mediator of early stimulation. We have conjectured that kinesthetic stimulation may be especially important because it is often used to restore the infant to an optimal state. When the infant is crying, it may soothe; when the infant is quiescent, it may be used to arouse him/her.

In regard to some of the other environmental variables related to our measures of mastery motivation, several studies have found variables similar to ours to be related to later development. Responsiveness of the mother was related to later infant competence (Ainsworth, Blehar, Waters, & Wall, 1978; Morgan, Busch, Culp, Vance, & Fritz, in press; Yarrow et al., 1975). Sensitive responsiveness to the infant has also been related to secure attachment (Ainsworth et al., 1978) which in turn seems to be related to attention span and persistence at tasks (Main, 1973; Matas, Arend, & Sroufe, 1978). Variety of social stimulation was related to several cognitive and cognitive-motivational functions in infants (Gaiter, Morgan, Jennings, Harmon, & Yarrow, in press; Morgan et al., in press; Yarrow et al., 1975). As in the present study, Yarrow, Klein, Lomonaco, and Morgan (1975) found that cognitive-motivational variables may be better predictors during infancy of later cognitive functioning than pure cognitive measures.

Although the theoretical writings of Piaget (1952), White (1959), and Hunt (1965) emphasize that motivation for competence plays a central role in cognitive development, there has been little empirical verification. Cognitive development has been studied extensively during infancy, but motivation has remained largely in the realm of theory. The paucity of research on infant motivation has been due in part to the lack of measures. The study represents a first step in correcting that deficiency.

We have developed tasks and measures to assess one aspect of early mastery motivation—persistence. Our findings suggest that early cognitive development and mastery motivation are closely, almost inextricably, linked. There seems to be a reciprocal relationship between persistence and competence in infancy. Infants who work assiduously at perfecting their skills may become more competent; in turn, competent infants derive greater satisfaction from working on skills, and thus are more likely to practice them. It does not seem to be simply a circular process, but a sequential and hierarchial one in which mastery motivation facilitates consolidation of skills and leads to the emergence of new ones.

REFERENCES

Ainsworth, M. D. S., Blehar, M. C., Waters, E. and Wall, S. (1978). *Patterns of Attachment: A Psychological Study of the Strange Situation*. New York: Erlbaum.

Bronson, W. C. (1974). Competence and the growth of personality. In *The Growth of Competence*, K. J. Connolly and J. S. Bruner, eds. New York: Academic Press.

Gaiter, J. L. (1973). *Differential Training and Transfer of Detour Behavior in 10-Month-Old Infants*. Unpublished doctoral dissertation, Brown University.

Gaiter, J. L., Morgan, G. A., Jennings, K. D., Harmon, R. J. and Yarrow, L. J. (In press). Variety of cognitively-oriented caregiver activities: Relationships to cognitive and motivational functioning at 1 and 3½ years of age. *Journal of Genetic Psychology*.

Gordon, I. J., Moreno, P., Rand, C., Beller, E. K., Lally, J. R., Freiberg, K. and Yarrow,

L. (1974). Studies in socio-emotional development in infancy. *JSAS Catalog of Selected Documents in Psychology*, 4:120. (Ms. No. 762).

Gregg, C. L., Haffner, M. E. and Korner, A. F. (1976). The relative efficacy of vestibular-proprioceptive stimulation and the upright position in enhancing visual pursuit in neonates. *Child Development*, 47:309–314.

Harter, S. (1978). Effectance motivation reconsidered: Toward a developmental model. *Human Development*, 21:34–64.

Hunt, J. McV. (1965). Intrinsic motivation and its role in psychological development. In *Nebraska Symposium on Motivation* (Vol. 13), D. Levine, ed. Lincoln, NE: University of Nebraska Press.

Korner, A. F. and Thoman, E. B. (1970). Visual alertness in neonates as evoked by maternal care. *Journal of Experimental Child Psychology*, 10:67–78.

Jennings, K. J., Harmon, R. J., Morgan, G. A., Gaiter, J. L. and Yarrow, L. J. (1979). Exploratory play as an index of mastery motivation: Relationships to persistence, cognitive functioning, and environmental measures. *Developmental Psychology*, 15:386–394.

Main, M. (1973). *Exploration, Play and Level of Cognitive Functioning as Related to Mother-Child Attachment*. Unpublished doctoral dissertation, Johns Hopkins University.

Matas, L., Arend, R. A. and Sroufe, A. L. (1978). Continuity of adaptation in the second year: The relationship between quality of attachment and later competence. *Child Development*, 49:547–556.

Morgan, G. A., Busch, N. A., Culp, R. E., Vance, A. K. and Fritz, J. J. (1982). Infants differential response to mother and experimenter: Relationships to maternal characteristics and infant functioning. In *Attachment and Affiliative Systems: Neurobiological and Psychobiological Aspects*, R. Emde and R. J. Harmon, eds. New York: Plenum Press, 245–262.

Morgan, G. A., Harmon, R. J., Gaiter, J. L., Jennings, K. D., Gist, N. F. and Yarrow, L. J. (1977). A method for assessing mastery motivation in 1-year-old infants. *JSAS Catalog of Selected Documents in Psychology*, 7:68. (Ms. No. 1517).

Piaget, J. (1952). *The Origins of Intelligence in Children*. New York: International Universities Press.

Ulvund, S. E. (1980). Cognition and motivation in early infancy: An interactionistic approach. *Human Development*, 23:17–32.

Watson, J. S. (1966). The development and generalization of "contingency awareness" in early infancy: Some hypotheses. *Merrill-Palmer Quarterly*, 12:123–135.

Wenar, C. (1976). Executive competence in toddlers: A prospective, observational study. *Genetic Psychology Monographs*, 93:189–285.

White, B. L. (1975). Critical influences in the origins of competence. *Merrill-Palmer Quarterly*, 21:243–266.

White, R. W. (1959). Motivation reconsidered: The concept of competence. *Psychological Review*, 66:297–333.

Yarrow, L. J., Klein, R P., Lomonaco, S. and Morgan, G. A. (1975). Cognitive and motivational development in early childhood. In *Exceptional Infant 3: Assessment and Intervention*, B. Z. Friedlander, G. M. Sterritt and G. E. Kirk, eds. New York: Brunner/Mazel 491–502.

Yarrow, L. J., Rubenstein, J. L. and Pedersen, F. A. (1975). *Infant and Environment: Early Cognitive and Motivational Development*. New York: Halsted Division, Wiley.

Yarrow, L. J. and Pedersen, F. A. (1976). The interplay between cognition and motivation in infancy. In *Origins of Intelligence*, M. Lewis, ed. New York: Plenum, 379–399.

PART III: LANGUAGE, COGNITION, AND LEARNING

15

Psychology and Education

Ann M. Clarke

Department of Educational Studies, University of Hull, England

The invitation to write a contribution on psychology for the anniversary number of this *Journal* is both an honor and a considerable responsibility. Inevitably an author must be selective of topics in order not to seem tedious, or to exceed the allocated space, while at the same time attempting to give an account of the subject which should be both acceptable to psychologists yet comprehensible to colleagues in other branches of education.

Psychology in the English-speaking world is firmly rooted in a tradition of empirical science with a positivist orientation. Perhaps its most important contribution to educational theory has been through the use of certain agreed procedures, many of which we share with clinical medicine. It is no accident that some of the more important contributions to the methodology of human science are to be found in the two *Handbooks of Research on Teaching* and are reflected in the style of many articles published in journals which incorporate educational psychology in their title. This is not to imply a necessary superiority of this approach to all problems, but to suggest that it is an essential way of specifying relevant questions and designing research which should yield both some coherent answers and also indicate further questions to be tackled.

The selection of topics for discussion here reflects both the author's commitment to this orientation in psychology, and also something of the range of educational problems which have been researched within a developing conceptual context. Education is an area in which appro-

Reprinted with permission from the *British Journal of Educational Studies*, 1982, Vol. XXX, No. 1, 43–56.

priately a number of different philosophical positions may be adopted; it is also one in which may be found dogmatic advocates of child rearing and teaching methods which range from the cranky to the antediluvian. Obviously it is important that both values and methods should be freely debated. However, if opinions are not subject to critical scrutiny and proper evaluation, then not only may one opinion appear as good as any other, but we risk falling prey either to anarchy or to mindless fashion. It is important that a wide range of approaches to educational practice should be attempted, but it is equally necessary that the sophisticated methods of evaluation research should be routinely used.

THE BACKGROUND

Thirty years ago educational psychology in this country was dominated by Sir Cyril Burt, although he was in the process of retiring from the Chair of Psychology at University College, London, held since 1931 when he moved from what is at present known as the London Institute of Education. Godfrey Thomson in Scotland also enjoyed high prestige, and their combined influence significantly affected both research and practice in this area. Human ability was to be explored by means of factor analytic studies, and applied psychologists were encouraged to construct and use standardized tests of intelligence and attainment to assess individual differences which were assumed to be largely constitutional in origin and relatively unchanging in rate of individual development. Although Burt understood and wrote extensively about the effects of social disadvantage on children, he gave to practicing educational psychologists a model which assumed their function to be the diagnosis of defects which were predominantly to be found in the child rather than as a consequence of an ongoing transactional process between biological endowments and the social environment, including the school.

Across the Atlantic a somewhat similar tradition developed from the work of Goddard who had first introduced the Binet test there, and others such as Yerkes and Terman who were concerned with the prediction of achievement in the armed forces, industry and education. The mental testing movement gathered momentum, attracting many able scientists and also shrewd businessmen.

However, there was in addition a different and very powerful force achieving rapid development in America, namely experimental psychology. The experimenter, instead of measuring the average mind and its variance, attempted to measure the effect of some specified environmental change; in an endeavor to emulate the vigor of the physical sciences he resorted to the controlled conditions of the laboratory, using as subjects animals who could (unlike humans) be bred and reared in a predetermined manner. Learning theories were almost exclusively American and for a long time were largely the product of theoretical models based on elegant experimental work in the area of conditioning. For these psychologists a deliberate manipulation of the environment resulted in demonstrable and often important changes in the organism's behavior; small wonder, then, that J. B. Watson in 1930 chanced his arm with the statement; "Give me a dozen healthy infants, well-formed, and my own specified world to bring them up in and I'll guarantee to take any one at random and train him to become any type of specialist I might select—doctor, lawyer, artist, merchant-chief and, yes, even beggarman and thief, regardless of his talents, penchants, tendencies, abilities, vocations, and race of his ancestors."

Much later Skinner declared "Don't test—teach!" and set about developing an educational technology based on the use of Thorndike's Law of Effect which he referred to as the law of *positive* reinforcement, (i.e., stimulus-response sequences which were satisfying in their consequences were thereby strengthened). In his book *The Technology of Teaching*[1] he argued that there was too much about schools that was negative, leading to passive compliance among pupils, rather than active learning, and, further, that teachers often unwittingly reinforced unruly and maladaptive behavior by drawing attention to it. Moreover, it appeared that by appropriate use of positive reinforcement and "time-out" procedures every kind of desirable behavior from problem solving to creative activities could be elicited and encouraged, while sloth, aggression and deceit would be reduced in a brave new world.

With these traditions pervading university departments of psychology, it is not surprising that in the main educational psychologists in the USA looked to the social context as the most important factor in pupil learning, many of them dismissing, often absurdly, cognitive and emotional factors as contributors. Furthermore, the experimental analysis of behavior became a major focus of endeavor among researchers in human as well as animal laboratories, resulting in a shift of emphasis from factorial studies of interrelationships to controlled experiments which demanded different research strategies and statistical design.

THE GENEVAN SCHOOL

Meanwhile in Geneva another theoretical approach had been developed which was to be espoused by many psychologists who shared an equal distaste for both psychometrics and behaviorism. Piaget's theory presented for the first time a process model of development concerned to account for cognitive changes from infancy to adult life; it was destined to have a profound influence on educational thinking in many parts of the world. As is well known, Piaget's genetic epistemology was based in the conceptual framework of a zoologist concerned with the manner in which organisms adapt to their environment, a process which he considered as occurring through an active interaction between biological structures and environment by means of assimilation and accommodation. He explicitly disassociated himself from behaviorism, arguing that the concept of association, which the various forms of associationism from Hume to Pavlov and Hull had used and abused, had been obtained only by artificially isolating one part of the general process defined by the equilibrium between assimilation and accommodation (Piaget, 1970).[2] He was equally critical of those environmentalists who sought to accelerate children through the stages, cautioning against a false optimism which some educational psychologists had encouraged in teachers. Genuine optimism, in Piaget's opinion, would consist in believing in the child's capacities for invention.

NATURE AND NURTURE

To many psychologists and educators a developmental theory which assumes an interaction between biological and social factors, while at the same time describing the maturational process in terms of clearly delineated stages, had considerable appeal. By contrast, others whose training was in psychometrics were attracted to a different methodological approach, namely a statistical estimation of the relative importance of genetic and environmental factors in accounting for differences in ability. Barbara Burks (1928)[3] was probably among the first to place a value of 80% as the genetic contribution to IQ differences, an estimate based on the results of a large scale and carefully planned adoption study. Others were to follow her lead, but not always with as much care, and unfortunately rather little attention was paid to the *nature* of environmental factors which might influence the developing child, or indeed, apart from Piaget's rather speculative conjectures, *how* these interacted with developing biological structures. The environment (together with errors of measurement) was accorded the *remainder* after the heritability percentage had been estimated. There was, however, an important exception to the neglect of environmental factors, mentioned by Freeman, Holzinger and Mitchell (1928)[4] and vigorously elaborated by the Iowa school in the 1930s, namely the allegedly critical significance for later development of environmental events in the first few years of life. This theory became, with the publication in 1949 of D. O. Hebb's *Organization of Behavior*,[5] and in 1951 of Bowlby's influential monograph *Maternal Care and Mental Health*,[6] the focus of considerable empirical study, mostly, but not exclusively, using animals.

The methodological problems inherent in most of the researches investigating child development, and many using animals, were overlooked when social policies relating to young children were formulated, the most famous being the Head Start program in America which aimed to give children from disadvantaged domestic environments enriched opportunities prior to school entry at the age of six. The assumption was that if children were to be shielded from later educational failure, preschool intervention was certainly necessary if not sufficient. When careful evaluation of the outcome of these programs indicated no advantage accruing to the children after three years in primary school, now known as the "washout" effect, one professor felt able in 1969 to write from the Department of Education at Berkeley, "Compensatory education has been tried and it apparently has failed" (Jensen, 1969).[7]

Jensen then proceeded to account for the substantial disparities in educational attainment across social classes and ethnic groups in terms of genetically determined differences in IQ, and concluded that for the vast majority of children in American schools it would not be possible substantially to boost the IQ and scholastic achievement. He did, however, concede that differences in attainment are more affected by social influences than are intelligence test scores. The article in the *Harvard Educational Review* resulted in a furious response in many quarters, particularly from those concerned with the education of disadvantaged children. "Jensenism" became a term of abuse, and some researchers started to look very critically at the quality of the empirical evidence on which the conclusions were based. In this connection the extensively cited researches by the late Sir Cyril Burt were (belatedly) pronounced fraudulent to an extent not as yet fully established (Kamin, 1974;[8] Gillie, 1976;[9] Hearnshaw, 1979;[10] Clarke and Clarke, 1980[11]). The scientific credentials of Britain's most prominent educational psychologist were at least diminished if not demolished, and his supporters on both sides of the Atlantic suffered a considerable blow.

However, sophisticated researchers, including Jensen, had gained from this unhappy affair, and they proceeded carefully to collect and evaluate evidence, much of it published in the last decade, which points to the following conclusions with respect to IQ scores:

1) biological relatives show significantly greater resemblance than do adopted relatives reared in the same social milieu;
2) social factors unrelated to biological differences have as yet not been shown to contribute, except relatively trivially, to variations in intelligence in families representing a wide spectrum of environments, excluding, however, the socially deprived;
3) the environment can be shown to have deleterious effects where circumstances are exceptionally disadvantageous;
4) removal of children from disadvantaged environments to favorable circumstances results in improvement in cognitive functioning;
5) as yet no early period in development has been identified which can be considered critical in the sense that the demonstrated effects of social disadvantage are irreversible, provided there is total ecological change.

Intelligence can justifiably be seen as a product of biological and social factors in interaction. In environments which are above a certain undefined threshold, almost certainly the vast majority in an advanced society, genetic factors are most readily inferred as major causes of intellectual differences, while below the threshold the environment may, to an unknown extent, be inferred as suppressing potential development. The nature of the transactions which serve to accelerate or retard development during the first fifteen years of life and thereafter are, however, as yet quite inadequately understood, but several large scale longitudinal studies have already been initiated with a view to clarifying some of the issues. The analysis offered here is based upon a consideration of a very large number of research reports which as yet have not been satisfactorily summarized in a single review. Each point is separately supported by several careful and recent studies too numerous to list.

COGNITIVE VIEWS OF LEARNING

As already mentioned, during the middle part of this century, behaviorism became the major theoretical model for American researchers interested in learning, with important applications in the form of programmed instruction and educational technology. However, the rise of behaviorism was accompanied by a considerable neglect of cognitive psychology across the Atlantic, although in Britain F. C. Bartlett had initiated important research at Cambridge into factors influencing the reception and retention of meaningful discourse, and had inspired a generation of students many of whom are today, in parallel with colleagues abroad, developing sophisticated models of human information-processing.

To this reviewer, one of the more exciting areas in educational psychology is the study of factors which influence the reception and retention of meaningful prose material, an activity which occupies perhaps more time in classrooms than any other. The radical initiator of this movement was David Ausubel whose first paper on the use of advance organizers was published in 1960 and who in the introduction to his lengthy text *Educational Psychology: A Cognitive View* (1968)[12] stated that he was not prepared to consider topics such as child development, adjustment, personality and group dynamics except insofar as they bear on and are *directly* relevant to classroom learning. Further, since educational psychology is an immensely complex subject, there would be no attempt to simplify and water down the material to be presented; Ausubel maintained that his aim was to furnish the prospective teacher with the basic psychological sophistication needed for classroom teaching. He proposed "assimilation theory," which has many elements in common with Bartlett's position with respect to "schemata," and in essence proposes that learning involves relating new, potentially meaningful material to an assimilative context of existing knowledge. Thus the conditions of meaningful assimilative learning are that the new material must be received; the learner must possess, prior to learning, a meaningful context for integrating the new material; and he must actively use this context to integrate the new information with old.

Ausubel introduced the concept of advance organizers to provide a conceptual bridge between existing knowledge and new material, by presenting the novel ideas at a high level of generality and abstraction. Early experimental work suggested that the effects of advance organizers were greatest for those of relatively low ability or poor background knowledge and the differences obtained between groups with and without the use of organizers were chiefly due to students of this kind.

Latterly, however, as so often is the case with new strategies for promoting learning, a somewhat confused and confusing situation has arisen with a sufficient number of experimenters finding no difference between "treated" and "untreated" groups for Barnes and Clawson (1975)[13] to conclude that "advance organizers as presently constructed, generally do not facilitate learning." The fact that two recent reviewers (Mayer, 1979[14] and Luiten et al., 1980[15]) disagree with the former assessment does little to mitigate the unsatisfactory nature of many of the researches and their reporting. In addition, the majority of those participating in these brief learning experiments have been college students. Perhaps, as with compensatory education, advance organizers have not failed, but have as yet not been systematically tried in contexts where they might be effective.

A somewhat similar situation is to be found in the literature on so called mathemagenic behaviors introduced by Rothkopf (1965).[16] The most often researched of these activities, designed to promote learning, are note-taking and the effect of inserted questions in prose passages. Insufficient effort has been devoted to analyzing the relative efficacy of different kinds of question in relation to various types of subject matter and the level of conceptual knowledge of the students. Furthermore, although as is the case with advance organizers small positive effects have been demonstrated in most experiments, learning *time* has usually not been controlled, leaving open an alternative interpretation of the results. Nevertheless, despite the inadequacies, a start has been made, and it must be hoped that more sophisticated experiments will in future yield insights into cognitive processes during learning activities which are urgently needed to improve strategies available to classroom teachers, particularly in connection with children of average ability. The evidence for biological factors interacting with the social environment during development to create the conditions for attainment at any point in time suggests that there is likely to be an interaction between the state of maturation and the most effective methods of enabling children to advance, a point of view corroborated in researches reviewed by Cronbach and Snow (1977).[17]

Often it seems that a failure to comprehend the complexity of the ongoing processes is at the root of the apparently conflicting results of attempts to observe or measure some brief intervention of the "main effect" variety. Furthermore, the emphasis on recall of large amounts of factual material (sometimes verbatim) has often seemed at variance with an important educational objective, namely the acquisition of new concepts or principles. A major contribution to an advance of this kind was presented in a recent symposium on learning processes and strategies in the *British Journal of Educational Psychology*. Two of the contributors, Marton and Säljö,[18,19] argued that a description of *what is learned* is more important than a summary of *how much is learned*. They presented students with substantial passages of prose and obtained information both on their comprehension of the discourse and also on the strategies used in processing. The authors were able to categorize the answers into those showing evidence of attention to learning the text itself, a reproductive strategy, or surface-level processing, and those which were concerned with comprehension of principles, deep-level processing. Attempts were made to modify processing strategies by means of inserted questions, and the conclusion reached was that the demand characteristics of assessment procedures have a considerable impact on how students proceed: Learning can be technified and runs the risk of being reduced to a search for the type of knowledge expected on the test. There is a clear implication here that thinking and proper understanding can be encouraged or discouraged according to how the pupil expects the material to be assessed. Watts and Anderson (1971)[20] had shown that deeper processing was encouraged by questions requiring the application of a text example to an unfamiliar situation, and distinguished between questions which measure true comprehension and those merely requiring textual repetition. Anderson (1972)[21] found that the vast majority of questions used in learning experiments failed to assess comprehension, and further that in those experiments in which depth of processing was manipulated by the insertion of questions demanding deep processing, retention and delayed recall were significantly increased. It appears to be much easier to produce questions demanding factual answers than problems requiring some deeper level of understanding for their solution, but it also seems likely that it would pay teachers to devote time and reflection to their routine methods of assessing their pupils' learning. A theoretical framework for studies in this area is provided by Craik and Lockhart (1972)[22] and Craik and Tulving (1975)[23] whose elegant experiments on depth of processing provide important insights into factors affecting learning and memory.

LEARNING TIME

As already noted, some of the experiments reporting superior learning as a function of changes in the structuring of material failed to control for time. A vast literature suggests that, of many factors available for teacher manipulation, this may be the single most significant in pupil learning, provided a clear distinction is made between available time and time-on-task, as Bloom (1980)[24] has put it. It seems likely that many children are not enabled effectively to utilize the time they are by law compelled to spend in school, resulting in serious waste of potential both to themselves and to the community. Investigations using a variety of procedures to determine the amount of time a student spends overtly or covertly engaged in learning suggest that the percentage of engaged time is highly related to subsequent measures of achievement. In turn, time-on-task is largely determined jointly by the quality of instruction, teacher-pupil relationships and the extent to which pupils have the cognitive prerequisites to accomplish tasks. Bennett (1976)[25] identified time spent on work-related activities as an important difference between formal and informal classrooms, a conclusion reiterated by Bell et al. (1976)[26] who believed that primary school children in an informal classroom wasted much of their time in aimless wandering, watching movements of other classes and interacting without useful purpose with their own classmates. Rutter et al. (1979)[27] from their study of senior high schools found that attainment and adjustment were related to classroom management strategies and that "one of the hallmarks of successful class management is keeping pupils actively engaged in productive activities rather than waiting for something to happen," a statement greatly amplified by some of the painstaking researches on the successful use of behavior modification in schools collated by O'Leary and O'Leary (1972),[28] Thoresen (1972)[29] and Merrett (1981).[30]

TEACHER-PUPIL INTERACTIONS

No review of the contribution of psychologists to education would be complete without consideration of the important, if diverse, researches on *teacher-student relationships*, to use the title of Brophy and Good's book (1974),[31] although space precludes the detailed discussion which the topic deserves.

In recent years a major stimulus to the extensive study of attitudinal and motivational factors in the social ecology of the classroom appears to have arisen from Rosenthal and Jacobson's *Pygmalion in the Classroom* (1968),[32] although this particular investigation into the effects of teacher expectation on pupil performance had too many methodological defects to be acceptable as valid evidence for the effect. A summary of the major criticisms has been compiled by Elashoff and Snow (1971).[33] In this country Pidgeon (1970)[34] reviewed a wide range of research into factors bearing on pupil motivation, including several studies of his own, arguing, among other things, that the general atmosphere of schools, or what Rutter would call their ethos, may differentially affect pupils' motivation and therefore their collective achievements.

Examination of the question of the extent to which individual teachers' attitudes hinder or help pupils of different ability levels or social background has been fraught with the usual difficulties surrounding experimental research in social psychology—particularly the problem of deceiving teachers so that they were unaware of the purpose of the research, which in some studies appears to have been ineffective and may have a bearing on the frequent failures to demonstrate the effect. The studies reported by Schrank (1968 and 1970)[35,36] and by Seaver (1973)[37] are among those which avoided the difficulty, and in each case showed a *small* effect of expectation on performance with US airmen and primary schoolchildren respectively. Seaver's method was ingenious in using existing school documents relating to young children whose older siblings either had or had not been taught by the same teacher who, hypothetically, in the former case might have formed an expectation based on knowledge of the achievement of an older sibling. He also raised the possibility that expectation effects might be as much pupil- as teacher-generated, and very recently the effect of student expectation on teachers has been explored (see for example Feldman and Prohaska, 1979).[38]

The better designed studies in the area of teacher-pupil interactions have been particularly useful in distinguishing between outcome and process variables, although it must be confessed that very few researchers have managed to provide evidence on both measures within the same study. It is increasingly apparent that many of the differences in teacher-pupil interactions in mixed ability classrooms are generated by the pupils (see, for example, Brophy and Good 1970),[39] thus providing important evidence on how children differentially contribute to their own learning environments. Dusek (1975)[40] in an important review article has made the distinction between *teacher expectation* which is a natural and often beneficial phenomenon and *teacher bias* in which children whose potential for learning does not apparently differ are accelerated or retarded by virtue of social or racial prejudice.

HOME AND SCHOOL

The question of the relative importance of school and home effects on attainment and social adjustment continues to provoke controversy. Recently a group of psychologists have called attention to an important variation among homes which can, at least to some extent, be harnessed as an educational resource: parental teaching. J. Hewison and the late Jack Tizard (1980[41] and forthcoming[42]) have reported a project which is outstanding in its methodological sophistication, provocative in the evaluation of results, and heartening as an object lesson in productive partnership between administrators, schools and research workers. Starting with the solidly based correlations between tests of academic attainment and various demographic characteristics associated with parental social status, they aimed to discover whether differences in reading achievement *within* a working-class population could be related to differences in children's home backgrounds. The usual modest correlations were obtained between reading attainment and various measures which included aspects of mothers' language and their attitudes to education. One factor, however, unexpectedly was found to be by far the most powerful predictor, namely whether mothers regularly heard their children read, in other words effectively coached them. The difference between pupils with and without this advantage amounted to almost one standard deviation, and could not be accounted for merely as a correlate of other influential factors including IQ, although the coached children were substantially brighter than those who were not. Two further important points emerged: first, that the total amount of help children received over several years was relevant, and second, that nearly half of the samples of working-class parents spent time helping their children with the mechanics of reading although none had been encouraged by the schools.

The next important question was, of course, whether an advantage accruing to some pupils by virtue of their parents' initiative could be reproduced in families where this had not occurred naturally. With the cooperation of the Heads and teachers in six primary and junior schools in the London borough of Haringey two types of intervention were employed for a two-year period. In one experimental condition teachers invited parents to hear their children read, books were supplied and regular checks made; in another condition an additional teacher was employed in the school to accelerate reading skills. Allocation to experimental or carefully designated control conditions was on a random basis, and the scoring of the standardized reading tests was done by experienced teachers unconnected with the intervention.

The results indicated that in this disadvantaged area of London, which included an immigrant population, inviting parents to coach their children produced a very significant effect in one school although not in another, while in neither school receiving additional teacher help was there any gain in reading accruing to the experimental pupils.

These findings are consistent with the results of intervention research which suggest that unless parents become involved with an ongoing process, gains for children are likely to be both limited and ephemeral.

IN CONCLUSION

Inevitably some topics to which educational psychologists have contributed have been omitted from this essay, including the area of backwardness and mental retardation which remain a focal point of interest and concern to this author. Had I indulged all my personal predilections a section on delinquency and maladjustment would have been included, together with a consideration of the school's potential role in helping troubled children from disadvantaged backgrounds. Unfortunately, several important research reports have had to be excluded, and with them the names of respected colleagues and friends. My endeavor has been to sketch a broad outline of psychologists' contributions to mainstream education, and to suggest that there is a gradually changing outlook which should serve us well in the future.

Among the more important changes in orientation are a better recognition of the complex interrelations of biological and many social factors which underlie various developmental trajectories, and strongly influence attainment and adjustment during the school years and later. Developmental psychology is increasingly perceived as life-span psychology in which there is always some potential for change in a majority of the population, sometimes in an upward and sometimes in a downward direction.

There is an awareness of the limitations of laboratory studies for defining accurately events in the field, leading to a greater sophistication in the design of experiments in classrooms, youth clubs, leisure centres and elsewhere, together with the use of quasi-experimental designs which make use of naturally occurring events. There is an increasing preoccupation with the investigation of *processes* as well as *outcomes* in the investigation of both cognitive and social-emotional characteristics. The fact that as yet research has not advanced very far in producing a proper understanding of the former in relation to the latter should not diminish the importance of investigating across both time and space.

It seems increasingly evident that children react differently to the same social or educational context, in many cases contributing directly to the nature of the environmental events which will in turn affect sequential transactions, in which the child may unwittingly affect his or her own development.

Perhaps it should not be assumed that each of the factors which can separately be shown to accelerate learning would, if added together, make a *vast* difference to most pupils' competence, although there is substantial reason to suppose they are important. Many of them are procedures naturally adopted by competent teachers, who modify their techniques according to the cognitive level of their pupils and the subject matter which is being taught. Thus they are probably correlated characteristics of inspired educators who will, in addition, form flexible judgments concerning their pupils, avoiding rigid expectancy effects and creating classroom climates in which children will have a maximal opportunity to develop. In discussing the apparent unpredictability of human development, the playwright Bertolt Brecht neatly makes the point that this is not because there are no determinants of personal characteristics, but rather that there are too many. This complexity is a challenge to both teachers and researchers.

REFERENCES

1. Skinner, B. F. (1968). *The Technology of Teaching*. New York: Appleton-Century-Crofts.
2. Piaget, J. (1970). Piaget's Theory, Chapter 9. In *Manual of Child Psychology*, P. H. Mussen, ed. New York: John Wiley.
3. Burks, B. (1928). The relative influence of nature and nurture upon mental development: A comparative study of foster parent-foster child resemblance and true parent-true child resemblance. *Yearbook of the National Society for the Study of Education*, Part 1, 27, pp. 219–316.
4. Freeman, F. N., Holzinger, K. J. and Mitchell, B. C. (1928). The influence of environment on the intelligence, school achievement, and conduct of foster children. *Yearbook of the National Society for the Study of Education*, Part 1, 27, pp. 103–217.
5. Hebb, D. O. (1949). *Organization of Behavior*. New York: Wiley.
6. Bowlby, J. (1951). *Maternal Care and Mental Health*. Geneva: W.H.O.
7. Jensen, A. R. (1969). How much can we boost IQ and scholastic achievement? *Harvard Educational Review*, 39:1–123.
8. Kamin, L. J. (1974). *The Science and Politics of IQ*. New York: Lawrence Erlbaum.
9. Gillie, O. (1976). Crucial data faked by eminent psychologist. *The Sunday Times* (London), 24th October.
10. Hearnshaw, L. S. (1979). *Cyril Burt, Psychologist*. London: Hodder and Stoughton.
11. Clarke, A. M. and Clarke, A. D. B. (1980). Comments on Professor Hearnshaw's "Balance Sheet on Burt." *A Balance Sheet on Burt*: Supplement to the *Bulletin* of the B.P.S., 33:17–19.
12. a) Ausubel, D. P. (1960). The use of advance organizers in the learning and retention of meaningful verbal material. *Journal of Educational Psychology*, 51:145–170.
    b) Ausubel, D. P. (1968). *Educational Psychology: A Cognitive View*. New York: Holt, Rinehart and Winston.
13. Barnes, R. B. and Clawson, E. V. (1975). Do advance organizers facilitate learning? Recommendations for further research based on an analysis of thirty-two studies. *Review of Education Research*, 45:637–659.
14. Mayer, R. E. (1979). Twenty years of research on advance organizers: Assimilation theory is still the best predictor of results. *Instruc. Sci.*, 8:133–167.
15. Luiten, J., Ames, W. and Ackerson, G. (1980). A meta-analysis of the effects of advance organizers on learning and retention. *American Education Research Journal*, 17(2): 211–218.
16. Rothkopf, E. Z. (1965). Some theoretical and experimental approaches to problems in written instruction. In *Learning and the Educational Process*, J. D. Krumboltz, ed. Chicago: Rand McNally, pp. 193–221.
17. Cronbach, L. J. and Snow, R. E. (1977). *Aptitudes and Instructional Methods: A Handbook for Research on Interactions*. New York: Irvington.

18. Marton, F. and Säljö, R. (1976). On qualitative differences in learning—I: Outcome and process. *British Journal of Educational Psychology*, 46(1):4–11.
19. Marton, F. and Säljö, R. (1976). On qualitative differences in learning—II: Outcome as a function of the learner's conception of the task. *British Journal of Educational Psychology*, 46(2): 115–127.
20. Watts, G. H. and Anderson, R. C. (1971). Effects of three types of inserted questions on learning from prose. *Journal of Educational Psychology*, 62(5): 378–394.
21. Anderson, R. C. (1972). How to construct achievement tests to assess comprehension. *Review of Educational Research*, 42(2): 145–170.
22. Craik, F. I. M. and Lockhart, R. S. (1972). Levels of processing: A framework for memory research. *Journal of Verbal Learning and Verbal Behavior*, 11:671–684.
23. Craik, F. I. M. and Tulving, E. (1975). Depth of processing and the retention of words in episodic memory. *Journal of Experimental Psychology: General*, 104(3): 268–294.
24. Bloom, B. S. (1980). *Better Learning in Schools: A Primer for Parents, Teachers and Other Educators*. New York: McGraw Hill.
25. Bennett, N. (1976). *Teaching Styles and Pupil Progress*. London: Open Books.
26. Bell, A. E., Zipursky, M. A. and Switzer, F. (1976). Informal or open-area education in relation to achievement and personality. *British Journal of Educational Psychology*, 43(3): 235–243.
27. Rutter, M., Maughan, B., Mortimore, P. and Ouston, J. (1979). *Fifteen Thousand Hours: Secondary Schools and Their Effects on Children*. London: Open Books.
28. O'Leary, K. D. and O'Leary, S. G. (1972). *Classroom Management: The Successful Use of Behavior Modification*. New York: Pergamon.
29. Thoresen, C. E. (1973). *Behavior Modification in Education*, The 72nd Yearbook of the NSSE. Chicago, IL: University of Chicago Press.
30. Merrett, F. E. (1981). Studies in behavior modification in British educational settings. *Educational Psychology*, 1:13–38.
31. Brophy, J. and Good, T. L. (1974). *Teacher-Student Relationships: Causes and Consequences*. New York: Holt, Rinehart and Winston.
32. Rosenthal, R. and Jacobson, L. (1968). *Pygmalion in the Classroom*. New York: Holt, Rinehart and Winston.
33. Elashoff, J. D. and Snow, R. (1971). *Pygmalion Reconsidered*. Worthington, OH: Charles A. Jones.
34. Pidgeon, D. A. (1970). *Expectation and Pupil Performance*. London: NFER.
35. Schrank, W. R. (1968). The labeling effect of ability grouping. *Journal of Educational Research*, 62(2): 51–52.
36. Schrank, W. R. (1970). A further study of the labeling effect of ability grouping. *Journal of Educational Research*, 63(8): 358–360.
37. Seaver, W. B. (1973). Effects of naturally induced teacher expectancies. *Journal of Personal Social Psychology*, 28(3): 333–342.
38. Feldman, R. S. and Prohaska, T. (1979). The student as Pygmalion: Effect of student expectation on the teacher. *Journal of Educational Psychology*, 71:485–493.
39. Brophy, J. and Good, T. L. (1970a). Teachers' communication of differential expectations for classroom performance. *Journal of Educational Psychology*, 61:365–374.
40. Dusek, J. B. (1975). Do teachers bias children's learning? *Review of Educational Research*, 45(4): 661–684.
41. Hewison, J. and Tizard, J. (1980). Parental involvement and reading attainment. *British Journal of Educational Psychology*, 50:209–215.
42. Tizard, J., Schofield, W. N. and Hewison, J. (In press). Collaboration between teachers in assisting children's reading. *British Journal of Educational Psychology*.

Part IV

SOCIAL ISSUES

It is a truism that stresses and threats generated by the social environment will have unfavorable effects on the psychological development of children. But how are we to place the threat of nuclear war, the threat to the destruction of civilization and all human life, within such a framework? This is not a question of some quantitative increase in stress and its consequences, but a qualitatively new ultimate horror which no previous generation has had to face or could even imagine. And, beyond this, the horror is created by our political leaders, whom we are taught to respect and trust, and yet who now appear to be controlled by irrational and even mad delusions that we can survive a nuclear war.

What are the effects on children of this socially engendered madness which threatens all human existence? What can mental health professionals do to mitigate this horror? These issues are addressed clearly and without recourse to unrealistic wishful thinking by two eminent psychologists, Sibylle Escalona and Milton Schwebel, who have devoted themselves both to study and action in this most fearful problem of our time. Their message is grim but not hopeless, and we need to hearken to the challenge they pose to all of us.

Rutter reviews with his usual comprehensiveness, clarity, and analytic incisiveness the question of how much we really know about prevention in the field of psychosocial disorders in children. His title "Myth and Substance" expresses his theme that the enthusiasm for prevention and the feeling that appropriate and early psychosocial interventions will have a lasting beneficial effect on mental health must be tempered with the reality that while a good deal is known about risk factors, less is known about precisely how to intervene to bring about the desired results. He cautions that at the same time that we must move ahead to implement what we know, we must simultaneously avoid both doing harm and wasting time and energies in well-meant activities that actually have no important effect. For this vital mental health goal, increased knowledge is necessary, knowledge which then must be translated into action.

245

Hobbs and Robinson point out that the emphasis of the significance of early infantile experience for later development led policymakers to concentrate public resources on compensatory educational programs for young, disadvantaged children. As laudatory and valuable as this policy was, it ignored the needs and possibilities of programs for later age groups. With the crystallization of a life-span perspective among developmental psychologists and psychiatrists in recent years, the potential effectiveness of programs for adolescents and young adults has become evident. This change in perspective has not as yet had an influence on public policy commensurate with its importance. The authors spell out the specific types of programs that can and should be implemented to develop the cognitive competence of adolescents and young adults.

In the final paper in this section Berlin considers the special emotional problems encountered by Native-American children caught between a hostile Anglo society and a not very powerful Native culture. He documents the specific consequences of this dilemma and outlines the strategies for intervention which make constructive change possible, though admittedly still very difficult. Berlin's analysis of the problems faced by Native-Americans emphasizes the need for such an approach to the mental health problems of specific populations at special risk for the development of emotional disorders if appropriate remedial programs are to be formulated and mounted.

16

Growing Up With the Threat of Nuclear War: Some Indirect Effects on Personality Development

Sibylle K. Escalona

Albert Einstein College of Medicine, New York

The effects of the nuclear peril upon youngsters in middle childhood are considered, with particular emphasis on the extent to which ego strengths and weaknesses are influenced by adult behavior. It is suggested that the adult response to a pervasive danger such as the nuclear arms build-up shapes children's views of the trustworthiness of adult society and defines the limits of their growth and development.

We know that nuclear weapons can destroy civilization as we know it, but the kind and the extent of devastation that would follow are beyond our comprehension, not because the facts are not available but because we cannot imagine what they mean in human and concrete terms. The physical, biological, and social destruction that would occur is so enormous that at first glance it seems trivial to worry about the psychological effect of living with the threat of nuclear war.

On second thought a better understanding of how people cope with an unprecedented danger brings us to the very heart of the matter. It is not the technological capability we are afraid of, it is how it may be used. It is people who design and build atomic weapons: it is people who

Reprinted with permission from the *American Journal of Orthopsychiatry*, 1982, Vol. 52, No. 4, 600–607. Copyright 1982 by the American Orthopsychiatric Association, Inc.

Presented at a symposium of Physicians for Social Responsibility/NYC, February 1982, New York.

deal with conflict and conflict resolution among nations. It is people who acquiesce to what is happening and who tolerate reckless so-called game plans that include the option of a first strike and the equally irrational and less questioned step of retaliatory nuclear attack. No one and nothing but people can oppose and counteract mounting tension among nations, can compel arms negotiations and can in a thousand ways act to avert the ultimate disaster. Nor is it necessary for the entire population to be roused to action. History shows that revolutions and other massive social changes have been set in motion by a determined minority of citizens. In retrospect we say, "the time was ripe." What ripened it? It was always that material and social circumstances had altered in fundamental ways and that a sufficient number of people responded to such objective changes by enforcing corresponding changes in social institutions and societal goals. In the present situation the people who matter most may well be those who are now children.

In beginning a consideration of the impact of the nuclear threat upon personality development I will state the conclusion I have reached: Growing up in a social environment that tolerates and ignores the risk of total destruction by means of voluntary human action tends to foster those patterns of personality functioning that can lead to a sense of power-lessness and cynical resignation. By the same token the development of those characteristics that can generate and support future-oriented collective social action is made more difficult in the present social climate. In short I believe that growing up fully aware that there may be no future, and that the adult world seems unable to combat the threat, can render the next generation less well equipped to avert actual catastrophe than they would be if the same threat existed in a different social climate. In his series of articles in the *New Yorker*, Jonathan Schell[3] asked "what it says about us and what it does to us that we are preparing our own extermination." As one part of his answer, he said that ". . . if we are dull and cold toward life in its entirety we will become dull and cold toward life in its particulars." This statement is reversible, and applies to the effect of nuclear danger upon children more precisely in its reversed form. Namely, if we are dull, cold, and uncaring about the events of our daily life we ultimately become dull and disengaged toward life in general. It is adult behavior and adult feelings in the private and public aspects of daily life that exert potent influence on character formation during childhood.

This perception is based on what is known about personality development. It is also based on what psychology and sociology have taught us about the effects of different kinds of stress upon behavior. Last but not least, it is based on what children say when invited to express their thoughts about the future, about nuclear power, and about their understanding of national and international affairs.

We know that not only adolescents but school-age children are aware of public issues, think about them, and are generally interested in the social institutions that govern adult life. This has been established through a variety of studies only a very few of which relate to the issue of nuclear power. The evidence cannot be reviewed here but I can say that all information so far obtained has confirmed children's awareness of public life. Different questions were asked, of different child populations, by different methods and by investigators holding different points of view. Total agreement on a fact under these circumstances is a rare event in our discipline. A few examples have to suffice. Judith Torney and her associates[5-7] are among those who studied children's conception of the body politic. They found, as have others, that young schoolchildren by and large tend to see their own country as ideal, far superior to all others, very powerful and protective. With advancing age presidents and prime ministers are no longer seen as infallible superheroes, but a naive trust in the power of social institutions and of one's own country generally remains unshaken. (Whether or not this is equally true in the 1980s is one of the many things we do not know.) Reading what children said in response to so many questions leaves no doubt that they interpret national and international affairs by drawing upon their personal experience, in particular, their experience in relation to the control of aggression, to rules and regulations generally, and to protection against danger. After the Cuban missile crisis a little boy said: "I thought Castro and Kennedy had made up so there won't be a war," much as a nine-year-old might refer to the settlement of conflict among children in the neighborhood. Several studies showed the degree to which children integrate their interpretation of world affairs with expectations of the future. During the early sixties, when air raid drills and the shelter building controversy acquainted children with the atom bomb, a group of us did a questionnaire study on this issue.[2] We carefully avoided any reference to the bomb or to war, and simply asked: Think about the world as it may be about ten years from now; what are some of the ways in which it may be different from what it is today? More than 70% of a total of 350 youngsters spontaneously mentioned the bomb—either by envisaging a gruesome existence underground, or in terms of possible wholesale destruction. Some larger studies—such as one conducted by Milton Schwebel,[1] and a very recent one by John Mack and others for the American Psychiatric Association[1]—asked directly

about nuclear power and what it meant to the older children and adolescents. Their results were congruent with early ones. The most characteristic attitude was well expressed by an articulate adolescent who
said, in part:

> Everything has to be looked at on two levels: the world with
> the threat of ending soon and life *with* a future . . . the former
> has to be blocked out for everyday functioning . . . but [the
> other] is always there on a much larger scale than individual
> deaths.

One could and should go on to show that, for children and adolescents,
optimism about a livable future largely depends on the degree to which
what they know about adults encourages trust in the rationality, good
will and effectiveness of the adult world.

One more thing has to be said. Those who grew up in the nuclear age
differ from previous generations in that they take for granted that the
threat is real and that it applies to all natural and social life on earth. In
this respect they are more clear-eyed and realistic than older adults. Not
because they are braver and brighter, but because their universe is not
the same as that of older generations. An example of what I mean will
be familiar to all who live with children. Children's perception of space
is not like ours. They automatically include other planetary systems and
distances reckoned in light years. What is to us an abstraction is immediate physical reality to them. Similarly a sudden, total void is within
the realm of what is possible to them. It should also be mentioned that
few, if any, children and adolescents live in fear of this threat, except
at moments of acute crisis, such as existed in the vicinity of Three Mile
Island for a while. And then the fear was not that the world would come
to an end but that they and their families might be hurt. Nor do I know
of any evidence to suggest that symptoms among emotionally disturbed
child patients focus on nuclear power. What, then, is the reason for
concern?

Most discussions of the topic deal with adolescence as the decisive
period, and rightly so. I shall focus on middle childhood. In adolescence
there occurs a sort of integration and consolidation into a well-defined
personality. Yet, identify formation, as Erikson has called this process,
depends heavily on development during the preceding phases. It is
roughly between the ages of six and twelve that children learn about the
world and develop what might be called an inner map of the social and
physical environment. (Schoolchildren still decorate the flyleaf of their

books with labels such as, "John Smith, 12 High Street, Middletown, USA, The World!") They come to view their own family and community as but a tiny part of a large structure that surrounds and supports personal experience. Similarly, they acquire time perspective. They know that their grandparents were children once and much of their life is focused on becoming an adult. They expect to found families, to hold jobs, to be part of a link that spans the generations forward into infinity.

With apologies for a schematic and highly selective reference to complex developmental processes, let me specify some of the developmental acquisitions that define middle childhood. It is then that children learn how to cope with challenges, demands, temptations, and apprehensions encountered in school and peer groups. They assume more responsibility for their own safety and well-being, and this involves dealing with social institutions beyond school—the monetary system, transportation, traffic rules and other aspects of the law, libraries, etc. To manage this, as well as to engage in academic learning, requires, among other things, that children learn to regulate their behavior from within. They develop internal structures and mechanisms that serve to control the expression of aggression, impatience, grief, and other strong impulses and emotions. Especially important are the ability and willingness to forego immediate wishes and satisfactions in order to achieve more important but distant goals. Psychologists speak of the capacity to delay gratification. In fact, psychosocial maturity is measured by the degree to which children have learned to control their temper, to endure disappointment and frustration, and by their perseverance in the pursuit of more distant goals. All this and more becomes possible only as children develop attitudes and values that become part of themselves (a process of internalization). All societies, and certainly ours, teach a set of values, an ideology so to speak. We tell children that conflicts are best settled by compromise and negotiation, not by fighting. If there is to be fighting it must be fair and, whatever happens, serious hurt and damage to the opponent must be avoided. Children are taught to think before they act and that this requires understanding of the other person's point of view. Selfishness and greediness are labeled as childish, while kindness and altruism are highly valued. Most children accept these teachings but test their truth and effectiveness against what they observe, not only in their family and neighborhood but in the world at large. Societal events are of interest to children precisely because there is a striking parallel between the functions of social institutions and issues that are relevant in their personal development. What is the judiciary for but to assure justice (which they call fairness)? What is the military for but to defend us against enemies? The police exist to protect persons and property. It can be shown that children, lacking full comprehension of what is involved, show the greatest interest in those aspects of society that deal with violence, conflict, and security—clearly because these concerns are close to home.

Children form their understanding of these topics on the basis of social reality as they perceive it. How adults manage their affairs is the only source of information, of aspiration, and of apprehension. I began this paper by saying that personality development, and especially the internal regulatory mechanisms, the preferred styles of coping, and the skills that are most readily developed, are affected by the total social climate. There is ample evidence to show that personality characteristics developed during childhood are predominantly those best suited to the adaptive requirements of the particular culture and society in which children grow. For one well known example: children who grow up in chronic urban poverty usually end up as excellent survivors in ghetto life. They have skills and strengths to adapt to that setting which those raised in middle-class environments cannot match. But these same children often do not have the motivation, the perseverance, the style of problem solving and reasoning that are best suited to achieve success in academic learning or in vocational careers in a technological society. The same principle operates across nations and continents. We transmit to children, or, better, they absorb and learn from us, what we are ourselves. Thus, what children see and sense about our individual and collective response to the nuclear threat and similar issues will have a strong bearing on the development of their potential ego strengths and ego weaknesses.

To children, as indeed to the rest of us, nuclear danger is but part of a total social atmosphere. What impresses children most is whatever most concerns and arouses the adults. Therefore, the nuclear issue is currently not a conspicuous foreground issue to most children, though it could easily become so were an acute crisis to occur. Yet the actions and attitudes of critical importance in this context are displayed in a thousand ways. Adults exhibit their way of coping with threats and violence, their manner of striving for power, their means of settling conflict. They do so vividly in relation to the fear of robbery and street violence, in relation to the use of money and the importance of possessions, in their attitudes concerning welfare, or other ethnic groups, or their boss. On the broader scene children do know that a build-up of defense, which they know is weapons, is presented by authority as a necessity for national security.

This account can only hint at some of the impressions children receive and give back to us when we listen to them—and it is not intended to convey a picture of how the total environment is perceived. I am identifying troublesome aspects of the complex whole, selected from those especially relevant to what it will take to keep our world going. One thing is sure: The values we instill in children are often contradicted by reality. If I may put some of this in childlike language, children have it on high authority that the only way for this nation to survive and prosper is to have the most and the biggest weapons, and further, that some other countries are all set to attach and demolish us, given half a chance. They hear little about negotiations or about respecting the needs and wishes of other nations. They observe that people rely on heavy locks and on handguns to protect themselves. They also see a strong reluctance to get involved when other people are in trouble. They note that these ways of coping are not especially effective. People are still being robbed and mugged and are still afraid. Through TV, and at times directly, children are more aware of the police as an armed force that subdues and jails criminals than of its protective functions, which are not highlighted for them. And they are very much aware of random violence as manifested, for instance, by crime, by terrorist activities, by highjackings, and the like. In many ways they perceive individuals and society as helpless and passive in the face of large forces. (They have no idea what inflation is but they know that it's something bad and that people cannot stop it.) The instances when energetic and at least partially successful constructive action does take place are seldom brought to their attention. Along with powerlessness and a sense of futility children see blind resentment, the use of violence or the threat of it, if not at home then in the larger world.

Psychologically speaking, one feature of the nuclear danger, which spreads throughout the social fabric in subtle ways, is especially important. Children respond with sensitivity to anything that is surrounded by a feeling of the uncanny and mysterious—a feeling such as that attached to our thoughts of nuclear disaster. The catastrophes of which we have experience are limited in time and space. In our lifetime millions have been killed in war and millions of Jews were slaughtered, and these events did leave their mark. But the thought that virtually all people in a huge area might suddenly die and sicken, and that survivors would have no life supports, leaves us with the prospect of something like a black hole or a vacuum. The fact, well understood by many children, that plants, water, and all organic life can at the same time be destroyed, touches upon deep and primitive fantasies of world destruction. Psychiatrists as well as poets know that such fantasies lie dormant in all human beings. It is as though a bizarre and for the most part unconscious fantasy that had been safe enough, because understood to be totally impossible, had become a fact, turning our perceptions and expectations inside out. This connection between the thought of nuclear war and a primitive inner dread lends an air of the uncanny and almost supernatural to much that is said about the topic.

What has been said thus far can be supported by facts. We cannot know the outcome of what is still in progress. Formulations have to be tentative, partial, and in the nature of informed guesses. Still, there are some things that can safely be said about the effect on ego functions and corresponding skills of aspects of the social milieu that have been sketched. It is clear that knowing that there may be no future makes everything provisional. (In the early '60s, schoolchildren thought it a good joke to ask, "What are you going to be *if* you grow up?") This awareness is likely to encourage an investment in the here-and-now. It weakens the readiness to invest energy and self-control in the attainment of distant goals. Involved are the functions of anticipation and long-range planning, as well as the motivation for learning skills that are not immediately applicable. Instead, talents and activities that are rewarding in and for themselves are cultivated. Among college students, interest in expressive and symbolic subjects such as drama, dance, and graphic arts is on the upswing, while many of the more traditional academic pursuits have become less attractive. We might also view in this same light the degree to which young people of all social strata have recently found popular music so central and involving. Note that I selected interests and talents that are valuable and healthy, but not crucial when it comes to concerted effort in behalf of any overriding social concern—preservation of civilization, and perhaps the species, being the single most important one. On another and deeper level there is reason to believe that a perception of adults as either weak and not much involved with broader issues, or else resorting to unreasoning blind resentment and uncontrolled hostile action, has an effect upon the developing sense of self. A perception of the self as competent, as an active agent, as having the power to alter things is invariably present not only in leaders but also in those who are able to participate and thus carry the momentum of organized collective action. Having a reasonable sense of self and others—the two are deeply intertwined—is a prerequisite for effective action.

In all societies and at all times in recorded history children have experienced and known about all of the weaknesses and all of the strengths of which individuals and societies are capable. A great variety of character structures and of achievements develop in any generation. This is as true now as it was before. But is it also true that many features of society and of the human condition are disproportionately highlighted and represented at present. Those aspects of social life of which children most easily become aware depict adults and their institutions as driven and constrained by impersonal forces too large to counteract or even comprehend. In addition, children are made more strongly aware of the fact that unmanageable destructive forces exist within people as well as outside. This is dramatized through the powerful medium of TV, an avenue of information that came to be central in the life of children only fairly recently. It says something about society at this point in history that even in entertainment programs violence and horror are major themes, and that it is no longer possible to tell the good guys from the bad ones by their actions. We are dealing with a shift in emphasis. Adolescents have always had ample cause to criticize their elders, but whereas they used to feel fairly certain that they could run things better, it's hard to be sure that the next wave will approach adulthood with that same confidence.

In sum, children are able to live with danger both of the acute and the anticipated uncertain sort. What has an impact on their development is their perception of the present and the future. To the extent that the present functioning of society conveys to children a picture of passive and evasive withdrawal, of fear of and belligerence toward other nations, and of not even trying to combat a host of evils both large and small—to that extent the effects of the nuclear peril upon us also affect the development of children. The adult response to ultimate danger is, to growing children, also the ultimate test of the trustworthiness of adult society.

REFERENCES

1. Beardslee, W. and Mack, J. (1982). The impact on children and adolescents of nuclear development. In *Psychosocial Aspects of Nuclear Development, Task Force Report #20*. Washington, D.C.: American Psychiatric Association, pp. 64–93.
2. Escalona, S. (1965). Children and the threat of nuclear war. In *Behavioral Science and Human Survival*, M. Schwebel, ed. Palo Alto, CA: Behavioral Science Press.
3. Schell, J. (1982). Reflections: The fate of the earth— II. *New Yorker* (Feb. 8):48–109.
4. Schwebel, M. and Schwebel, B. (1981). Children's reactions to the threat of nuclear plant accidents. *American Journal of Orthopsychiatry*, 51(2):260–270.
5. Torney, J. (1977). The international attitudes and knowledge of adolescents in nine countries: The IEA civic education survey. *International Journal of Political Education*, 1:3–20.

6. Torney, J. (1980). Middle childhood as a critical period for education about international human rights. In *Daring to Dream: Law and the Humanities in the Elementary School*, L. Falkenstein and C. Anderson, eds. Chicago: American Bar Association.
7. Torney, J. and Hess, R. (1971). The development of political attitudes in children. In *Psychology and Educational Practice*, G. Lesser, ed. Glenview, IL: Scott, Foresman and Co.

17

Effects of the Nuclear War Threat on Children and Teenagers: Implications for Professionals

Milton Schwebel

Rutgers University

Several studies of youngsters are cited as evidence of their pervasive awareness of the possibility of nuclear cataclysm. It is suggested that the nuclear threat is a contributing factor in anxiety and other disorders noted among these youth. The role of mental health and other professionals in educating and guiding youngsters, and in working with them to reduce the anxiety and alleviate its causes, is outlined.

Mental health and education professionals, confronted with behavior that all too often is inexplicable, cannot help but wonder about the influence of the threat of nuclear war. Having hung over the heads of several generations of children during years which saw an increase in family disruption, drug abuse, and heightened loneliness, as well as a decline in the quality of behavior and scholastic performance in the nation's schools, the threat must be considered as a possible contributor to those costly changes in contemporary life. The studies reported here represent only preliminary attempts to inquire about that relationship.

After the height of the Berlin crisis in 1961, but while it was still very much part of the daily news, some 3000 students were queried about

Reprinted with permission from the *American Journal of Orthopsychiatry*, 1982, Vol. 52, No. 4, 608–618. Copyright 1982 by the American Orthopsychiatric Association, Inc.

Presented at a symposium of Physicians for Social Responsibility/NYC, February 1982, in New York.

the threat of war and about civil defense.[14] During the first week of the Cuban crisis in 1962 about 300 high school students were the subjects of a parallel study.[14] They were asked the following questions: Do I think there is going to be a war? Do I care? Why? What do I think about fallout shelters? In the wake of the Three Mile Island nuclear plant accident in 1979, the responses of 368 elementary and secondary students, addressing parallel questions, were obtained.[15]

In sum, these young people said that in the event of a nuclear war they would have the most to lose. Time and again, in response to questions about nuclear conflict, they said—and they said it bitterly—that they would pay the biggest price. They would be denied a chance to live, to love, to work, to bear children and raise a family. They would lose, they felt, the largest portion of their lives, and they would miss the opportunity to enjoy the pleasures they had hardly even begun to taste.

This is what came from some 3500 students in response to questions. They were female and male; black, Hispanic, Oriental, and white; urban, suburban, and rural; and they were, at the time of questioning, in the second grade to the second year in college, though most were from fourth through twelfth grades and, in fact, in junior and senior high school.

THE RESPONSES

When young people were asked what they expected if there were to be a nuclear war, many of the responses were eloquent in their simplicity: "I will die." "We will all die." Most of those who had any hope that perhaps they themselves might live nonetheless felt that their fate would be as bad as death because, as one said,

> If I was in school when the bomb was dropped and I hid under some wall or something, and I came out alive and came home and found my family gone, disappeared with everything, who'd want to live anyway?

But even when they thought that there might be a chance that they and their families would be fortunate enough to survive, they saw through that, too; they did in the early 1960s, and they do now. Even though they were confused and sometimes talked about wanting to be safe and hoping that they would be safe, and maybe there would be bomb shelters that would save them, nonetheless they said:

> Supposing my family was lucky enough, even if we lived, we couldn't last. Animals and plants would be destroyed, and if they weren't, they'd be radioactive. Who could eat them?

The younger subjects are especially vulnerable. In a recent study on the reaction of children to nuclear plant accidents, those in the intermediate grades were more fearful than the older students. The fourth graders dreaded the dangers of nuclear plant accidents more than the senior high students did, and were more insistent that the nuclear plants be closed. Understandably, the younger ones are even less informed about the nature and behavior of radioactivity than the older ones, and their comments reveal their naivete. For example, they gave such responses as these, in connection with the consequences of nuclear plant accidents: "We'd probably have to run fast to stay ahead of the radioactivity." Or: "We should kill it, we should shoot it with a shotgun." But naive as these statements are, their images convey the terror these children associate with nuclear perils.

The ignorance of some of the older students just comes in more sophisticated packages. For example: "Bomb shelters should be available for us all." Sometimes the older student is speaking not so much out of ignorance about the dangers—ignorance about the possibility of survival—as out of an effort to deny the threat by postponing its likely occurrence to a distant future. "A nuclear war could break out," said one senior high school student, "in the far future."

The use of denial appeared in an interesting way some 20 years ago. When young people were questioned within the first three days after President Kennedy addressed the nation at the very height of the Cuban crisis in 1962, the world was teetering on the brink. Their responses about the expectation of nuclear war, compared with those of students a year earlier after the Berlin crisis had abated, revealed the use of denial under circumstances of helplessness in the face of great danger. Whereas after the Berlin crisis, in comparable groups of junior high school students, almost 50% expected there would be a nuclear war, now, a year or so later, during the Cuban crisis week at this time of great peril, fewer than 25% expected that there would be a nuclear war. The heightened threat of annihilation, it seems, nourished an irrational optimism, an insistent need to believe that there would be no war, nourished, that is, a denial of the obviously greater possibility of war.

When they were asked if they cared about the nuclear threat, their answers were emphatic:

Anyone who doesn't is insane.
Anyone who doesn't care is inhuman.
It's insulting even to be asked such a question.
It's a naive question.
Of course I care. Sometimes I cry when I think of it.
It keeps me awake at night.
It's so terrible I try not to think about it.

Generally they deal with their anxiety by trying one means or another to deny the existence of the threat:

If I allowed myself to think about it, I'd be miserable.

But when the thought of it, the knowledge of it, penetrated into their consciousness, then their reactions were manifold. They expressed bitter resentment against what some young people called the "old men who have lived and who control our government," and against adults in general for putting them in this position—bitter resentment against those who had had a full life and didn't really care about the young. For many of them knew what price they would have to pay. One high school student asked, "If I live, dare I bear children?' A sixth-grader in Tucson, which is ringed by missiles, said recently, in answer to the question about personal feelings: "I'm scared and mad."

Besides resentment, they feel helpless: "I'm outraged that the leaders can consider the world's population expendable," one high school junior said, "and there's just nothing I can do about it." The powerlessness that teenagers feel, at a time when they should be developing a sense of identity and a sense of mastery, came through frequently, no matter in what part of the country these questions were asked. The mix of emotions brings to mind a statement that Eleanor Roosevelt made many years ago: "War's greatest evil is the degradation of the human spirit."[12]

Living with the nuclear threat, feeling resentful, bitter, and helpless, are degrading to the spirit. They erode the hopes for a future. The feelings may well emanate from a form of double jeopardy. It is burden enough for human beings to discover, when we are young, that we have to die some day. We don't like it, we deal with it in many kinds of ways, but we have to face it. And we are reassured by the knowledge that we could really live a long life, by the fact that there are after all—and there always are—a lot of old people around. We are reassured even when some young children die. It's too much to deny children that reassurance—to expect them to accommodate to the threat of sudden extinction without paying a great price. One student said:

> It makes me start to think that the end of my time in life may not be as far off as I would like it to be.*

In order to deal with the anxiety, to deal with a life of double jeopardy, in a land, they feel, whose leaders and even adults don't care, they resort to different forms of accommodation. One of them is immediate gratification. If there's no tomorrow, they say, let me live for today:

> I'm constantly aware that any second the world might blow up in my face. It makes living more interesting.

Another one put it this way:

> It's terrifying to think that the world may not be here in a half-hour, but I'm still going to live for now.

We could ask what another adolescent, the victim of an actual Holocaust, would have said were she alive today. Anne Frank, living in a hideout with her own and another family—including the young man Peter, aged 17—wrote in her diary[7] after she had embraced Peter for the first time:

> Oh, Anne, how scandalous! But honestly, I don't think it is; we are shut up here, shut away from the world, in fear and anxiety, especially just lately. Why, then, should we who love each other remain apart? Why should we wait until we've reached a suitable age? Why should we bother?

A high school student, echoing Anne's thoughts, said in 1979:

> Sometimes, when I think that there may be no future at all, I feel just like letting myself go. Why wait?

---

*This and several other student comments were taken from a recent study of Beardslee and Mack.[2] The rest, from the author's studies, were obtained in 1961, 1962, 1979, and 1982.

Another response to the weight of anxiety that they carry reflects an illusion of power. We're not that much in danger, this point of view goes, because we'll win or we're smart enough to do them in before they get us. This macho attitude, which was hardly apparent in the early 1960s, and is even now the expression of only a small group of males, is very disquieting, especially after the Air Florida crash in Washington. In excerpts reported by the *New York Times* it was evident that the officers, especially the copilot, were acutely anxious about the ice on the wings. They laughed and joked as men do trying to mask their fears before combat. The copilot seemed to be suggesting that they leave the take-off line-up, and said, among other things:

> Boy, this is a losing battle here on trying to de-ice those things,
> it [gives] you a false sense of security, that's all that does.

On that afternoon another crew decided to leave its place on the take-off line to be de-iced again, but not this one. Would it have been unmanly to acknowledge and be guided by the fear? Would it have been weakness? To some of the subjects in our several studies, it seems, it is unmanly to show that one is frightened, to suggest that we are at an impasse, in a "no-win" situation, unmanly to hold any but a superior, controlling position, and trigger-ready to use our arms first. The illusion appears in the responses of some but not many sophisticated and academically able high school students. Still it is chilling to have them say:

> We have the intelligence to use the bombs only when absolutely necessary.

Another form of response to nuclear anxiety is a narcissistic one. A small but distinct portion of the 1979 sample of students exhibited this quality by responding in a noticeably different way from the 1960 sample. In the 1960s, in frequent responses, the young people would say in effect: We find it abhorrent that people should suggest that you keep a rifle in your bomb shelter so you can kill anyone who wants to come in. Over and over, with only rare exception, they found this suggestion terribly immoral. But today, in response to questions about nuclear plant accidents, shortly after one at Three Mile Island, there were some—a minority, but still too many—who said, "Why should I care? It didn't happen in New Jersey, it happened in Pennsylvania." Or: "Why should I care if something like this happens in California?" It is possible, of course, that the difference is simply the result of a sampling bias, either in the 1960 studies or the recent one. On the other hand, perhaps this indifference to the welfare of others reflects a wider social change in the past 20 years evidenced also by a self-interested disregard for others, first highlighted in connection with the Genovese murder which many witnessed but did not report to the police out of fear of "becoming involved."

The final reaction to the nuclear threat is what some students refer to as nervousness, tension, and pressure. In considering the sources of these symptoms, one is aware that a nuclear threat hardly exists in isolation. It coexists with a diversity of international and domestic conflicts, involving economic and political power, and personal ones as well. The threat is in fact a product of these conflicts and, again, contributes to them; yet because of its extraordinary nature, it seems likely to have a major impact on mental condition. In commenting about the world of the future, some juniors and seniors in New Jersey, in individual interviews, talked about problems at home and with relationships and said the following:

> I don't look forward to the future. We're all antsy these days. There's too much tension, too much hassle. I hope there will be a lot less unhappiness in the future. Maybe people will be more caring, but not until we have a terrible upheaval. There's so much tension now from the uncertainty in the world, maybe if there were no threats of war, people would have friendlier interactions.

And one high school student in Massachusetts said:

> I refuse to bring up children in a world of such horrors and dangers of deformation.

For years many of us believed that sustained unemployment had a profound effect on mental health. This was no more than a hypothesis, however, until Brenner[4] in 1973 reported substantial evidence of the association between unemployment and such dire human consequences as suicide, mental hospital admissions, alcoholism, and, in fact, general mortality. It is knowledge such as this that leads us to wonder about and investigate the consequences of the sustained threat of nuclear disaster.

Collectively, then, young people tell us that the nuclear threat is too terrible to contemplate; when they do think about it, they feel resentful and helpless. They learn to cope with life today either by living for the moment, by persuading themselves that they are on the winning side—the surviving side, that is—by postponing the nuclear holocaust to a far-distant future, by putting hope in bomb shelters, by expecting part of this country and its people to survive, or, probably most of the time, by keeping the nuclear threat out of mind.

THE ROLE OF THE PROFESSIONAL

Knowledge about the needs of school-aged children and adolescents is persuasive that the role of professionals (mental health specialists, educators, clergy, etc.) is first and foremost to reassure children in the most formidable way, by actions in support of reducing the nuclear threat, wherever they perform their role: in school or college; in church, synagogue, or mosque; in clinic, agency, or mental health center; in newspaper, publisher's, or TV programmer's office, trade union, art studio, and at home; wherever the young need to know that there are adults struggling to see that reason prevails in human affairs—strong adults, whom they can depend upon, who will give them the feeling of caring about them, adults who can serve as models, adults who care as much about the nuclear threat as their children do, and who let them know that they're afraid and that they care and that they mean to do something about it—in other words, adults who don't themselves deny the peril, who have courage enough to work to change some prevailing practices in their own organizations—a tough job to do in most, if not all, organizations—and to include the nuclear threat as an issue central to their professional activity. The role means that they help young people acquire the knowledge and skills necessary for effective participation in community affairs.

What in particular should they learn? What attitude is constructive? What might be set as the criterion against which to evaluate the effectiveness of adult effort? To answer that, I want to highlight one particular feature that separates a small portion of the young whom I have studied from the rest. This group finds the arguments for nuclear armament incredible, and while they know the threat of a holocaust is very real, they find it so extraordinarily absurd that it too seems incredible. To their great advantage they are perceptive enough to recognize the perilous delusions; they understand that we are being victimized by claims that the world can tolerate a little nuclear war, and that we are more secure when we have the capacity to destroy the enemy ten times or a hundred times over rather than once. In terms of self-efficacy they are fortunate because they have not been deceived—have not allowed them-selves to be deceived. Yet it is painful to realize that some of one's leaders and some adults are mad, just as it is terribly painful to discover that one's parents are mad. But not so painful as being caught up oneself in the irrationality, powerlessness, and accompanying degradation. It is better by far, because then one can come to understand what keeps the threat of a nuclear holocaust alive, and one can do something reasonable and effective about it.

People's inability or refusal to credit their senses is not new; others before us have resisted allowing themselves to make the unthinkable thinkable. Paul Fussell,[8] in his book on the First World War, commented that

> . . . the problem for the writer trying to describe the elements
> of the Great War was its utter incredibility.

The world had never known industrialized mass trench warfare with its efficient mechanized butchery day in and day out over a few feet of land. The world had never known that form of absurdity. Writers could not assimilate what their senses were experiencing; it was too incredible to accept as real.

The more one resists accepting the absurd as an acceptable reality, in fact, the more one can resist the madness. Anne Frank wrote about the incredibility of the world she experienced. By contrast with the nuclear holocaust, and the carnage perhaps of billions, hers was a "minor" hol-ocaust since only six million died, but it still leaves us stupefied with disbelief. Her diary entry[7] of May 3, 1944, written three months before she was arrested and sent to Bergen-Belsen, contains the following:

> Yes, why do they make still more gigantic planes, still heavier
> bombs and, at the same time, prefabricated houses for re-construction? Why should millions be spent daily on the war
> and yet there's not a penny available for medical services,
> artists or for poor people? Why do some people have to starve,
> while there are surpluses rotting in other parts of the world?
> Oh, why are people so crazy?

During the Cuban crisis, a few students asked how grown people, leaders, could be "so crazy," could bring the people of the world to the abyss. Referring to Hiroshima, one said in 1979:

I remember feeling sad and bitter belonging to a race that would do such things.

For more than 35 years, since the Allied troops liberated the concentration camps, many people have asked themselves time and again: Why did we ignore the Holocaust? Why did the world sit it out? Surely professionals have been among them. If they are to serve young people in connection with the psychological effects of the nuclear threat, they would have to stop beating their breasts and wringing their hands because there is nothing that can be done about that Holocaust but study and remember it and assist the surviving victims. It can't be reversed, and we hardly wish, by example or other form of instructions, to encourage children to be obsessed with reversing the irreversible. However, we can abort the one that's in the making, as millions of people are seeking to do; and as professionals, we had better not be timid about it. A "limited" nuclear war is as mad and immoral as a limited Nazi Holocaust. To say it forcefully again and again, and to give young children the opportunity to see that for themselves, will validate their impulses and give them strength.

Despite differences among professional groups that work with the young, the similarities are considerable, and the principles proposed here are generally applicable. In brief they are:

1. Professionals see to it that they themselves are well-informed about the dangers, the potential consequences, their own reactions to the threat of nuclear war, and those of children and adolescents.

2. Professionals set as their goal that young people be informed, and be helped to deal with their reactions, through knowledge about adult action to protect them and the world from nuclear war, and about actions they might take appropriate to their age.

3. Professionals work at improving the methods of serving the young in this connection, among others in detecting those most in need of adult intervention.

To concretize these principles, we can start with the school setting and examine a number of actions that those working in the schools can take (and insofar as the particular measures permit, students and parents could profitably be involved): Get the professional organizations to include nuclear threat as one of their professional concerns incorporated in meeting agendae and in committee activities. Obtain support for in-service programs for school board members, school administrators, and teachers to acquaint them with the physical, biological, and psychological consequences of the threat. Encourage PTAs to institute programs of their own. Seek to establish, as a minimum, at least a two-week unit of work in science and social science for the program of every child in junior high schools to insure that they have the opportunity to learn the basic facts about the bombs and the threat. (Though it is difficult to estimate the extent to which those facts are already incorporated in programs in schools, one expert opinion[11] is that in all probability at most five percent, and more likely one percent, of young people get some organized and systematic instruction in them—other than a current events discussion—but primarily in elective courses in the senior high school and usually for students who have other opportunities to learn about those matters.) Organize committees of teachers to consider ways of integrating material into the curriculum and to make some of the work interdisciplinary in nature. Include nuclear threat issues in auditorium programs, calling on organizations such as Physicians for Social Responsibility for appropriate resources. Work at the state level as well to develop interest in both experimental and collaborative programs on a state-wide basis. Work with publishers in connection with school texts; surely they need that. Use the arts related to peace and the threat of nuclear war, perhaps dance, rock concerts, and exhibits of graphic art. Develop a system to get acquainted with the new resources that are rapidly becoming available, such as those through organizations like Educators for Social Responsibility.*

The role of the educator in exposing social realities is, to make a gross understatement, not a simple one. There are many objections to educating children about the nuclear threat. First is the tendency to deny the threat. It hasn't happened so far, one adult reassured himself, forgetting, or perhaps just ignorant of the effort that had gone into preventing it from happening during past crises; countless people had worked at controlling the situation. Second, there will be claims that it will arouse the anxieties of the young. One student, when asked about that, said:

---

*See, for example, *The War Game*, a movie simulaton of a nuclear attack on London; also, the Facing History and Ourselves Project, for access to information about events in history usually unavailable to students; both, and other materials, available through Educators for Social Responsibility, Box 1041, Brookline Village, Mass. 02147. Some general guiding principles in bringing information on nuclear dangers to children have been published previously.[13]

> We *should* be anxious. We've been lucky so far. How long can that go on? I put it out of mind, I guess we all do. We shouldn't.

Of course children are anxious, or at least they are made anxious when crises occur and when the news reports, if not the anxieties of adults themselves, set off their own alarm responses.[10] Third, there will be resistance on the grounds that there is no room in the curriculum. Recently, a student in a private secondary school that prides itself on the quality of its programs, said she would really like to discuss the issues but her teachers explained there wasn't the time if they were to cover all the work. Anyone acquainted with the history of the American school since World War II can genuinely sympathize with the argument that we have dumped on schools every conceivable social problem, reduced the time available for the established curriculae, and then blamed them for the declining student performance. We can hardly expect the schools to solve the problems of the nuclear threat. However, this topic is not some unrelated extra. It *is* the curriculum; it's science and history, literature and economics and drama. It's their life experience, a source of relevance and of motivation for students. The fourth objection is that the children are too young to comprehend anything about the nuclear threat, a strange objection considering that third and fourth graders have some horrible images about the dangers, even if distorted ones. However, we have reason to believe that any topic, no matter how complex, can be treated at a level appropriate to almost any age group.[5] Of course, as far as the early elementary grades are concerned, we would be particularly sensitive to their anxiety and would convey to them what efforts we are making to protect them. The fifth objection is an important one: It is unpatriotic to raise questions or encourage reading and discussion that lead students to find the policies of some of their government leaders to be irrational and indefensible. In fact, the contrary is correct; if our children are to develop as reasonable people and intelligent citizens, they need to be able to be critical. This, we must assert and insist, is the American way in its best tradition.

Children can be helped immeasurably by learning about competition and cooperation and, in particular, the psychological knowledge about what enhances a cooperative relationship. It is important for them to learn how essential it is to be able to appreciate the perspective of the other person, the other side, not only in international relations but in family relations as well, in relations between people, in relations between the sexes; to develop trust through social interaction, to have a stake in the other's welfare, a husband and a wife, as well as the Soviet Union and the United States.

So far applications have been made from the perspective of the school. There are obvious counterparts in other settings, e.g., the child, youth, and family serving organizations where mental health professionals can also make the nuclear war threat an ongoing agenda item at staff and association meetings and a consideration in assessing the sources of un-accountable anxiety. Professionals can also give special attention to the research necessary to identify those types of children who are particularly vulnerable to the periodic crises of brinkmanship. Some studies[1,10] are helpful in indicating the stressfulness of the early years when children feel particularly helpless, and in identifying conditions that appear to contribute to susceptibility to the deterioration of functioning, and those influences and conditions that seem to establish the capacity to cope with the environment and stress. Other studies[16] are suggestive of tempera-mental differences that may account for vulnerability. And some propose ways of training individuals in the use of roping skills.[9] (In addition, an early study by Escalona[6] addresses related issues.)

The application of the principles enumerated above, about addressing the psychological consequences of the nuclear war threat, is nowhere needed more than on television, that major educational force in the lives of children: and television, which is filled with so much brutality, need show no timidity concerning the brutality of programs devoted to nuclear war and the nuclear threat—only care that the programs explore the issues in rational ways with sound information and with no false hopes. But with realistic hope—hope based on ongoing programs of education for the people of our country, ongoing programs unrelentingly pursued. For if we survive, the nuclear threat that each new generation inherits is going to be a factor in the forseeable future. Instead of it being a source of terror and trauma, it can, with adult assistance and with adults as models, be transformed into social learning experiences that help rather than impede children's developing sense of identity, their mastery and strength.[3] That action could give them more reason to expect and to plan for a future, more desire to be an adult.

The young people who voice hope for survival, and who say they want to live and make a better world, echo the words Anne Frank[7] wrote the month before she was taken. She talked then about her circumstances, which were such as to shake anyone's ideals:

> It's really a wonder that I haven't dropped all my ideals, be-cause they seem so absurd and impossible to carry out. Yet

I keep them, because in spite of everything I still believe that people are really good at heart. I simply can't build up my hopes on a foundation consisting of confusion, misery, and death. I see the world gradually being turned into a wilderness, I hear the ever-approaching thunder, which will destroy us too. I can feel the sufferings of millions and yet, if I look up into the heavens, I think that it will all come out right, that this cruelty too will end and that peace and tranquility will return again.

Anne had only the heavens to look to, and a memorable work to write. We professionals must do more than look to the heavens.

REFERENCES

1. Anthony, E., Koupernick, C. and Chiland, C., eds. (1978). *The Child in His Family.* New York: John Wiley.
2. Beardslee, W. and Mack, J. (1982). The impact on children and adolescents of nuclear development. In *Psychosocial Aspects of Nuclear Development, Task Force Report #20.* Washington, D.C.: American Psychiatric Association, pp. 64–93.
3. Bandura, A. (1977). *Social Learning Theory.* Englewood Cliffs, N.J.: Prentice-Hall.
4. Brenner, M. (1973). *Mental Illness and the Economy.* Cambridge, MA: Harvard University Press.
5. Bruner, J. (1960). *The Process of Education.* Cambridge, MA: Harvard University Press.
6. Escalona, S. (1965). Children and the threat of nuclear war. In *Behavioral Science and Human Survival.* M. Schwebel, ed. Palo Alto, CA: Behavioral Science Press.
7. Frank, A. (1953). *The Diary of a Young Girl.* New York: Pocket Books.
8. Fussell, P. (1975). *The Great War and Modern Memory.* New York: Oxford University Press.
9. Meichenbaum, D. and Cameron, R. (1982). Stress-inoculation training: Toward a general paradigm for training coping skills. In *Stress Prevention and Management,* D. Meichenbaum and M. Jarenko, eds. New York: Plenum Press.
10. Murphy, L. and Moriarty, A. (1976). *Vulnerability, Coping and Growth.* New Haven: Yale University Press.
11. Nelson, J. (1982). Professor of Social Education, Rutgers University. Personal communication.
12. Roosevelt, E. (1953). Introduction. In *The Diary of a Young Girl,* A. Frank. New York: Pocket Books.
13. Schwebel, M. (1963). Students, teachers and the bomb. *National Education Association Journal.*
14. Schwebel, M. (1965). Nuclear cold war: Student opinion and professional responsibility. In *Behavioral Science and Human Survival.* Palo Alto, CA: Behavioral Science Press.
15. Schwebel, M. and Schwebel, B. (1981). Children's reactions to the threat of nuclear plant accidents. *American Journal of Orthopsychiatry,* 51(2):260–270.
16. Thomas, A. and Chess, S. (1977). *Temperament and Development.* New York: Brunner/Mazel.

18

Prevention of Children's Psychosocial Disorders: Myth and Substance

Michael Rutter

Institute of Psychiatry, London

A critical appraisal of primary prevention of children's psychosocial disorders indicates that our knowledge on this topic is limited and that there are few interventions of proven value. Nevertheless, there are possibilities for effective prevention. Myths associated with unwarranted claims for the value of prevention are reviewed in terms of unproven assumptions that: (1) prevention cuts costs; (2) prevention in childhood will improve adult health; (3) improved living standards will reduce mental illness; (4) sensible interventions can only be beneficial; (5) providing people with information leads to preventive action; (6) the main issue in prevention is implementing what we know; (7) the best approach is to tackle the basic cause; and (8) the crucial issue is to identify that one basic cause. Principles of causation are discussed and a model of causative influences is used to consider potentially effective primary prevention policies with respect to those directed at (a) individual predisposition; (b) ecologic factors; (c) influences on opportunity and situation; and (d) current stresses and strengths. It is concluded that a good deal is known about risk factors and the areas in which primary prevention might be effective, but that less is known concerning precisely how to intervene in order to bring

Reprinted with permission from *Pediatrics*, 1982, Vol. 70, No. 6, 883–894. Copyright by the American Academy of Pediatrics, 1982.

Presented as the Aldrich Award Lecture to the American Academy of Pediatrics, New Orleans, Nov. 1, 1981.

about the desired results. There is a potential for effective primary prevention but, so far, it remains largely unrealized.

To most people it seems obvious that prevention must be a good thing, and it is no surprise that the literature is full of books and articles with ringing phrases urging that more be done in the field of prevention. But how much do we really know about prevention in the field of psychosocial disorders of childhood? And is it necessarily the benign and helpful enterprise that it is usually portrayed to be? In his assay on meddling Lewis Thomas[1] took a rather skeptical view. He argued:

> Intervening is a way of causing trouble. . . . Whatever you propose to do, based on common sense, will almost inevitably make matters worse rather than better. You cannot meddle with one part of a complex system from the outside without the almost certain risk of setting off disastrous events that you hadn't counted on in other, remote parts. If you want to fix something you are first obliged to understand, in detail, the whole system. . . . Even then, the safest course seems to be to stand by and wring hands, but not to touch.

That sounds both destructive and discouraging and it contrasts starkly with the present great enthusiasm for prevention and the general feeling that appropriate and early psychosocial interventions ought to have a lasting beneficial influence on mental health and social functioning. But is this so, and are we yet in a position to advocate major preventive programs? Is the notion of effective prevention a myth or does it have substance? Critical appraisals of preventive policies have generally concluded that our knowledge on primary prevention is extremely limited and that there are very few interventions of proven value.[2-7] Nevertheless, also they emphasize that there are possibilities for effective prevention.

PROBLEMS IN PRIMARY PREVENTION

There are several key problems in carrying out successful primary prevention. First, there is a considerable gap between the identification of a damaging factor and knowledge on how to eliminate or reduce its effect.[8] Thus, it has long been clear that severe family discord puts children at an increased risk for conduct disorders and delinquency. But it is quite another matter to know what can be done to increase family harmony. Second, with but few exceptions, short-term improvements in a chronically depriving situation will rarely have long-term benefits.[9] To be effective in influencing ultimate levels of development, either the interventions must involve a lasting change (as is the case, for entirely different reasons, with both immunization and adoption), or the improved experiences will need to be available throughout the child's period of growth. The very best of summer camps for preschool children cannot be expected to have any substantial long-term benefits. Third, even when an effective measure is available, there may be problems in ensuring that it reaches all target populations. For example, effective means of contraception have been available for some years and their use has undoubtedly led to major changes in patterns of family building. On the other hand, there has been much less success in reducing unwanted births among teenagers.[5] Fourth, although for the most part "critical periods" of development do not exist, and thus it's never too late to intervene, nevertheless patterns of disadvantage and failure once established tend to persist. Accordingly, there is a need to start interventions early in children's lives.

Last, all programs of prevention must take into account the cost-benefits ratio.[7] This requires an assessment of the importance of the behavioral disorder that they are meant to influence; the likelihood of the measure making a real difference; the number of people who can be reached by the method of intervention; the disadvantages that come as side effects (almost no effective intervention is free of these); political and ethical considerations (such as the loss of personal freedom in the imposition of remedies); and the cost of the preventive measures in terms of finance, resources, and personnel. With these considerations in mind, before discussing the various possibilities of action that are open to us, let me consider some of the myths (or at least unproven assumptions) about prevention.

MYTHS

Prevention Cuts Costs

The first myth is the economic argument that necessarily effective prevention will cut medical expenditure. At first sight, it seems self-evident that this must be so. If you prevent a disease, then the costs of treating it are eliminated. However, that argument assumes that there is a fixed number of illness episodes, and that if you could prevent one, no other will come to take its place. Experience with physical disease immediately indicates that this argument is false. We have been enormously successful in preventing a number of the killing infectious diseases of childhood but medical costs have risen year by year. The point is that if people do not die of childhood illnesses, then they are likely to go on to suffer from many of the chronic illnesses of old age. No, we should not introduce prevention in the false hope that it will save money.

Effective Prevention in Childhood Will Improve Adult Health

The next myth is in many ways an extension of the first—namely, the notion that effective prevention in childhood will in some way improve adult mental health. Although early actions may be of some long-term benefit, it is important to recognize that many adult mental disorders do not have their roots in childhood and also that if we remove one set of environmental hazards, another set may well come to take their place. Just as the elimination of smallpox in childhood has had no effect on cardiovascular disease in adult life, so the reduction of emotional disturbance in childhood may make no difference at all to, say, schizophrenia or manic depressive psychosis in adulthood.

Improvements in Living Standards Will Reduce Mental Illness

The third myth is of a different kind. A common plea from social scientists or clinicians of liberal persuasion is for the nation to improve living standards in the expectation that this will improve mental health. This expectation is almost certainly false. Of course, we should work to eliminate poverty and to raise standards of housing, but that is because they are worthwhile goals in themselves, and not because their attainment will reduce rates of psychosocial disorder. But why is this a myth? Surely it is likely to help? After all, everyone knows that psychosocial problems of many kinds are much more common among the seriously deprived. Yes, indeed that is the case, but the causal inference is an uncertain one.[5,6] The association is based on cross-sectional data, and historical analyses give a rather different picture. In both Britain and North America there has been a major improvement in living standards during the course of the last 100 years. But these social gains have been accompanied by a worsening in many indices of disorder. Juvenile delinquency rates have increased greatly, and psychiatric conditions such as suicide and attempted suicide, anorexia nervosa, and alcoholism have also become more frequent among young people.[5,6] Unfortunately, the general expectation that raising living standards will improve mental health is misplaced. (It could be that the crucial feature is not the absolute level of affluence but rather the range of incomes or extent of inequality,[10] as there has been little diminution in the disparities between top and bottom incomes over this century. However, few data are available to test that hypothesis.)

Sensible, Humane Interventions Can Only Bring Benefits

The next myth is that sensible humane measures are bound to bring some benefits even if they do not eliminate the problem. Regrettably, that too is false. In the first place there are many basically sensible interventions that have proved to be of no benefit; for example, individual counseling as a means of preventing delinquency. From the original Cambridge-Somerville study[11] through the work of Tait and Hodges[12] to Craig and Furst[13] and others, this mode of intervention has consistently shown no benefits.[6] On the other hand, it may be argued that even if it did not help, at least it did not harm. But even that is not always the case. For example, there is some suggestion that the Cambridge-Somerville interventions may have had a slight effect in predisposing to a worse outcome,[14] and there are community-based behavioral treatments known to benefit delinquents but which are associated with an increased risk of delinquency when applied to predelinquents.[15] Or again there is the well known attempt by Cummings and Cummings[16] to educate a community in greater understanding and tolerance toward mental patients which seemed paradoxically to reduce acceptance of psychiatric disorder.

Provision of Information on Risks Will Lead to Preventive Action

A further myth is that the provision of greater information concerning serious risks and hazards in itself will lead people to take appropriate preventive action. Would that were the case, but unfortunately often it is not.

There are several problems in this connection. However, one of the most important is that human behavior is not wholly rational and that a knowledge of risks does not necessarily mean that people will take the appropriate action to avoid the consequences. For example, although health information has had some effect on smoking by adults, most antismoking campaigns in secondary schools have been singularly unsuccessful.[17,18] Telling youngsters that smoking will lead to cancer many years later is not sufficient to cause them to stop smoking.

Main Issue in Prevention Is Implementing What We Know

A commonly held belief, but one that constitutes a myth, is that the main issue in prevention is implementing what we know. The implication is that a combination of apathy, political obstruction, and special pleading has stopped effective prevention from being carried out.[19,20] Clearly, there have been political obstructions of various kinds and it is important that these be dealt with. But the main problem is that in most instances we do not know what to do. This assertion of ignorance may seem to be a curious statement in the light of the vast increase in knowledge over the last half century which has led to a fairly good understanding of many of the major risk factors. But what we do not understand nearly so well is the mechanisms that underlie the statistical associations, and even when we do understand those mechanisms, we have a very poor knowledge of how to prevent the risk factor arising or having its adverse effect.[8] Indeed, there is a danger that we may precipitously rush into the wrong action just because we do not understand why something is a risk. The claim by the World Health Organization in the early 1950s[21] that day care inevitably caused permanent mental damage to children is an obvious case in point. The recommendation to eliminate day care was based on the increasing awareness that children could suffer from "maternal deprivation" and it seemed prudent to avoid these risks. The trouble arose from the false assumption that day care necessarily involved deprivation. As we know now, day care can be beneficial, neutral, or harmful in its effects depending on the age and other characteristics of the child, and on the quality and nature of the care provided.[22,23]

Always Tackle the Basic Biologic Cause

A rather different myth is that it is always best to tackle the basic biologic cause, whatever that may be. Obviously, in the field of child psychiatry, there are many conditions that do not have a straightforward biologic cause of the kinds characteristic of internal medicine. But even when there is such a cause, it is not self-evident that it provides the best mode of intervention. For example, there are now many studies to show that children who suffer severe chronic malnutrition have impaired cognitive development.[24] It would seem obvious that the solution lies in feeding the children adequately so that their intellectual growth will proceed normally. Of course, it is desirable to feed the children. But what has been shown is that the provision of a better range of experiences and of personal interaction in the home may have at least as great an effect as the provision of food.[24,25] The point seems to be that malnutrition acts not only through direct effects on the brain (these do occur), but also in terms of the effects on interpersonal interaction. Weak, sickly children tend not to get the sort of experiences they need.

Crucial Issue Is to Identify the One Basic Cause

A further myth of a similar kind is that the crucial issue in prevention is the identification of the one basic cause of each disorder. Medicine teaches that there is a single basic cause for most conditions: the tubercle bacillus causes tuberculosis, and abnormalities in the production of insulin cause diabetes. The approach has paid off richly as the identification of specific causes has led to the development of specific remedies.[26] In psychiatry, too, it is likely that specificities of this kind may be discovered for some of the main disease states, although few examples have been found up to now. However, it is important to recognize that this is not the only causal question that can be posed.

Principles of Causation

First, the notion of a basic fundamental cause often requires a rather arbitrary decision on what to regard as the beginning.[5,9] This may be illustrated by considering the syndrome of so-called "deprivation dwarfism." This is a condition found in young children who usually come from grossly disturbed families and who are of extremely short stature. At first it was thought that a lack of love impaired growth even when the intake of food remained adequate. This now seems not to be the case, at least in most instances. The answer is more humdrum: the children have not received enough to eat. To that extent, the dwarfism is "caused" by starvation. However, that leaves open the question of why the children had not been adequately fed. The answer often lies in parental neglect, or the child's depression following chronic stress. Therefore, it could be said that parental neglect or lack of love is the real cause. But that only puts the question back one stage further. Why did the parents neglect the child? The answer may lie in current social disadvantage or in adverse childhood experiences that failed to provide the proper basis for parenting. Are these then the causes? Or do we also need to ask why this child was deprived rather than his brother? Perhaps the answer to that question lies in his temperamental makeup or the fact that his birth had been unwanted. Of course, in a sense all of these variables are causes, and appropriate action requires an understanding of the process as a whole.

The second point is that multifactorial causation is the rule for most psychosocial disorders. Of course, to some extent that is true with medical conditions generally. An example serves to emphasize how the most effective mode or point of intervention varies according to both the state of knowledge and the environmental circumstances. Tuberculosis is due to infection by the tubercle bacillus, and specific means of prevention and treatment are now available. However, malnutrition may also play a part in predisposition as shown by the fact that tuberculosis is still so common in parts of Asia and that it was rife in concentration camps during World War II. Improved standards of nutrition, and of public hygiene generally, might well do much to reduce susceptibility to tuberculosis if more specific remedies were not available; and even when they are available, a combined approach may be most effective of all.

The third point is that causation tends to be thought of in terms of the "who" question; that is, the reason why one person has a disorder or problem rather than another. That is a most important causal question. But it is not the only one, and in some circumstances it may not even be the most important. For example, we may need to ask the "how many" question.[9] The implications of the distinction are evident in the example of unemployment. The answer to the "who" question, i.e., why this man is unemployed rather than that one, comes down to personal factors in large part. Those who are old, who lack work skills, who have chronic physical incapacities, or who show marked personality disorders are the ones most likely to be left without jobs. On the other hand, these factors have little or nothing to do with the "how many" question, e.g., why the unemployment rate in many Western countries has risen so catastrophically over recent years. Here the answer is more likely to lie on the national or international economic situation, in political decisions, and in regional job opportunities. Whether the same applies in the mental health or social fields is uncertain. But, for instance, it may well be that the reasons why the delinquency rate has increased so much since World War II are different from the reasons why George becomes delinquent and Peter does not.[6]

The last point with respect to principles of causation is that in planning services it is not enough to know the reason why the disorders arise; we must also understand why they continue, and why they do or do not lead to functional impairment. For example, some 2.5% of the population are intellectually retarded insofar as they have a measured IQ

< 70. But only some of these people require special schooling because of educational difficulties or failure; others cope satisfactorily in ordinary school classes. Many boys have a propensity to behave in disruptive or disturbing ways. But whether this actually results in vandalism, or truancy, or scuffles in class depends on the school environment they experience.

It is evident that the concept of causation involves a variety of different processes and a range of points at which intervention may be effective (Figure). The types of causal processes may be summarized in the form of a model with four main headings: individual predisposition, ecologic

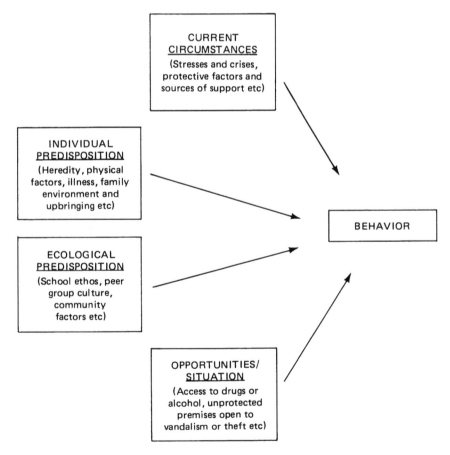

Figure. Simplified model of causative influences.

or group predisposition, current stresses or supports, and the prevailing situation or opportunities.

Individual predisposition may be shaped by genetic variables and by influences in the physical and psychosocial environment. Thus, in addition to hereditary factors as they apply to personality, intelligence, and mental illness, there are the effects of perinatal complications, postnatal trauma, or concurrent physical illness. But also, an individual's predisposition will have been influenced by the form of upbringing he has received—by the environment stresses and traumas experienced as a child, by the kind of love and discipline provided by his parents, by the values he has been taught, and by the social skills he has acquired.

Second, there is a different set of predisposing influences of a kind that apply to groups rather than to individuals. These may be subsumed under the general heading of ecologic predisposition. This would cover, for example, the effects of the social environment provided by schools. There is good evidence that children's behavior is strongly influenced by the ethos of the school they attend. Much the same applies to other social settings. Thus, young people's behavior is much influenced by the characteristics of the peer group of which they are a part,[6] and by the social role expectations relevant to the situations in which they find themselves. Also, under this same heading, there is a whole range of community and subcultural influences, together with the effects of the mass media, in increasing or decreasing the acceptability of particular forms of behavior.[5,6]

Third, a person's current circumstances must also be taken into account in terms of the stresses and supports for the individual. This heading would cover those acute life events such as the death of a parent, the loss of a job, a quarrel with girl friend, or public humiliation at school which may precipitate depression or a suicidal attempt or an act of vandalism. Also it would include those protective factors and sources of support (such as good, confiding relationships at home, or the satisfactions and high self-esteem associated with accomplishments in school or on the sports field), that may enable the young person to survive the crisis and cope successfully with the life stresses he is experiencing.

Last, there is the situation or the opportunities prevailing at the time. Thus, a girl may have become depressed because of her genetic predisposition, her susceptibility as a result of attending a school in a disintegrating neighborhood in which morale is low and the precipitating influence of the death of her best friend in a road accident. However, whether this results in suicide may also be influenced by whether or not lethal drugs are readily accessible to her at the time. Similarly, whether a troubled teenager becomes an alcoholic will be influenced by the cost and availability of alcohol; and whether a potentially disruptive adolescent engages in vandalism may depend on his being in the vicinity of a poorly lit street with an empty building left unsupervised and already identified as being a suitable target by the existence of broken windows left unrepaired.

Of course, these four sets of variables are not truly separate. There are complex interactions between them. Nevertheless, they provide a convenient way of considering possible modes of preventive intervention.

Last Myth: Possibilities of Prevention

The last myth is that we know so little that there is nothing we can do. There are dangers that ill-thought-out interventions may do more harm than good, and certainly there is a very considerable risk that we are going to promise far more than we can achieve. But these are reasons for caution and for thinking before we act, not reasons for not acting at all. Admittedly what we know is limited, but there are some things we can do now and it is our responsibility to see that the few effective interventions at our disposal are implemented.

PREVENTIVE POLICIES DIRECTED AT INDIVIDUAL PREDISPOSITION

In the field of psychosocial disorders the aim of policies directed at individual predisposition has usually been to provide some kind of experience that, it is hoped, will give the child strength to counter chronic stresses and disadvantages with which he/she has had to cope in growing up. There have been many unsuccessful attempts to intervene in this way. Nevertheless, there are some things that can be done.

General Health Measures

There is good evidence that young people with any form of organic brain dysfunction (such as cerebral palsy, epilepsy, or encephalitis) or with mental retardation have a much increased rate of psychosocial disorders.[27,28] Any measures that reduce the incidence of these conditions should have psychosocial benefits. In this connection there are a variety of actions that may be taken, but as most of these are well known,[7] I will not dwell on them here.

Prevention of Unwanted Births

Children whose birth was not wanted by their parents, or who were born to teenage mothers, or who were brought up in single-parent households, or who grow up in very large families are all subject to a substantially increased risk of psychosocial problems. Much could be done to reduce the disadvantage experienced by all these groups, but also it is important to reduce the number of unwanted births. This is no straightforward matter. The free availability of family planning services is one important step but it is not enough. Those most likely to produce unwanted children (young single people and those with personal and social problems) are those least likely to avail themselves of services. Usually it is not that they positively wish to conceive a child or that they have ethical objections to contraception, but rather that their difficulty in planning a family is merely one facet of a general feeling of hopelessness and inevitability, or of a pervasive lack of foresight in planning all aspects of their lives. Conflicts over sexuality and sociocultural attitudes also play a part in the lack of use of services. For these reasons, family planning must form part of a wider community service that is educational in its broadest sense.[5]

Provision of Continuity in Good Quality Parenting

Children who repeatedly go in and out of children's homes or foster homes or who live with their own parents in a severely unstable and unsettled family environment tend to have a high rate of psychosocial problems in adolescence. The same applies to young people who are reared in institutions with multiple changing caretakers.[29] Those from a similar background who are adopted or who receive long-term fostering in an ordinary family environment are much more likely to develop normally.

Accordingly, in the case of young children whose parents seem unlikely even to look after them at all adequately, an early decision should be taken with respect to adoption or long-term fostering.[5] It is not in the child's interest for there to be vacillation and indecision while he shuffles to and fro from his parents into and out of foster care; nor is it in his interest to remain for long periods in an institution in the forlorn hope that the parents who abandoned him and who now only visit sporadically will one day take him back. Children require stability and continuity in parenting. It is important that their needs be paramount in such circumstances. Adoption is the one intervention in early childhood that really makes a major environmental change that is often of long-term benefit to the child. Obviously there must be stringent legal safe-guards to ensure that children are not compulsorily removed from their parents without it being shown in court that this is a necessary step to ensure the child's well-being. As accurate knowledge on the likelihood of children being damaged by particular types of inadequate parenting is limited, there needs to be caution in advising that such removal is necessary. Also such removal should not take place (unless it is essential to preserve life), without strenuous and well-thought-out efforts made first to improve family circumstances and to help the parents in their task of child rearing. Such safeguards are essential both because of the great difficulties in making state provision of a quality that is up to even the average conditions in the ordinary family, and to protect parents from discriminatory intervention. Nevertheless it is not helpful for chil-dren to remain with parents who reject them, and cannot look after them properly, and who repeatedly give them up to foster care for short periods. In these circumstances it may be well to recognize that things are not going to improve and that it will be preferable for the child to receive long-term fostering to be adopted.

A related issue is the need to improve the quality of children's homes in order to meet the young children's psychosocial needs. It has proved possible to make residential nurseries for preschool children stimulating and interesting places with plenty of joint activities between staff and children. No longer need there be intellectual impairment associated with an institutional upbringing. However, it has proved much more difficult to ensure any kind of continuity in parenting. All too frequently the pattern is of a very large number of different and changing care-takers concerned with any one child during the preschool years. This is not a pattern conducive to normal social development[29] and ways must be found to improve this aspect of institutional life for young children. Of course an institutional upbringing should never be a first choice, but regrettably it is likely that there will always be circumstances in which no other alternative is available. We should strive to find better ways of dealing with family breakdown, but also we must take steps to ensure that, for those children who experience it, being brought up in a chil-dren's home is as positive and beneficial in its effects as we can make it.

Admission to Hospital

Repeated hospital admissions, especially in young children already experiencing chronic family adversity, is associated with an increased risk of psychosocial problems in later childhood and adolescence. Although the precise mechanisms whereby this leads to long-term disorder remain uncertain, a variety of steps can be taken to diminish the likelihood of psychological damage. These include, not only the provision of daily visiting or the opportunity for a parent to remain with the child during his stay in hospital and the improvement of conditions in the hospital itself,[29] but also various means of better preparing the child for hospitalization, as several controlled evaluation studies have demonstrated.[30,31]

Day Care and Working Mothers

In recent years more mothers of young children have been going out to work, and more young children have been experiencing various forms of day care. Professionals have reacted to this trend in different ways, some wanting to reverse the trend by paying mothers to stay at home with their children and some wanting to meet the needs by a major expansion in the state's provision of day care facilities. Yet others have seen the need to bring fathers more into child care or to provide more part-time work for women. The available research data do not allow any empirical basis for a choice between these and other alternatives, although certainly it is clear that the quality of care is crucial.[22,23]

For that reason there is everything to be gained from efforts to improve children's experiences in day care facilities of all kinds, whether they be day care centers, day nurseries, play groups, nursery schools, or private baby-sitters. Thus it is important that there be continuity in the staff who care for the children, so that each child has only a limited number of primary caretakers. But also there needs to be a sufficient number of staff to provide the children with play and conversation, with an adequate range of experiences and learning opportunities. The second immediate need is to ensure that the day care experiences enhance, rather than diminish, the parent-child interaction at home. This is not just a matter of including parents in the day care activities; this may not be possible with working parents, and indeed their presence at the central nursery may detract from their effective functioning if they are made to feel inexpert in contrast to the professionals looking after their children. Rather it is a recognition that day care should be viewed in terms of its effects on family life as a whole, and not merely as an experiential "input" to the child. Also it needs to be seen as an opportunity, if properly taken, to help parents better enjoy their children, understand their needs, and know how to play and talk with them. Many studies provide valuable leads on what may be done in this connection, but the merits and demerits of different approaches remain to be evaluated.

Three other areas of potentially effective prevention in relation to individual predisposition must be mentioned. It is well established that children being reared by mentally ill or criminal parents have a considerably increased risk of psychosocial problems. Much of the risk seems to stem from family difficulties, discord, and disturbance associated with the parental problems. Obviously, this provides an opportunity for preventive action but knowledge is lacking on how best to intervene effectively.

It is also well established that there are reasonably strong links between educational retardation and delinquency or other disturbances of conduct.[6] Although the mechanisms involved are both multiple and poorly understood, one factor seems likely to be the effect of severe reading difficulties in predisposing to emotional and behavioral problems through the experience of scholastic failure and its accompanying stigma. Insofar as that is the case, the effective prevention or remediation of reading and other scholastic difficulties should have psychosocial benefits, although this is yet to be demonstrated. Unfortunately, little is known about the best means of remedial treatment for children with severe reading retardation, and further research is much needed in this area.

It is obvious from all that I have said up to now that we should aim for an enhanced public awareness of children's needs, and that in particular we should do more to improve parental skills and sensitivities. Many parents fail to enjoy their children because they do not know how to play and talk with them; and discipline is a cause of strain and discord because parents set about it in the wrong ways. However, although that is generally recognized and accepted, there is considerable disagreement on just what to do about it. Clearly there is no one "right" way. The two most striking features of child care manuals over the years have been, first, that professionals have usually expressed considerable certainty at any one time on the best method of child rearing, and second, that their recommendations change each decade or so. Rather than a "best buy" on the techniques to follow, it is a question of appreciating the implications of individual differences; of understanding the meaning of children's sensitivities and signals; of developing coping strategies of learning when to persist and when to desist; of monitoring what is done to see if it works, and if not, why not; and most of all, of maintaining harmonious relationships in the home with respect to the different personalities, and different ways of doing things in the family. How should that be accomplished? Several studies[32-34] have produced valuable leads but no well-tested general answer is available.

Ecologic interventions constitute the second type of preventive measure. Human ecology refers to the study of the mutual interactions between man and his environment; it deals with systems rather than with individuals; and it is concerned with social groups in terms of their features as groups, rather than as unconnected individuals.[5,35] The implication is that groups have a life and force of their own that is both more than, and different from, the sum of the separate effects of the individuals in them. Ecologic interventions, in turn, are those that are best seen with respect to their impact on groups and the interaction of those groups within environmental settings. Perhaps the most obvious application of this approach is to schools, because they constitute social organizations with a recognizable boundary and purpose, and because research findings have shown that schools have important effects on young people's behavior and attainments.[36]

The first issue with respect to prevention possibilities arises from the observation that pupil outcomes tend to be worse in schools with a particularly high proportion of intellectually less able children. This is not just another way of saying that outcomes are usually less good for less able children (although obviously they are); but rather that for children of any level of ability outcomes tend to be less good if the bulk of the school population consists of children of below average intelligence. The implication is that there are considerable disadvantages in an educational system that allows such an uneven distribution of children that some schools have enrollments with a heavy preponderance of the intellectually less able. The findings point to the major drawbacks of either a community school system or an open market system. In the long term it is likely to be best when communities are sufficiently socially mixed so that community schools would fairly automatically get a reasonably balanced enrollment. Socially deprived ghettos have many other disadvantages and, quite apart from the benefits of schooling, it seems highly desirable that towns be planned to avoid that development. In the shorter term, there is no alternative to local authorities maintaining a degree of control over admissions to school to ensure a fair parity between enrollments. So far as possible this should be done in keeping with parental and child choice. This cannot happen so long as some schools are markedly inferior to others. The most urgent requirement is to improve the quality of schooling generally, and especially to upgrade the worst schools. If this happens, parental choice is unlikely to work against the need to make enrollments of different schools comparable.

A further issue is that the skilled management of classroom groups constitutes a crucial element in successful schooling, and moreover, that schools vary greatly in the support and guidance provided to teachers. There is a need for better in-service training, in which probationary teachers observe their senior colleagues at work and benefit from the comments and advice of those who have observed them teach.

Third, there is the most crucial question of all with respect to schooling, that of implementing change and maintaining success. Given that we have a notion of some of the features that make for successful schooling (these concern the social ethos or climate of schools as well as improved teaching methods and approaches), what needs to be done to ensure that the right kinds of changes are brought about in schools that are currently experiencing difficulties? The issue is a complicated one and further research will be needed before we can have a really satisfactory set of answers.

The main bulk of evidence on schooling suggests that the benefits are most likely to come from improvements in the social organization of schools and classes as a whole—through the setting of appropriately high standards of behavior and work, the provision by teachers of good models of behavior, the opportunities for pupils to take responsibility and to participate in the life of the school, the ample use of praise and encouragements, harmonious teacher-pupil relationships, and a sufficient staff consensus on the values and aims of the school as a whole. However, there is the further question of whether there is merit in preventive programs specifically designed to foster mental health or to alleviate emotional/behavioral difficulties at an early stage. There are a few studies that offer promise of benefits from programs of this kind[37,38] but, others have shown a lack of effect[39] and, at present, it remains unclear whether these constitute a worthwhile investment.[6] The matter warrants further investigation.

The idea of involving "the community" in preventive and therapeutic interventions of various kinds has become somewhat fashionable in recent years. There are now a handful of studies of various community development projects.[6] It is uncertain how much has been achieved in most of these, but certainly they include examples of constructive action. However, the ultimate value of this style of intervention remains to be determined.

There is good evidence indicating the importance of area influences in determining levels of child psychopathology.[6,9] In general, rates of problems tend to be high in inner city areas and lower in small towns. But there are exceptions to this tendency and it is not yet known what are the key variables.[40] Further research is urgently needed. The opportunity for primary prevention is undoubtedly present, but until the mechanisms or key variables can be identified, the opportunity for effective intervention remains potential rather than actual.

Various writers have argued that the concentration of high-risk families in any particular neighborhood affects the overall crime rate. In other words, a teenage boy from a high risk family is more likely to be delinquent if living in an area with a conglomeration of similar families than if he lives in a more mixed housing development. In fact, empirical data for adequate testing of these ideas are largely lacking.[6] It is apparent that the ways in which families with problems are distributed among neighborhoods may well influence the behavior of teenagers in those families; but there is a paucity of evidence on which to base policy recommendations. Nevertheless, the monitoring of natural experiments in terms of varying housing policy should provide both an answer and a guide to future housing policies.

There can be little doubt that, if skillfully employed, some types of propaganda can have sizeable effects on both attitudes and behavior (as shown for example by the success of sales campaigns in persuading mothers in developing countries to use powdered milk). It would be reasonable to suppose that it ought to be possible to harness this power in the interests of health education. However, the results up to now have been rather disappointing. The explanation almost certainly is not that the mass media cannot have an effect on the behavior of parents and children, but rather that we have not set about it in the right way.

PREVENTION THROUGH INFLUENCES ON OPPORTUNITY AND SITUATION

The field of prevention through interventions designed to affect opportunity and situation is one which has been long been part of police thinking with respect to crime;[6] but up until recently it has played little part in thinking about psychiatric problems. However, it is probable that the approach is more relevant than has usually been appreciated.

For example, there is good evidence from historical trends that the cost of alcoholic drinks bears a strong relationship to the per capita annual consumption of alcohol, which in turn is strongly related to the extent of alcoholism and of alcohol-related diseases. There are many reasons for supposing that the correlation represents a causal link. As the general level of alcohol consumption increases, so does the proportion of the population who suffer from alcoholism rise in parallel. Of course many factors will influence how much alcohol people will consume, but both economic influences (that is, through pricing) and formal controls (as through licensing) seem to play a part. There is a mass of evidence from data in many different countries that the price of alcohol is a major determinant of how much people drink. The implication is that if taxation is used to ensure that alcoholic drinks are relatively expensive, it is likely that this will limit the amount of alcohol that people consume, and this in turn will limit the extent of alcoholism. The evidence on the effects of licensing controls (such as those restricting the sales of alcohol to certain times, to certain stores, or to people above a particular age) is less clear-cut. It appears that major relaxations or tightening of controls probably do have some impact on alcohol consumption. For example, there was a 50% increase in alcohol consumption in Finland between 1968 and 1970 when extremely restrictive licensing controls were abruptly relaxed. Conversely, alcohol consumption in Britain fell by half during World War I when government restrictions were increased in an attempt to deal with the nation's lessened productivity that seemed to stem from excessive drinking. It is uncertain whether the growth of supermarket sales of alcoholic drinks has encouraged their purchase as part of routine weekly shopping, and hence has increased consumption; but it may well have done so.

In much the same way, access to drugs is likely to be of some importance in relation to the levels of drug abuse, and of successful and attempted suicide, all of which have been increasing among children and adolescents.[5] The very substantial reduction in the toxicity of domestic coal gas in Britain led to a dramatic decrease in suicides due to coal gas poisoning, and in the population as a whole it probably also led to an overall reduction in deaths due to suicide. Since the early 1960s there has been a marked decrease in self-poisoning by barbiturates and a threefold increase in posionings by psychotropic drugs, almost certainly reflecting changing patterns of prescribing habits. The present extremely high rate of prescribing of drugs acting on the CNS may well make self-poisonings more likely, both as a result of potentially toxic drugs being left lying around in a large proportion of households, and through the creation of an attitude of reliance on drugs to solve personal problems. Moreover, the extent to which prescribed drugs kill if taken in excess may well constitute one factor that plays a part in deciding whether an attempted suicide becomes a completed suicide. The greater safety of many of the more modern drugs probably is an advantage in this connection. Steps to persuade doctors to reduce prescriptions to a more acceptable level and steps to increase the safety of drugs would likely be beneficial.

The availability of addictive drugs is also likely to be of importance in the spread of drug abuse. There is evidence that the rates of use and abuse of any particular drug depend on the availability of that drug. Moreover, strict drug legislation has been effective in some cases. Effective control of the availability of addictive drugs should help to limit drug abuse.

Not much evidence is available on the value of diversionary measures in relation to prevention. On the other hand, high delinquency areas are often those with a striking lack of leisure facilities; delinquency rates go up during periods when adolescents are out of school and have no organized activities; unemployed adolescents are particularly likely to become involved in crime. Although the benefits remain unproved, it is desirable that adequate leisure facilities should be available in all areas where young people live and congregate.

Examples of the protective efficacy of physical design features[5,6] include the marked reduction in car thefts brought about by steering wheel locks, and the limiting of telephone booth vandalism in Britain through the extensive strengthening of equipment. It is not known how generally effective protective measures of this kind are, nor is it clear how often they serve only to "displace" vandalism from one site to another. Clearly not much is likely to be gained if one part of a public area is made vandal resistant while the immediately adjacent area is left unprotected. However, there seems to be a strong opportunistic element in vandalism committed by adolescents, and if the opportunities are not readily available, damage may not take place.

Research has shown that vandalism tends to be less in schools in which the buildings are well maintained and the decorations are kept in good condition.[36] Adolescents seem more likely to cause damage to property that has already been damaged or which appears abandoned or uncared for. There is an interesting report that when a London underground station that had been free of damage for many years had one ceiling panel broken, 30 more were broken in the following three weeks.[41] Satisfactory evidence is lacking, but the strong impression is that neglect leads to vandalism and that the rapid repair of damage may prevent further destruction.

Finally, under the general heading of influences and opportunity there is the crucial matter of surveillance. This is not just a question of supervision by police, caretakers, and the like. It is also clear that the role of the general public may be crucial.[6]

For example, there is the question of housing design. As Oscar Newman[42] put it,

> In a high rise building in which over a hundred families share an entry it is virtually impossible to distinguish neighbor from intruder or for anyone to attempt to enforce an acceptable mode of behavior or to feel comfortable about questioning the presence or activities of others.

The key physical variable seems to be the number of people involved in sharing a defined environment. The smaller the number of families sharing a facility, whether it's a demarcated portion of a project or the access and circulation space within a circumscribed portion of a multi-family building, the stronger are the feelings of possession, and ultimately of concern and responsibility. It should be appreciated that the main issue here is not space, although space helps, but design. High density neighborhoods can be built in a way that ensures that the streets and grounds are linked to specific dwellings (rather than left in the public domain), and that the building entries and accompanying space serve only a limited number of families.

There is also the separate issue of getting people in the community to take more interest and responsibility for the care of public facilities. In this connection there are some interesting examples of local efforts that appear to have been successful in reducing delinquency.[5] For example, there are several instances of contingency contracts in schools. There was one in Britain in which the pupils' side of the bargain was to keep the lavatories free of damage and graffiti for one summer term. In return, if they succeeded in doing that, Capital Radio would provide a disco. To most people's surprise, the scheme appeared to succeed. Or there is an example of a school in America in which the student body was provided with a set sum of money to cover window breakage, with the agreement that the student body could keep what was left over after payments for window repairs. The result was a dramatic reduction in window breakage.

Little systematic evaluation of preventive policies that affect opportunities has been undertaken up to now. Nevertheless, even from the slender leads so far available, it does appear that these approaches contain the possibilities of actions that could make a worthwhile (although limited) impact on certain forms of adolescent problems. The leads are worth following further.

CURRENT STRESSES AND STRENGTHS

The fourth potential area of intervention concerns current circumstances with respect to the level of stresses experienced, the coping methods possessed by children, and the protective or ameliorating factors that are available. It might be thought that this would be the major area for preventive action in that (at least in theory) it has the most direct connection with the development of disorders. However, surprisingly little is known about the role of stresses as precipitants of children's problems of any type,[43] and hence there is no ready point at which to obtain leverage for action. There is no doubt that further research is needed, both on the role of stresses and on the influence of protective factors. But regrettably, no immediate policy recommendations can be made with respect to preventive interventions in this field.

Of course, a considerable clinical literature has built up around the notion of crisis intervention as a means of preventing psychiatric problems. The idea has enormous appeal; in theory, it is brief, effective, strengthening, health-oriented, and capable of widespread community application. Unfortunately, apart from the already discussed actions in connection with hospital admissions there is very little evidence that it works. Indeed, the one study undertaken by Polak and colleagues[44] to evaluate crisis intervention following the sudden death of a family member (a situation in which there is good evidence that it is indeed a relevant stress) showed no benefits at all. Of course that does not mean that other forms of crisis intervention could not work, but it does imply that our level of knowledge in this area is not yet at a stage when it is possible to make recommendations on a community-wide application of this approach. The same applies to the availability of a supporting social network. There is good evidence for the importance of social supports in protecting people from emotional disturbance,[3,43] but little is known about the value of attempts to provide such supports for those individuals who lack them. The potential is there for prevention but it is yet to be realized.

SUMMARY

It is all too evident that the area of primary prevention of psychosocial disorders of childhood is indeed a minefield involving both the dangers of actually doing harm and the parallel danger of spending time and energies in well-meant activities that actually have no important effect. It is important that we do not oversell what can be achieved, because if we do, there is almost certain to be a backlash that will jeopardize the few effective modes of intervention that we do have at our disposal now.

The difficulty is not that there are no leads available. To the contrary, there are a multitude of leads. We know a good deal about the risk factors and the areas in which preventive intervention might be effective. What we know much less about is precisely how to intervene in order to bring about the results we desire. The implication is that we should move ahead to implement what we do know; to undertake systematic research, both to understand better the nature of children's stresses and their successful coping with them, and also to develop more effective methods of intervention; and finally to evaluate what we do. We should be optimistic for the future, but there is no easy road to success. Much needs to be done and much can be done, but there is no patent nostrum for the ills of society.

REFERENCES

1. Thomas L. (1979). On meddling. In *The Medusa and the Snail: More Notes of a Biology Watcher*. New York: Viking Press, pp. 110–111.
2. Bolman, W. M. and Bolian, G. C. (1979). Crisis intervention as primary or secondary prevention. In *Basic Handbook of Child Psychiatry: Prevention and Current Issues, Vol. 4*, I. N. Berlin and L. A. Stone, eds. New York: Basic Books, pp. 225–254.
3. Eisenberg, L. (1981). The research framework for evaluating the promotion of mental health and prevention of mental illness. *Public Health Report*, 96:3.
4. Graham, P. J. (1977). Possibilities for prevention. In *Epidemiological Approaches in Child Psychiatry*, P. J. Graham, ed. London: Academic Press, pp. 377–397.
5. Rutter, M. (1980). *Changing Youth in a Changing Society: Patterns of Adolescent Development and Disorder*. London: Nuffield Provincial Hospitals Trust, 1979. Cambridge, MA: Harvard University Press.
6. Rutter, M. and Giller, H. (1982). *Juvenile Delinquency*. Harmondsworth, Middlesex: Penguin Books, in press.
7. World Health Organization. (1977). *Child Mental Health and Psychosocial Development: Report of a WHO Expert Committee*. WHO Technical Report Series No. 613, Geneva: WHO.
8. Rutter, M. (1978). Research and prevention of psychosocial disorders in childhood. In *Social Care Research*, J. Barnes and N. Connolly, eds. London: Bedford Square Press.
9. Rutter, M. and Madge, N. (1976). *Cycles of Disadvantage*. London: Heinemann Educational Books, Ltd.
10. Braithwaite, J. (1979). *Inequality, Crime and Public Policy*. London: Routledge & Kegan Paul.
11. Powers, E. and Witmer, H. (1951). *An Experiment in the Prevention of Delinquency: The Cambridge-Somerville Youth Study*. New York: Columbia University Press.
12. Tait, C. D. and Hodges, E. F. (1962). *Delinquents, Their Families and the Community*. Springfield, IL: Charles C Thomas.

13. Craig, M. M. and Furst, P. W. (1965). What happens after treatment? *Social Service Review*, 39:165.
14. McCord, J. (1978). A thirty year follow-up of treatment effects. *American Psychologist*, 33:284.
15. O'Donnell, C. R., Lydgate, T. and Fo, W.S.O. (1979). The Buddy system: Review and follow-up. *Child Behavior Therapy*, 1:161.
16. Cummings, E. and Cummings, J. (1957). *Closed Ranks*. Cambridge, MA: Harvard University Press.
17. Holland, W. W. and Elliot, A. (1968). Cigarette smoking, respiratory symptoms and anti-smoking propaganda. *Lancet*, 1:41.
18. Thompson, E. L. (1978). Smoking education programs 1960–1976. *American Journal of Public Health*, 68:250.
19. Segal, J. (Ed.) (1975). *Research into the Service of Mental Health: Report of the Research Task Force of the National Institute of Mental Health*. DHEW Publication No. (ADM) 75–236. Washington, DC: Government Printing Office.
20. Keniston, K. and The Carnegie Council on Children (1977). *All Our Children*. New York: Harcourt, Brace, Jovanovich.
21. WHO Expert Committee on Mental Health (1951). *Report on the Second Session 1951*. Geneva: World Health Organization.
22. Belsky, J., Steinberg, L. P. and Walker A. (1982). The ecology of day care. In *Nontraditional Families: Parenting and Child Development*, M. Lamb, ed. Hillsdale, NJ: Lawrence Erlbaum.
23. Rutter, M. (1981). Social/emotional consequences of day care for preschool children. *American Journal of Orthopsychiatry*, 51:4.
24. Cravioto, J. and Arrieta, R. (1983). Malnutrition in childhood. In *Developmental Neuropsychiatry*, M. Rutter, ed. New York: Guilford Press, in press.
25. Grantham-McGregor, S., Stewart, M. and Powell, C., et al. (1979). Effect of stimulation on mental development of malnourished children. *Lancet*, 2:200.
26. Dollery, C. (1979). *The End of an Age of Optimism*. London: Nuffield Provincial Hospitals Trust.
27. Rutter, M., Tizard, J. and Whitmore, K. (1981). *Education, Health and Behaviour*. London: Longmans, 1970; Huntington, NY: Robert E. Krieger Publishing Co., Inc.
28. Rutter M. (1981). Psychological sequealae of brain damage in children. *American Journal of Psychiatry*, 138:1533.
29. Rutter, M. (1981). *Maternal Deprivation Reassessed*, 2nd edition. Harmondsworth, Middlesex: Penguin Books.
30. Ferguson, B. F. (1979). Preparing young children for hospitalization. A comparison of two methods. *Pediatrics*, 64:656.
31. Wolfer, J. A. and Visintainer, M. A. (1979). Prehospital psychological preparation for tonsillectomy patients: Effects on children's and parents' adjustment. *Pediatrics*, 64:646.
32. Cullen, K. J. (1976). A six-year controlled trial of prevention of children's behavioral disorders. *Journal of Pediatrics*, 88:662.
33. Gutelius, M. F., Kirsch, A. D. and MacDonald, S., et al. (1977). Controlled study of child health supervision: Behavioral results. *Pediatrics*, 60:294.
34. Dickie, J. R. and Gerber, S. C. (1980). Training in social competence: The effect on mothers, fathers and infants. *Child Development*, 51:1248.
35. Bronfenbrenner, U. (1979). *The Ecology of Human Development: Experiments by Nature and Design*. Cambridge, MA: Harvard University Press.

36. Rutter, M., Maughan, B. and Mortimore, P., et al. (1979). *Fifteen Thousand Hours: Secondary Schools and Their Effects on Children*. Cambridge, MA: Harvard University Press.

37. Cowen, E. L. (1971). Emergent directions in school mental health: The development and evaluation of a program for early detection and prevention of ineffective school behavior. *American Scientist*, 59:723.

38. Rose, G. and Marshall, T. F. (1974). *Counselling and School Social Work: An Experimental Study*. London: Wiley.

39. Kellam, S. G., Branch, J. D. and Aggawal, K. C., et al. (1975). *Mental Health and Going to School: The Woodlawn Program of Assessment, Early Intervention and Evaluation*. Chicago: University of Chicago Press.

40. Rutter, M. (1981). The city and the child. *American Journal of Orthopsychiatry*, 51:610.

41. Central Policy Review Staff (1978). *Vandalism*. London: HMSO.

42. Newman, D. (1975). Reactions to the "defensible space" study and some further findings. *International Journal of Mental Health*, 4:48.

43. Rutter, M. (1981). Stress, coping and development: Some issues and some questions. *Journal of Child Psychology and Psychiatry*, 22:323.

44. Polak, P. R., Egan, D. and Vandenbergh, R., et al. (1975). Prevention in mental health: A controlled study. *American Journal of Psychiatry*, 132:146.

19

Adolescent Development and Public Policy

Nicholas Hobbs and Sally Robinson

Vanderbilt University

Emphasis by psychologists on the importance of early experience led policy makers in the 1960s and 1970s to concentrate public resources on compensatory educational programs for young, disadvantaged children. Research on the reversibility of early cognitive deficits and on the remediation of poor school achievement suggests that an expanded national investment in developing the cognitive competence of adolescents and young adults is warranted. Public policy should encourage schools, youth-serving agencies, business and industry, and the military to provide educational programs that stress general problem-solving abilities and basic academic skills, rather than trade skills alone. Demographic observations underscore the importance of such a policy for the strength of the nation.

The thesis of this article is that current public policies concerned with human resource development are based on erroneous assumptions about cognitive development and that research of the past decade supports an expanded national investment in teaching cognitive skills to adolescents and young adults in schools, business and industry, and the military.

Reprinted with permission from *American Psychologist*, 1982, Vol. 37, No. 2, 212–223. Copyright 1982 by the American Psychological Association. Reprinted by permission of the publisher and author.

This article was presented by Nicholas Hobbs, the recipient of the 1980 Distinguished Professional Contributions to Public Service Award, at the meeting of the American Psychological Association, Los Angeles, August 1981.

Four strands in the development of thought about age, experience, and cognitive development are discernible. The strands are not precisely sequential but, rather, weave their way through the fabric of our understanding of cognitive competence.

1. First, there was the largely prescientific or philosophical emphasis on the importance of early experience in shaping development.

2. This was followed (in the 1920s–1940s) by research-based observations (as well as speculative comment) on the ontological development of behavior and its emergent character, with experience playing largely a triggering role, a theme given contemporary emphasis by ethologists and psychobiologists.

3. Then from the 1940s to the present, emphasis shifted back to the importance of the early years, this time buttressed by hundreds of investigations and pressed by advocates who profoundly influenced public policy.

4. Finally in the last decade there has emerged (or reemerged) a life-span perspective on age, experience, and cognitive competence, which has not yet had an influence on policy commensurate with its importance.

EMPHASIS ON EARLY YEARS

The importance of the early years in shaping the development of the individual is widely accepted. Few concepts are so generally endorsed; the notion has become embedded in the culture, with support from many quarters. Leon Yarrow (1961) writes: "The significance of early infantile experience for later development has been reiterated so frequently and so persistently that the general validity of this assertion is now almost unchallenged" (p. 459). The concept has had a profound effect on public policy in the United States, especially in the last two decades.

The prepotency of early experience was assumed by educational philosophers, including Plato, Quintillian, Locke, Rousseau, Mill, Pestalozzi, and Froebel (cited by Clarke & Clarke, 1976). An emerging science of behavior carried forward the philosophers' view. Itard (1932), inspired by Rousseau, attempted to educate "The Wild Boy of Aveyron," and his failure was well-known, strengthening the popular belief that early experience deficits are not reparable. Freud (1938) dramatized the enduring effects of early experience in his clinical studies of the effects of early trauma on adult character structure. The public remembered his dramatic cases relating early experience to adult neurosis but overlooked his biological determinism. John B. Watson's (1928) behaviorism reinforced the Freudian contention; his "give me a dozen healthy infants" promise was widely quoted in the Sunday supplements in the 1920s, and his ideas on early childhood profoundly affected child-rearing manuals such as the federal government's *Infant and Child Care*.

THE "UNFOLDING" EMPHASIS

Interestingly enough the first early and rigorous experiments from psychological and physiological laboratories suggested that experience, early or late, is of little importance in behavioral development; these studies suggested that behavior unfolds as a consequence of structural development, more or less independently of experience. Coghill (1929) demonstrated that the orderly cerebro-caudal development of the salamander was paralleled by the emergence of behavioral capabilities; he asserted that experience did not affect the process. Carmichael (1926, 1927, 1928) anesthetized salamanders to prevent early practice in swimming; later put in clean water, the salamanders swam with age-appropriate skill. Cruze (1935) studied the effect of practice on the pecking efficiency of chicks raised in darkness and concluded that the pecking response unfolded automatically and that a more mature chick required less practice than a younger one to perfect the response. Shirley (1931, 1933) reached similar conclusions about the motor development of young children. Myrtle McGraw (1935) taught identical twins to swim, one earlier than the other; the delayed learner learned faster than the one with early practice and caught up quickly. Dennis and Dennis (1940) showed that Hopi Indian babies, traditionally immobilized on a carrying board for the first year of life, walked at the appropriate age with little practice. In the 1930s the IQ was considered immutable by most psychologists; Wellman, Skeels, and Skodak were ridiculed for suggesting otherwise (McNemar, 1940). Experiments with children in schools by Gates and Taylor (1925), Gesell and Thompson (1929), and Hilgard (1932, 1933), and others emphasized the importance of maturation in learning; for example, children learn to read more rapidly at seven than at four. Generalizations drawn from such studies led to two or three decades of educational policy emphasizing the unfolding of the child and the avoidance of overstimulation in the early years. For example, a study (Thomson, 1934) described as "an experiment that may revolutionize the traditional idea that reading must begin with the first grade" concluded:

As reading requires the use of accurate and abstract powers, it was recommended that an age level of six or seven years chronologically be attained before children were offered definite reading opportunities. For it seemed evident that though children have sometimes learned to read a year earlier, such learning was attended by much nervous strain, resulting in the growth of undesirable social and emotional habits and in the loss of many longed-for experiences with "things." (p. 445)

See also Morphett and Washburn (1931).

RENEWED INTEREST IN EARLY EXPERIENCE

Then the pendulum swung, pushed by new developments in research and theory. Dennis and Dennis (1941) revised their views on the basis of further observations of the development of twins reared with good physical care but with minimum stimulation. The problem was that although some behaviors appeared without apparent antecedent experience, others did not. Gradually psychologists began to join with philosophers in emphasizing the importance of early experience for full development of the individual. Among the studies that led to this new (but old) position were such diverse investigations as the following: Burtt's (1932) study of the long-term memory of Greek read to his son between the ages of 15 months to 3 years and tested at 18 years; Cruze's (1935) further experiments on the effect of stimulation of chicks' pecking behavior; Hunt's (1941) study of early food deprivation and adult hoarding behavior in the rat; McGraw's (1939) follow-up study of the effects of motor training in infancy; Spitz's (1945, 1946a, 1946b) clinical studies of anaclitic depression in institutionalized orphaned infants and its reported long-term effects; Goldfarb's (1943a, 1943b, 1943c, 1944, 1945, 1947) follow-up study in adolescence of 15 pairs of children, one of the pair institutionalized early and the other placed in a foster home; Bowlby's (1951) classical accounts of maternal deprivation and its effect on the subsequent mental health of the individual; Hess's (1958, 1964) and Lorenz's (1965) studies of imprinting; Dennis and Najarian's (1957) comparison of institutionalized infants with those who had more opportunity for stimulation; Harow and others' (Harlow, Harlow, Schlitz, & Mohr, 1971; Harlow, Schlitz, & Harlow, 1969) studies of the effects of early maternal deprivation on the social and sexual behavior of the adult rhesus monkey; Dennis's (1960) observations of motor development of children in an orphanage; Rosenzweig and others' (Krech, Rosenzweig, & Bennett, 1962; Rosenzweig & Bennett, 1976; Rosenzweig, Krech, & Bennett, 1960; Rosenzweig, Krech, Bennett, & Diamond, 1962) studies of early experience and brain mass in rats; Bettelheim's (1967) clinical accounts of infantile autism that treated as causal inadequate mothering during a "critical period" in early development; and to bring this far-from-complete catalogue of studies to a close, O'Connor's (1980; O'Connor, Vietze, Sherrod, Sandler, & Altemeier, 1980) recent studies on infant-mother bonding in the first hours of life, which report correlations with subsequent parent–child relationships, including the possibility of predicting child abuse. Hunt (1979) has recently provided a highly valuable summary and synthesis of early experience and psychological development. The general academic wisdom of the 1970s is well stated by Bettye Caldwell (1973): "Considerable research evidence has converged to suggest that the first three years of a child's life represent the most important period for primary cognitive, social, and emotional development and it is during this period that the environment will exert maximum effect for either facilitation or inhibition of the child's genetic potential for development" (p. 24).

EARLY YEARS AND PUBLIC POLICY

Evidence for the importance of early experience for later development was brought together and persuasively interpreted in two books that had a profound impact on public policy. One was J. McV. Hunt's *Intelligence and Experience* (1961) and the other was Benjamin Bloom's *Stability and Change in Human Characteristics* (1964). They provided, along with Michael Harrington's (1962) book on poverty, intellectual inspiration for important aspects of the Great Society programs. Hunt (1961) summarized the emerging view this way: "It is no longer unreasonable to consider that it might be feasible to discover ways to govern the encounters that children have with their environments, *especially during their early years of development*, to achieve a substantially faster rate of intellectual development and a substantially higher adult level of intellectual capacity" (p. 363; emphasis added). Gray and Klaus (1965; Klaus & Gray, 1968), in their early intervention studies, demonstrated effective ways to govern children's encounters with their environments. Sargent Shriver knew firsthand of their pioneering work and, as a consequence, was ready to intervene early in the lives of disadvantaged children as a major strategy in the War on Poverty.

Public policy from the Johnson years to the present reflects, for the most part, the assumption that the early years are the important years for intellectual development and that there is little to be gained by efforts to enhance cognitive competence after childhood. Head Start, for children ages three to five, is the nation's single most comprehensive child development program, costing about $820 million a year. When early research dampened some of the confidence in the efficacy of Head Start, the remedy was to start earlier and then to follow-up in the elementary school years. Thus Home Start, Parent and Child Development Centers, and Follow-Through were initiated. The federal government's largest investment in the schools of the nation is through Title I of the Elementary and Secondary Education Act, passed in 1965 as part of the War on Poverty. It provides funds for compensatory education for economically and educationally disadvantaged children, again with a focus on the early years. Seventy-five percent of the $2⅓ billion appropriated for the annual (1978–1979) support of Title I programs goes to children in grades 1–6 and 7% to children in preschool programs, whereas only 18% goes to students in grades 7–12.

In the early 1970s, in response to public concerns about alienated and disruptive youth, three national panels (Brown, 1973; Coleman, 1974; Martin, 1976) concluded that high schools contribute to the alienation of some youth and recommended that educational alternatives, that is, jobs or job training, be provided for adolescents not responding to schooling. Several states have lowered, and others are considering legislation to lower, the upper limit of the compulsory school age, usually from 16 to 14, thus reversing a trend of 150 years to extend schooling upward (Stipek, Note 1). The possibility of reforming secondary schools to nurture cognitive development seems not to have been sufficiently considered as a possible solution, probably because of the belief that by the adolescent years, it is too late to make any difference in the development of cognitive competence.

Federal support for youth training and employment programs increased dramatically during the last two decades, authorized through the Manpower Development and Training Act (1962), the Economic Opportunity Act (1964), the Comprehensive Employment and Training Act (1973), amendments to the Vocational Education Act (1976), the Career Education Incentive Act (1977), and the Youth Employment and Demonstration Projects Act (1977), later subsumed under the now defunct Comprehensive Employment Training Act (CETA) program (National Commission for Employment Policy, 1979). In these programs as well as in programs to increase the competence of adolescents and young adults in business and industry, emphasis is placed almost entirely on the development of specific job-related skills and not on the development of general cognitive competence. The same is true of training programs in the military.

EVIDENCE FOR THE CONTINUED MODIFIABILITY OF ORGANISMS

We now review the evidence for the continued development of cognitive competence beyond the childhood years and for the possibility of repairing developmental deficits resulting from early trauma or deprivation in mice and humans. The review, in our judgment, opens up new vistas for remedial and compensatory interventions in later childhood and adolescence and offers a new foundation for public policy in human resource development.

Novak and Harlow (1975; Suomi & Harlow, 1972) have demonstrated that the earlier reported devastating effects of early isolation on adult adjustment in monkeys can be reversed by appropriate interventions. Cairns and Nakelski (1971) have reported similar findings with mice. Hess (1972) has shown that ducklings imprinted to follow a human can quickly be taught to follow a mallard, long after the critical imprinting period. Davis (1940, 1947) and Koluchová (1972, 1976) studied the effects of remedial programs on children raised in extreme isolation and found, contrary to Itard's experience, that they were remarkably responsive and achieved essentially normal levels of intellectual functioning. A number of investigators, including Clarke and Clarke (1954, 1959), Rutter (1971, 1972), Skodak and Skeels (1949), Skeels (1966), Lewis (1954), and Rathburn, Di Virgilio, and Waldfogel (1958) studied children who were moved from unfavorable environments (such as an institution for the mentally retarded or refugee camps for orphaned children) to favorable environments (such as foster-home placement) and reported substantial gains in cognitive development and general adjustment. Kagan and Klein (1973) studied infants and children living in an isolated, subsistence farming village in the highlands of Guatemala. The Guatemalan children were substantially delayed in development by American norms but by age 10 had achieved competencies comparable to American children. On the basis of his studies and others cited, Kagan (1976) concludes:

> The data offer no firm support for the popular belief that certain events during the first year can produce irreversible consequences in either human or infrahuman infants. If one limits the discussion to universal cognitive competencies, in

> contrast to culturally specific skills, it appears that a slower
> rate of mastery of the universal abilities during the first two
> years places no serious constraints on the eventual attainment
> of many of the competencies of pre-adolescence. (p. 121)

It is widely believed in the United States that early labeling of children has a long-lasting, damaging effect on them (Schur, 1971). Actually the evidence for this belief is essentially nonexistent; what we do have evidence for is the deleterious effects of the consequences of labeling. For example, long-term placement of a child in an impoverished learning environment, such as an institution for the mentally retarded, may seriously limit cognitive development (M. T. Hobbs, 1964). But even these long-term effects are in some measure reversible (Tizard & Rees, 1974).

Results of studies of formal efforts to modify the course of cognitive development in childhood through compensatory education programs were initially disappointing. A couple of years after Project Head Start got underway, studies began to appear suggesting that its effects were modest and transient, fading away in the early years of school. So, too, with early studies of the effectiveness of Elementary and Secondary Education Act (ESEA) Title I programs. These negative studies influenced political sentiments of the time responsive to the idea that "nothing works." In 1969 President Nixon expressed the sentiment of the times in his educational message to the Congress: "We must stop letting wishes color our judgments about the educational effectiveness of many compensatory programs—despite some dramatic and encouraging exceptions—there is growing evidence that most of them are not yet measurably improving the success of poor children in school." Now we have evidence that cognitive competence, academic aptitude, and staying power in school can be increased in childhood. We would cite Heber and Garber (1975), Frank Porter Graham Center (1981), Lazar and Associates (Note 2, Note 3), Bronfenbrenner (1974), and especially the important recent book by Gray, Ramsey, and Klaus (1981). The recently completed and impressive study of ESEA Title I programs by the National Institute of Education (1978) is of utmost practical importance in demonstrating that compensatory programs can work on a widespread nonexperimental basis. The question now seems to be not whether cognitive competence can be taught but under what circumstances it can be taught.

From the weight of evidence reviewed thus far, we reach these tentative conclusions:

1. That the early years are important for the development of the

human individual, but that this does not mean that later years are unimportant;

2. That the concept of critical ages for the influence of experience on
cognitive development of the human is fragile;

3. That the child is remarkably resilient and resistant to adverse environmental effects, if not prolonged indefinitely; and

4. That early deprivations in experience can be repaired, but that it
takes sustained or even ingenious effort to do so.

None of these conclusions bears directly on the modifiability of cognitive
competence in adolescence, but they do clear the ground of presup-
positions that interventions must be initiated at very early ages to be
effective. Unfortunately the widely accepted belief in the crucial importance of the early years in human development has influenced not only
public policy but research programs as well. Research bearing on the
modifiability of cognitive functioning in adolescence and the early adult
years is scarce, but we believe it is sufficient to call for a reordering of
research priorities as well as to suggest new public policy strategies.

COGNITIVE DEVELOPMENT AND MODIFIABILITY IN ADOLESCENCE

We turn now to an appraisal of the adolescent years with respect to
the effects of experience on the development or acquisition of (a) intelligence, (b) academic skills, and (c) general problem-solving competence. It would be interesting if this appraisal of potential for cognitive
development in adolescence could be supported by quotations from educational philosophers back to Plato, as was possible for the so-called
formative years. Instead we must recognize that adolescence is a recent
phenomenon closely linked to social and economic conditions of the last
century in the United States and Europe, a period of delay in the transition from childhood to adulthood. Whereas the onset of adolescence
is signaled by relatively clear-cut biological events, the ending is a poorly
defined social event, responsive to current expectations for schooling,
work, and marriage. Formal rites of passage to mark emergence from
adolescence are conspicuously absent in Western culture. Bakan (1971)
dates the philosophical beginning of adolescence from the following
statement in Rousseau's (1762/1966) novel *Emile*, "We are born, so to
speak, twice over; born into existence, and born into life; born a human
and born a man" (p. 172). Perhaps adolescence offers a second chance.
We must balance our optimism with two caveats, however: (1) Research
on cognitive functioning in adolescence is limited, and many studies are

flawed by almost insurmountable sampling problems, and (2) to reiterate one of the conclusions reached after reviewing intervention programs in early childhood: "early deprivations in experience can be repaired, but . . . it takes sustained or even ingenious effort to do so." In assessing the promise of the adolescent and young-adult years for enhancing competence, we must avoid the error made by psychologists in the early 1960s in promising too much too soon with regard to intervention programs in early childhood. Indeed, we shall see if we are intelligent enough to profit from experience in those efforts to contribute to public policy.[1]

1. *Intelligence.* Numerous early studies (Bayley & Oden, 1955; Freeman, 1936; Jones & Conrad, 1933; Owens, 1953, 1966; Shock, 1951; Thorndike, 1948) have shown that intelligence as measured by conventional tests continues to rise in early adolescence, begins to level off in later adolescence and early adulthood, roughly from 16 to 22 years of age, and then to decline in later years, with conspicuous individual differences in rates of decline. More recent studies done from a life-span developmental perspective have seriously challenged the inevitability of decline in intelligence in later years (Birren & Schaie, 1977). Schaie and Strother (1968a, 1968b) demonstrated that earlier reports of decreases in intelligence after adolescence can be accounted for in large part by cohort differences and that when the same group of adolescents is followed over time, performance on intellectual tasks continues to improve into the adult years. Baltes and Schaie (1976) have emphasized the plasticity of intelligence in adulthood and the need to study the effects of alternative contexts on intellectual functioning. Nancy Bayley (1970) and others have convincingly demonstrated that the decline in intelligence scores in later years is less for people who continue to engage in work requiring the use of intellectual abilities than for those not so engaged. Since intellectual development is demonstrably affected by experience in childhood and in later life, it is not unreasonable to expect experience to affect intelligence in the adolescent years, though research demonstrating this is sparse. Two studies of large cohorts in Sweden (Husen, 1951; Harmquist, 1968) suggest that higher intelligence is associated with staying in school to an extent that cannot be accounted for by differential dropout rates.

---

[1]This section draws heavily on excellent papers by Deborah J. Stipek (Note 1) and by Mary Carol Day (Note 4).

2. *Academic skills.* As for the acqusition of basic academic skills—the ability to read, write, spell, and do arithmetic—without which intelligence simply cannot be exercised in a complex society, current evidence is considerably more promising than evidence from earlier studies. The profoundly influential assessments of Coleman (Coleman, Campbell, Hobson, McPortland, & Mood, 1966) and of Jencks (1972) led to the pessimistic conclusion that formal schooling can do little to repair the academic deficits engendered by impoverished family backgrounds. Such impoverished children are "born to fail," to use Mia Kellmer Pringle's (1971) powerful construction. The evidence now seems to be that they are indeed born to fail in traditional schools, but skillfully designed and executed compensatory education programs from preschool through high school can more than repair early deficiencies. We base this conclusion on the impressive, nationwide evaluation by the National Institute of Education (1978) of Title I programs of the Elementary and Secondary Education Act of 1965. This thoroughgoing study demonstrated that academic skills can be taught efficiently at any age up through adolescence. But school programs must respond with imagination and tenacity to the challenge of overcoming early deficiencies; they must give children and adolescents the basic skills necessary to get and keep a job, to negotiate with society's institutions, and to live satisfactory and satisfying lives. Evaluation of scattered demonstrations such as those funded by the California Demonstration Projects Act suggests what characteristics of curricula, teaching methods, and other aspects of schooling are effective with students in secondary schools (Larson & Dittman, 1975; Tinto & Sherman, Note 5). One appealing approach to teaching basic skills to older children and adolescents, especially those not culturally attuned to academic learning, is to transfer to regular classrooms strategies and techniques developed in special education (Hobbs, Bartel, Dokecki, Gallagher, & Reynolds, 1979).

We find especially heartening the comprehensive studies of secondary schools in England by Michael Rutter and his associates (Rutter, Maughan, Mortimore, & Ouston, 1979). They found that adolescents learn well in some schools and poorly in other schools and that the major source of the variance was the character of the schools:

> The differences between schools in outcome were systematically related to their characteristics as social institutions. Factors as varied as the degree of academic emphasis, teacher actions in lessons, the availability of incentives and rewards, good conditions for pupils, and the extent to which children

were able to take responsibility were all associated with outcome differences between schools. All of these factors were
open to modification by the staff, rather than fixed by external
constraints. . . . The total pattern of findings indicates the
strong probability that the associations between school process
and outcome reflect in part a *causal* process. In other words,
to an appreciable extent children's behavior and attitudes are
shaped and influenced by their experiences at school and, in
particular, by the qualities of the school as a social institution.
(pp. 178–179)

3. *General problem-solving ability.* Thus far our discussion embraces intellectual development as measured by conventional intelligence tests,
which do not capture transformations in cognitive capacity from childhood to adolescence, such as those underscored by Piaget's developmental theory (Inhelder & Piaget, 1958). Piaget posits a qualitative shift
in the nature of intelligence in the adolescent years, from the concrete
operational stage of childhood to the formal operational stage of adolescence. The adolescent becomes capable of formal thought, that is, the
ability to treat events abstractly, to subordinate the real to the possible,
to use metaphor in construing the world, to engage in hypothetico-de-
ductive thought, to manipulate combinatorial systems, to use internalized
speech, to think about thinking, to use namable strategies for problem
solving, and to monitor his or her own thought. The changes that begin
to occur around 11–12 years of age "constitute a major revolution in the
individual's way of thinking about the world, and these changes continue
to occur throughout the period of adolescence" (Day, Note 4, p. 1).
Adolescent thought appears to be more like adult thought than like the
thought of the child, thus making adolescence a period of crucial importance for the nurturance of general cognitive competence.

Yet not all adolescents achieve the ability to distance themselves from
a problem and address it with formal problem-solving strategies; indeed,
some people never achieve an adequate level of formal operational ability. Elkind (1973) has suggested, on the basis of his clinical work, that
experience may play a large role in the differential application of formal
operations. He has identified two types of low-income adolescents who,
as a result of their experience, prematurely structure their intelligence
or elaborate their intellectual abilities in alternative ways not usually
assessed by standard measures. Other adolescents may fail to demonstrate latent competence in formal operations because they do not recognize what strategies or knowledge are appropriate to a given situation

(Day, Note 4, p. 7). Preliminary conclusions to be held with varying levels of confidence until the research base has been more firmly established suggest:

1. The preformal stages in Piaget's developmental scheme may be acquired without schooling, but experiences like those provided in secondary schools are necessary to develop formal operational ability (Ashton, 1975; Cole & Scribner, 1974; Goodnow, 1962; Goodnow & Bethon, 1966; Luria, 1971; Pellufo, 1967; Scribner & Cole, 1973; Sharp, Cole, & Lave, 1979). "Formal schooling . . . appears to increase one's ability to engage in second-order processes, e.g., to deliberately invoke mnemonic strategies for memorization, to think about and formulate into a rule the manner in which a problem has been solved and then to transfer the rule to other problems, and to describe to others the cognitive activities that have been employed on a task" (Day, Note 4, p. 48).

2. The achievement of formal operational competence is related to success in learning scientific and mathematical concepts (Collis, 1971; Lawson & Nordland, 1977; Lawson & Renner, 1975) as well as in other domains where systematic thought is required, such as the humanities (Peel, 1971). These subjects, as currently taught, do not always encourage the development of second-order thinking (Chiappetta, 1976).

3. Although studies available are few in number, they do suggest that formal operational strategies can be taught to adolescents and, in some instances, to preadolescents (Bloom & Broder, 1950; Danner & Day, 1977; Lawson & Wollman, 1976; Siegler, Liebert, & Liebert, 1973; Day, Note 4).

Although the research evidence is as yet limited, we conclude that the "transformation in thought" that occurs in the adolescent years is essential for coping with the intellectual tasks of a complex society, that the transformation does not occur automatically, that schooling without specific instruction in formal operational procedures nonetheless is essential for their development, and that formal operational procedures can be taught deliberately. In this set of observations rests, it seems to us, an exciting opportunity for exploration of the possibility of substantially raising the level of cognitive competence of adolescents and young adults in the nation.

THE WORK OF FEUERSTEIN

We have noted the paucity of research on cognitive development in adolescence (Elkind, 1975). The resulting deficit in knowledge has severely constrained public investments in compensatory education programs beyond the childhood years. Reuven Feuerstein, Israeli psychologist, promises to remedy this knowledge deficit through his own research and through the stimulation his ideas will bring to the field. Feuerstein has recently published two books (1978, 1979) reporting 25 years of research on cognitive development in older children, adolescents, and young adults. Inspired by Jean Piaget and André Rey at Geneva, Switzerland, Feuerstein initiated work leading to "a radical shift from a static to a dynamic approach in which the test situation was transformed into a learning experience for the child" (in the Learning Potential Assessment Device) and, ultimately, to a formal instructional program (the Feuerstein Instrumental Enrichment Program) designed "to change the cognitive structure of the retarded [read as *delayed* or *ineffectual*] performer and to transform him into an autonomous, independent thinker, capable of initiating and elaborating ideas." We quote from the foreword to the book *Instrumental Enrichment*:

> Although Feuerstein's work is based on extensive experience with Israeli adolescents who were retarded in intellectual performance for reasons associated with their diverse cultural origins, disrupted lives, and limited opportunities to learn, he in fact provides the foundation for a general theory of cognitive competence, coupled with a technology for assessing learning potential and for repairing functional deficits in the cognitive process. Feuerstein is concerned generally with the ability to learn and solve problems; with why this ability fails to develop in the absence, during early childhood, of systematic learning mediated by a caring adult; and how, much later than generally thought possible, identified cognitive deficits can be remedied by a formal instructional program. Thus the significance of his work extends substantially beyond its implications for programs for retarded performers—to, for example, general programs of child care and parent education, as well as to programs to enhance the cognitive competence of adolescents. (Hobbs, 1979)

Concurrently with the development of Feuerstein's thought, Luis Alberto Machado of Venezuela (1980) began to urge steps to narrow the gap between human potential and human achievement. In 1979 Venezuela established a Ministry of State for the Development of Human Intelligence and appointed Machado to head it.

Feuerstein's methods have been used extensively in Israel in clinics, schools, and the defense forces. Recently published research shows that Israeli soldiers who completed the Instrumental Enrichment program performed significantly better on conventional tests of intelligence and achievement than did a comparison group that received a traditional educational enrichment program and, further, that in a follow-up study, the Instrumental Enrichment group continued a linear gain in cognitive competence for 2½ years without instruction. The structural changes induced by Instrumental Enrichment appear to be continuous and cumulative (Feuerstein, Miller, Hoffman, Rand, Mintzker, & Jensen, 1981).

Feuerstein's theories and methods are undergoing large-scale tests in the United States and Canada, directed by H. Carl Haywood (Arbitman-Smith & Haywood, 1980; Haywood & Arbitman-Smith, 1981). The research program, though extensive, is far from complete. The record is not yet in and conclusions must be guarded, but the early studies are promising and they do permit one, as Haywood says, "to speak in a soft voice" of the effectiveness of Instrumental Enrichment programs. They tend to fortify the conclusions of the Clarkes (Clarke & Clarke, 1976) that "the worse the early social history, the better the prognosis for change" (p. 72) and that "what one does for a child at any age, provided it is maintained, plays a part in shaping his development within the limits imposed by genetic and constitutional factors" (p. 273).

CONCLUSIONS AND IMPLICATIONS FOR PUBLIC POLICY

We couch our conclusions in quotations from others who have committed themselves deeply to understanding cognitive development in childhood, adolescence, and the adult years:

First, Feuerstein (1979): "Except in the most severe instances of genetic and organic impairment, the human organism is open to modifiability at all ages and stages of development" (p. 9).

Then, Clarke and Clarke (1976): "The whole of development is important, not merely the early years. There is as yet no indication that a given stage is clearly more formative than others; in the long-run, all may be important" (p. 272).

Then, Zigler and Cascione (1977):

> It is a mistake to try to isolate some critical (magical?) period in the life of the child where intervention will be particularly effective. With other developmentalists, we are impressed with the growth process that takes place from conception

through adolescence. We feel that there are programs appropriate for each period in this segment of the life span and that the dovetailing of such programs holds the greatest promise for any society committed to the optimal development of its children. (pp. 248–249)

And finally, Brim and Kagan (1980):

The conception of human development presented in this volume differs from most western contemporary thought on the subject. The view that emerges from this work is that humans have a capacity for change across the entire life span. It questions the traditional idea that the experience of the earlier years, which have a demonstrated contemporaneous effect, necessarily constrain the character of adolescence and adulthood. . . . There are important growth changes across the life span from birth to death. Many individuals retain a great capacity for change, and the consequences of the events of early childhood are continually transformed by later experience, making the course of human development more open than many have believed. (p. 1)

What are the implications of these conclusions for public policy? We judge that they call for a measured and patient, yet imaginative, response to nurture cognitive competence in the adolescent and young-adult years in the interest of the common good as well as of individual fulfillment. We suggest:

1. That a substantially augmented investment be made in basic research on the nature and uses of intelligence, guided by a developmental or lifespan perspective on the acquisition of cognitive competence under varied circumstances in childhood, adolescence, and the adult years;

2. That experimental curricula be developed for junior and senior high schools to provide systematic assessment of cognitive skills and sustained instruction in the processing of information and in general problem-solving strategies and skills, following the leads of Piaget and Feuerstein but not limited to these, in a variety of settings and with diverse groups of adolescents, and that the experimental curricula be evaluated for both immediate and long-term effectiveness;

3. That basic academic skills, without which intelligence cannot be effectively exercised in a complex society, be taught in secondary schools

for all adolescents with deficits, without regard to socioeconomic status, by expanding opportunities for compensatory education under Title I of the Elementary and Secondary Education Act of 1965 and other means, and that there be established a continuing research program to assess the effectiveness of a variety of methods of teaching basic skills to adolescents and young adults;

4. That educational alternatives programs for adolescents (i.e., jobs or job training) not abandon education, but that they include a substantial component of general cognitive training as well as instruction in basic academic skills so essential for coping in the modern world; academic skills should be taught using methods appropriate for adolescents;

5. That business, industry, and the military establish experimental programs to teach general cognitive competence and basic academic skills as well as job-related skills to adolescents and young adults, and that these programs be rigorously evaluated for their short- and long-term effectiveness in increased efficiency and productivity.

Now, is there any conceivable circumstance in these arduous times that could render these recommendations anything other than a self-serving exercise of academicians and developmentalists hungry for research support? Is there some compelling force that transcends our narrow interests and commands public action as well as our more private commitment? We think there is. It is to be found in shifts in the demographic composition of the population of the country. It is possible to predict with more certainty than life usually permits that in the decades ahead, composition of the work force will change dramatically. There will be many more older workers (the baby-boom adults) and many fewer younger workers, who are needed for their vigor, creativity, and recent educations. The empty school benches of today will become the empty work benches of tomorrow. The productive capacity of the nation as well as its military security and the security of dependent groups, especially old people, will depend on our foresight and ingenuity in compensating for loss in numbers of younger workers by a commensurate increase in their competence (Espenshade & Serow, 1978). We may be at an inversion point in history when children and adolescents will once again be recognized as economic assets and therefore be accorded a measure of concern not now evident in our national policies for human resource development. And if the thesis of this article is sustained by further research, we will gain a second chance: We can help the adolescents we neglected as children achieve the compentence required to discharge effectively the heavy responsibilities they will bear.

REFERENCE NOTES

1. Stipek, D. J. (1978). Adolescents—Too young to earn, too old to learn? Compulsory school attendance and intellectual development. Unpublished manuscript, University of California, Los Angeles.
2. Lazar & Associates (1977). Consortium on Developmental Continuity. *The persistence of pre-school effects* (Final rep. of Grant 18-76-007843, Administration for Children, Youth, and Families, OHDS, DHEW). Washington, D.C.: ACYF.
3. Lazar & Associates (1978). Consortium on Longitudinal Studies. *Lasting effects after pre-school* (Final rep. of DHEW Grant 90C-1311). Denver, Colo.: Education Commission of the States.
4. Day, M. (1979). Adolescent thought: Theory, research, and educational implications. Unpublished manuscript, University of Houston.
5. Tinto, V. and Sherman, R. (1974). *The Effectiveness of Secondary and Higher Education Intervention Programs: A Critical Review of the Research* (Rep. to U.S. Office of Education, Contract OEG-74-3580). New York: Teachers College.

REFERENCES

Arbitman-Smith, R. and Haywood, H. C. (1980). Cognitive education for learning-disabled adolescents. *Journal of Abnormal Child Psychology*, 8:51–64.

Ashton, P. (1975). Cross-cultural Piagetian research: An experimental perspective. *Harvard Educational Review*, 4:475–506.

Bakan, D. (1971). Adolescence in America: From idea to social fact. *Daedelus*, 100:979–995.

Baltes, P. B. and Schaie, K. W. (1976). On the plasticity of intelligence in adulthood and old age: Where Horn and Donaldson fail. *American Psychologist*, 31:720–725.

Bayley, N. (1970). Development of mental abilities. In *Carmichael's Manual of Child Psychology*, 3rd edition, P. H. Mussen, ed. New York: Wiley, 1970.

Bayley, N. and Oden, M. H. (1955). The maintenance of intellectual ability in gifted adults. *Journal of Gerontology*, 10:91–107.

Bettelheim, B. (1967). *The Empty Fortress: Infantile Autism and the Birth of the Self*. New York: Free Press.

Birren, J. E. and Schaie, K. W. (Eds.) (1977). *Handbook of the Psychology of Aging*. New York: Van Nostrand Reinhold.

Bloom, B. S. (1964). *Stability and Change in Human Characteristics*. New York: Wiley.

Bloom, B. S. and Broder, L. (1950). *Problem-solving Processes of College Students*. Chicago: University of Chicago Press.

Bowlby, J. (1951). *Maternal Care and Mental Health* (Monograph 2). Geneva, Switzerland: World Health Organization.

Brim, O. G. and Kagan, J. (1980). *Continuity and Change in Human Development*. Cambridge, MA: Harvard University Press.

Bronfenbrenner, U. (1974). *Is Early Intervention Effective? A Report on Longitudinal Evaluations of Pre-School Programs* (Vol. 2). Washington, D.C.: U.S. Government Printing Office (DHEW Publication No. CHD 74-25).

Brown, F. (1973). *The Reform of Secondary Education* (Report of the National Commission on the Reform of Secondary Education). New York: McGraw-Hill.

Burtt, H. E. (1932). The retention of early memories. *Journal of Genetic Psychology*, 40:287–295.

Cairns, R. B. and Nakelski, J. S. (1971). On fighting in mice: Ontogenetic and experimental determinants. *Journal of Comparative and Physiological Psychology*, 74:354–364.

Caldwell, B. M. (1973). Infant day care. In *Child Care—Who Cares?*, P. Roby and S. Chisolm, eds. New York: Basic Books.

Carmichael, L. (1926). The development of behavior in vertebrates experimentally removed from influence of external stimulation. *Psychological Review*, 33:51–58.

Carmichael, L. (1927). A further study of the development of behavior in vertebrates experimentally removed from the influence of external stimulation. *Psychological Review*, 34:34–77.

Carmichael, L. (1928). A further experimental study of the development of behavior. *Psychological Review*, 35:253–260.

Chiappetta, E. (1976). A review of Piagetian studies relevant to science instruction at the secondary and college level. *Science Education*, 60:253–261.

Clarke, A. D. B. and Clarke, A. M. (1954). Cognitive changes in the feebleminded. *British Journal of Psychology*, 45:173–179.

Clarke, A. D. B. and Clarke, A. M. (1959). Recovery from the effects of deprivation. *Acta Psychologica*, 16:137–144.

Clarke, A. M. and Clarke, A. D. B. (1976). *Early Experience: Myth and Evidence.* New York: Free Press.

Coghill, G. E. (1929). *Anatomy and the Problem of Behavior.* Cambridge, England: Cambridge University Press.

Cole, M. and Scribner, S. (1974). *Culture and Thought: A Psychological Introduction.* New York: Wiley.

Coleman, J. S. (1974). *Youth: Transition to Adulthood* (Report of the Panel on Youth of the President's Science Advisory Committee). Washington, D.C.: U.S. Government Printing Office.

Coleman, J., Campbell, E., Hobson, C., McPortland, J. and Mood, A. (1966). *Equality of Educational Opportunity.* Washington, D.C.: U.S. Department of Health, Education, and Welfare.

Collis, K. F. (1971). A study of concrete and formal reasoning in school mathematics. *Australian Journal of Psychology*, 23:289–296.

Cruze, W. W. (1935). Maturation and learning in chicks. *Journal of Comparative Psychology*, 19:371–409.

Danner, F. W. and Day, M. C. (1977). Eliciting formal operations. *Child Development*, 48:1600–1606.

Davis, K. (1940). Extreme social isolation of a child. *American Journal of Sociology*, 45:554–565.

Davis, K. (1947). Final note on a case of extreme isolation. *American Journal of Sociology*, 32:432–437.

Dennis, W. (1960). Causes of retardation among institutional children. *Journal of Genetic Psychology*, 96:47–59.

Dennis, W. and Dennis, M. G. (1940). The effect of cradling practice upon the onset of walking in Hopi children. *Journal of Genetic Psychology*, 56:77–86.

Dennis, W. and Dennis M. G. (1941). Infant development under conditions of restricted practice and minimum social stimulation. *Genetic Psychology Monographs*, 23:149–155.

Dennis, W. and Najarian, P. (1957). Infant development under environmental handicap. *Psychological Monographs*, 71:1–13.

Elkind, D. (1973). Borderline retardation in low and middle income adolescents. In *Theories of Cognitive Development: Implications for the Mentally Retarded*, R. M. Allen, A. D. Cortazzo, and R. P. Toister, eds. Coral Gables, FL: University of Miami Press.

Elkind, D. (1975). Recent research on cognitive development in adolescence. In *Adolescence in the Life Cycle*, S. E. Dragastin and G. Elder, Jr., eds. Washington, D.C.: Hemisphere.

Espenshade, T. J. and Serow, W. J. (Eds.) (1978). *The Economic Consequences of Slowing Population Growth*. New York: Academic Press.

Feuerstein, R. (1978). *The Dynamic Assessment of Retarded Performers*. Baltimore, MD: University Park Press.

Feuerstein, R. (1979). *Instrumental Enrichment*. Baltimore, MD: University Park Press.

Feuerstein, R., Miller, R., Hoffman, M. B., Rand, Y., Mintzker, Y. and Jensen, M. R. (1981). Cognitive modifiability in adolescence: Cognitive structure and the effects of intervention. *Journal of Special Education*, 15:269–287.

Frank Porter Graham Child Development Center (1981). Items 41, 58, 89, 90, 100, 107, 112, and 117. In *Bibliography of the Abecedarian Project and Project Care*, June 1981.

Freeman, F. A. (1936). Intellectual growth of children as indicated by repeated tests. *Psychological Monographs*, 47:20–34.

Freud, S. (1938). *The Basic Writings of Sigmund Freud*, A. A. Brill, ed. and trans. New York: Modern Library.

Gates, A. I. and Taylor, G. A. (1925). An experimental study of the nature of improvement resulting from practice in a mental function. *Journal of Educational Psychology*, 16:583–593.

Gesell, A. and Thompson, H. (1929). Learning and growth in identical twin infants. *Genetic Psychology Monographs*, 6:1–124.

Goldfarb, W. (1943). Effects of early institutional care on adolescent personality. *Journal of Experimental Education*, 12:106–129. (a)

Goldfarb, W. (1943). The effects of early institutional care on adolescent personality. *Child Development*, 14:213–223. (b)

Goldfarb, W. (1943). Infant rearing and problem behavior. *American Journal of Orthopsychiatry*, 13:249–266. (c)

Goldfarb, W. (1944). Effects of early institutional care on adolescent personality: Rorschach data. *American Journal of Orthopsychiatry*, 14:441–447.

Goldfarb, W. (1945). Psychological privation in infancy and subsequent adjustment. *American Journal of Orthopsychiatry*, 15:247–255.

Goldfarb, W. (1947). Variations in adolescent adjustment of institutionally-reared children. *American Journal of Orthopsychiatry*, 17:449–457.

Goodnow, J. J. (1962). A test of milieu differences with some of Piaget's tasks. *Psychological Monographs*, 86(36, Whole No. 555).

Goodnow, J. J. and Bethon, G. (1966). Piaget's tasks: The effect of schooling and intelligence. *Child Development*, 37:573–582.

Gray, S. W. and Klaus, R. A. (1965). An experimental pre-school program for culturally deprived children. *Child Development*, 36:887–898.

Gray, S. W., Ramsey, B. K. and Klaus, R. A. (1981). *From 3 to 20: The Early Training Project*. Baltimore, MD: University Park Press.

Harlow, H. F., Harlow, M. K., Schlitz, E. A. and Mohr, D. J. (1971). The effect of early adverse and enriched environments on the learning ability of rhesus monkeys. In *Cognitive Processes of Non-Human Primates*, L. E. Jarrad, ed. New York: Academic Press.

Harlow, H. F., Schlitz, K. A. and Harlow, M. K. (1969). The effects of social isolation on the learning performance of rhesus monkeys. In *Proceedings of the Second International Congress of Primatology* (Vol. 1), C. R. Carpenter, ed. New York: Karger.

Harmquist, K. (1968). Relative changes in intelligence from 13 to 18. *Scandinavian Journal of Psychology*, 9:50–82.

Harrington, M. (1962). *The Other America: Poverty in the United States*. New York: Macmillan.

Haywood, H. C. and Arbitman-Smith, R. (1981). Modification of cognitive functions in slow-learning adolescents. In *Frontiers of Knowledge in Mental Retardation,* (Vol. 1). P. Mittler, ed. London: I.A.S.S.M.D.

Heber, R. and Garber, H. (1975). Progress report II: An experiment in the prevention of cultural-familial retardation. In *Proceedings of the 3rd Congress of the International Association for the Scientific Study of Mental Deficiency,* D. A. Primrose, ed. Warsaw, Poland: Polish Medical.

Hess, E. H. (1958). Imprinting in animals. *Scientific American,* 198:81–90.

Hess, E. H. (1964). Imprinting in birds. *Science,* 146:1129–1139.

Hess, E. H. (1972). Imprinting in a natural laboratory. *Scientific American,* 227: 24–31.

Hilgard, J. R. (1932). Learning and maturation in pre-school children. *Journal of Genetic Psychology,* 41:36–56.

Hilgard, J. R. (1933). The effect of early and delayed practice on memory and motor performances studied by the method of co-twin control. *Genetic Psychology Monographs,* 14:493–567.

Hobbs, M. T. (1964). A comparison of institutionalized and noninstitutionalized mentally retarded. *American Journal of Mental Deficiency,* 69:206–210.

Hobbs, N. (1979). Foreword. In *Instrumental Enrichment,* R. Feuerstein, ed. Baltimore, MD: University Park Press.

Hobbs, N., Bartel, N., Dokecki, P. R., Gallagher, J. J. and Reynolds, M. C. (1979). *Papers on Research About Learning: Exceptional Teaching for Exceptional Learning* (Report to the Ford Foundation). New York: Ford Foundation.

Hunt, J. McV. (1941). The effects of infantile feeding-frustration upon adult hoarding in the albino rat. *Journal of Abnormal Social Psychology,* 36:338–360.

Hunt, J. McV. (1961). *Intelligence and Experience.* New York: Ronald Press.

Hunt, J. McV. (1979). Psychological development: Early experience. *Annual Review of Psychology,* 30:103–143.

Husen, T. (1951). The influence of schooling upon IQ. *Theoria,* 17:61–88.

Inhelder, B. and Piaget, J. (1958). *The Growth of Logical Thinking From Childhood to Adolescence: An Essay on the Construction of Formal Operational Structures.* New York: Basic Books.

Itard, J. M. G. (1932). *The Wild Boy of Aveyron,* G. Humphrey and M. Humphrey, trans. New York: Appleton-Century-Crofts.

Jencks, C. (1972). *Inequality: A Reassessment of the Effect of the Family and Schooling in America.* New York: Harper & Row.

Jones, H. and Conrad, H. (1933). The growth and decline of intelligence. *Genetic Psychology Monographs,* 13:223–298.

Kagan, J. (1976). Resilience and continuity in psychological development. In *Early Experience: Myth and Evidence,* A. M. Clarke and A. D. B. Clarke, eds. New York: Free Press.

Kagan, J. and Klein, R. E. (1973). Cross-cultural perspectives on early development. *American Psychologist,* 28:947–961.

Klaus, R. A. and Gray, S. W. (1968). The early training project for disadvantaged children: A report after the first five years. *Monographs of the Society for Research in Child Development,* 33(4, Serial No. 120).

Koluchová, J. (1972). Severe deprivation in twins: A case study. *Journal of Child Psychology and Psychiatry and Allied Disciplines,* 13:107–114.

Koluchová, J. (1976). The further development of twins after severe and prolonged deprivation: A second report. *Journal of Child Psychology and Psychiatry and Allied Disciplines,* 17:181–188.

Krech, D., Rosenzweig, M. R. and Bennett, E. L. (1962). Relations between brain chemistry and problem-solving among rats raised in enriched and impoverished environments. *Journal of Comparative and Physiological Psychology*, 55:801–807.

Larson, M. and Dittman, F. (1975). *Compensatory Education and Early Adolescence: Reviewing Our National Strategy* (Project No. 2158). Stanford, CA: Stanford Research Institute.

Lawson, A. E. and Nordland, F. H. (1977). Conservation reasoning ability and performance on BSCS Blue Version examinations. *Journal of Research in Science Teaching*, 14:69–75.

Lawson, A. E. and Renner, J. W. (1975). Relationships of science subject matter and developmental levels of learners. *Journal of Research in Science Teaching*, 12:347–358.

Lawson, A. E. and Wollman, W. T. (1976). Encouraging the transition from concrete to formal cognitive functioning—An experiment. *Journal of Research in Science Teaching*, 13:413–430.

Lewis, H. (1954). *Deprived Children*. London: Oxford University Press.

Lorenz, K. Z. (1965). *Evolution and the Modification of Behavior*. Chicago: University of Chicago Press.

Luria, A. R. (1971). Towards the problem of the historical nature of psychological processes. *International Journal of Psychology*, 6:259–272.

Machado, L. A. (1980). *The Right to Be Intelligent*, M. C. Wheeler, trans. New York: Pergamon Press.

Martin, J. H. (1976). *The Education of Adolescents: National Panel on High School and Adolescent Education*. Washington, D.C.: U.S. Government Printing Office.

McGraw, M. B. (1935). *Growth: A Study of Johnny and Jimmy*. New York: Appleton-Century-Crofts.

McGraw, M. B. (1939). Later development of children specially trained during infancy. *Child Development*, 10:1–19.

McNemar, Q. (1940). A critical examination of the University of Iowa studies of environmental influences upon the IQ. *Psychological Bulletin*, 37:63–92.

Morphett, M. V. and Washburn, C. (1931). When should children begin to read? *Elementary School Journal*, 31:496–503.

National Commission for Employment Policy (1979). *Expanding Employment Opportunities for Disadvantaged Youth* (Fifth Annual Report to the President and the Congress of the National Commission for Employment Policy). Washington, D.C.: U.S. Government Printing Office.

National Institute of Education (1978). *Compensatory Education Study* (Final rep.). Washington, D.C.: Department of Health, Education, and Welfare.

Novak, M. A. and Harlow, H. F. (1975). Social recovery of monkeys isolated for the first year of life: I. Rehabilitation and therapy. *Developmental Psychology*, 11:453–465.

O'Connor, S. (1980). Quality of parenting and the mother-infant relationship following rooming in. In *Parent-Infant Relationships*, P. Taylor, ed. New York: Grune & Stratton.

O'Connor, S., Vietze, P. M., Sherrod, K. B., Sandler, H. M. and Altemeier. W. A. (1980). Reduced incidence of parenting inadequacy following rooming-in. *Pediatrics*, 66:176–182.

Owens, W. A. (1953). Age and mental abilities: A longitudinal study. *Genetic Psychology Monographs*, 48:3–54.

Owens, W. A. (1966). Age and mental abilities: A second adult follow-up. *Journal of Educational Psychology*, 51:311–325.

Peel, E. A. (1971). *The Nature of Adolescent Judgment*. New York: Wiley.

Peluffo, N. (1967). Culture and cognitive problems. *International Journal of Psychology*, 2:187–198.

Pringle, M. K. (1971). *Deprivation and Education*, 2nd ed. London: Harlow, Longman.

Rathbun, C., Di Virgilio, L. and Waldfogel, S. (1958). The restitutive process in children following radical separation from family and culture. *American Journal of Orthopsychiatry*, 28:408–415.

Rosenzweig, M. R. and Bennett, E. L. (Eds.) (1976). *Neural Mechanisms of Learning and Memory*. Cambridge, MA: MIT Press.

Rosenzweig, M. R., Krech, D. and Bennet, E. L. (1960). A search for relations between brain chemistry and behavior. *Psychological Bulletin*, 57:476–492.

Rosenzweig, M. R., Krech, D., Bennett, E. L. and Diamond, M. C. (1962). Effects of environmental complexity and training on brain chemistry and anatomy: A replication and extension. *Journal of Comparative and Physiological Psychology*, 55:429–437.

Rousseau, J. J. (1966). *Emile*, B. Foxley, trans. New York: Dutton. (Originally published, 1972.)

Rutter, M. (1971). Parent-child separation: Psychological effects on the children. *Journal of Child Psychology and Psychiatry*, 12:233–260.

Rutter, M. (1972). *Maternal Deprivation Reassessed*. Harmondsworth, England: Penguin.

Rutter, M., Maughan, B., Mortimore, P. and Ouston, J. (1979). *Fifteen Thousand Hours: The Secondary Schools and Their Effects on Children*. Cambridge, MA: Harvard University Press.

Schaie, K. and Strother, C. (1968). A cross-sequential study of age changes in cognitive behavior. *Psychological Bulletin*, 70:671–680. (a)

Schaie, K. and Strother, C. (1968). The effect of time and cohort differences upon age changes in cognitive behavior. *Multivariate Behavioral Research*, 3:259–294. (b)

Schur, E. M. (1971). *Labeling Deviant Behavior: Its Sociological Implications*. New York: Harper & Row.

Scribner, S. and Cole, M. (1973). Cognitive consequences of formal and informal education. *Science*, 182:553–559.

Sharp, D., Cole, M. and Lave, C. (1979). Education and cognitive development: The evidence from experimental research. *Monographs of the Society for Research in Child Development*, 44(1–2, Whole No. 178).

Shirley, M. M. (1931). A motor sequence favors the maturation theory. *Psychological Bulletin*, 28:204–205.

Shirley, M. M. (1933). *The First Two Years* (2 vols.). Minneapolis: University of Minnesota Press.

Shock, N. W. (1951). Gerontology (later maturity). *Annual Review of Psychology*, 2:353–370.

Siegler, R. S., Liebert, D. E. and Liebert, R. M. (1973). Inhelder and Piaget's pendulum problem: Teaching pre-adolescents to act as scientists. *Developmental Psychology*, 9:97–101.

Skeels, H. M. (1966). Adult status of children with contrasting early life experiences: A follow-up study. *Monographs of the Society for Research in Child Development*, 31(3, Serial No. 105).

Skodak, M. and Skeels, H. M. (1949). A final follow-up study of one hundred adopted children. *Journal of Genetic Psychology*, 75:85–125.

Spitz, R. A. (1945). Hospitalism: An inquiry into the genesis of psychiatric conditions in early childhood. *Psychoanalytic Study of the Child*, 1:53–74.

Spitz, R. A. (1946). Anaclitic depression. *Psychoanalytic Study of the Child*, 2:313–342. (a)

Spitz, R. A. (1946). Hospitalism: A follow-up report. *Psychoanalytic Study of the Child*, 2:113–117. (b)

Suomi, S. J. and Harlow, H. F. (1972). Social rehabilitation of isolate-reared monkeys. *Developmental Psychology*, 6:487–496.

Thomson, J. L. (1934). Big gains from postponed reading. *Journal of Education*, 117:445–446.

Thorndike, R. L. (1948). Growth of intelligence during adolescence. *Journal of Genetic Psychology*, 72:11–85.

Tizard, B. and Rees, J. A. (1974). A comparison of the effects of adoption, restoration to the natural mother, and continued institutionalization on the cognitive development of four-year-old children. *Child Development*, 45:92–99.

Watson, J. B. (1928). *Psychological Care of Infant and Child*. New York: Norton.

Yarrow, L. J. (1961). Maternal deprivation: Toward an empirical and conceptual re-evaluation. *Psychological Bulletin*, 58:459–490.

Zigler, E. and Cascione, R. (1977). Head Start has little to do with mental retardation: Reply to Clarke and Clarke. *American Journal of Mental Deficiency*, 82:246–249.

20

Prevention of Emotional Problems Among Native-American Children: Overview of Developmental Issues

Irving N. Berlin

University of New Mexico School of Medicine

The Native-American child's achievement of developmental tasks may be seriously interfered with by the depression and alcoholism of the nurturing adults. Native-Americans are caught between a hostile Anglo society and a not very powerful Native culture. Generations of such conflict are in some cases being altered by more militant use of their ancient heritages along with finding ways to keep adolescents employed and a part of the community. Examples of early intervention and secondary prevention efforts at several development stages indicate that constructive changes are possible, though still very difficult.

Problem-solving approaches in education, which involve adolescents learning about child development through their engagement in early intervention programs, alter the adolescents' understanding of children, enhance cultural values, and provide adolescents with marketable skills.

Teaching Native-American paraprofessionals techniques of early identification and early intervention is one important step in prevention programming in the Native communities. Many communities are becoming oriented toward early intervention and secondary prevention. Health and mental health professionals who work with such

Reprinted with permission from the *Journal of Preventive Psychiatry*, 1982, Vol. 1, No. 3, 319–330. Published by Mary Ann Liebert, Inc., New York.

communities must acquire special knowledge and skills for teaching and collaboration.

INTRODUCTION

Anthropologists and sociologists document that the developmental tasks of infancy, childhood, and adolescence are similar in various societies and cultures. But facilitation of development is idiosyncratic to each culture. Among culturally widespread goals is the development of an adult who can contribute to the community by means of work and family roles, as well as the continuity of traditions.[1,2]

The enormous increase in substance abuse, alcoholism, accidental death, and suicide in the last decade among adolescents and young adults in many Native-American communities is of grave concern. A close examination of current developmental problems and failures is, therefore, important.[3-7]

At the 1981 American Indian Child Conference, a number of concerns were expressed by investigators and Native-American professionals and paraprofessionals from many tribes. Several tribal judges described their intense concern about the increasing number of alcoholic young parents with accompanying increase of child abuse. The Children's Code of the Navajo Nation is being rewritten with specific attention to issues of child abuse and neglect because of the enormous increase documented in cases brought to the court's attention. Tribal officials voiced their distress that the increase in alcoholism among adults, in child abuse, and in neglect of children would have serious effects on the mental health of future generations. Also some are concerned that because of the increase in fetal alcohol syndrome babies, the development and physical health of many children will be seriously impaired.[8,9]

Evaluation of the development of those young adults and adolescents who do well will help clarify some of the necessary and sufficient factors for optimal development. Such studies, added to our current knowledge, will help with planning for prevention and early intervention. Similarly, a serious concern to many tribes and communities is the understanding of factors that make for such different life outcomes and the implications for their prevention. To date such investigations have not been undertaken.[10-12] However, prevention strategies incorporating both developmental and epidemiological data are forthcoming from some pilot programs. These strategies point to intervention methods that can be effective now.

INTERFERENCES WITH NORMAL DEVELOPMENTAL TASKS:
SOME HIGHLIGHTS OF SPECIAL RELEVANCE

The infant's attachment to adults and establishment of trust in adults are seriously interfered with by inconsistent mothering by alcoholic and depressed young Indian mothers. An infant's constant irritability, crying, and sleeplessness signal the failure of regular and predictable attention to his or her needs.

Separation, individuation in the preschool child, and the development of language and motor skills make independence and satisfying one's curiosity possible. Abuse and neglect (which have the greatest incidence at this age) seriously delay and distort mastery of such developmental tasks.[10,13,14]

The schoolage child who has not suffered previous developmental disturbances still needs adults who are concerned with his or her learning to be successful academically. Extended family may substitute for alcoholic parents. However, cognitive development requires both personalized concern of adults and a stimulating educational system.[15-17]

Adolescent development, especially acquiring meaningful sexual and work roles and learning to become a concerned, caring, tender person is vital to marriage and parenting and requires adult models.[18-20] In many communities opportunities for work are rare. In some settings adults whose effective living would provide models for adolescents of both sexes are also rare. In addition, many of the most disturbed and depressed adolescents have suffered serious developmental disturbances since infancy or early childhood and are not able to take advantage of work opportunities and/or adult modeling; they require treatment.[12,21,22]

It is still rare for courts to use developmental criteria in making custody or adoption decisions. The ability of the adults to provide a supportive developmental environment at the child's present age and through succeeding developmental stages is rarely considered. The lack of such concerns by courts contributes to adopted Indian adolescents having twice the suicide rate of Indian adolescents raised with their families.[23-25]

SOME SOCIOCULTURAL DIMENSIONS OF ADOLESCENT PROBLEMS

In the Native-American and Eskimo cultures, as in society at large, child rearing has become an increasingly difficult task.

It is clear from a variety of studies on alcoholism, drug and P.C.P. abuse, glue sniffing, and suicide that adolescent depression is a common concern on many reservations and in many Pueblos.[3-7,26,27] For generations the Anglo society has had a purposive, destructive, and demeaning impact on Native-Americans. The current militant concern with establishing Indian culture and heritage as critical for survival has been encouraging to some adolescents and young adults. Many Native-Americans, however, find themselves in severe conflict. They are confronted with their parents' often hopeless and helpless attitudes, resulting from overwhelming impoverishment, discrimination, and society's concerted efforts to destroy Native-American cultural ties. They find that learning about and practicing the tenets of their heritage, although a potential filled with hope for a future as a people, does not alter their economic or social position.[28-34]

OPTIMAL DEVELOPMENT

The author's observations of infant and early child care in Native-American tribes from Alaska, the Pacific Northwest, and the Southwest make it clear that in many settings the infant is cherished, loved, and handled with tenderness. A variety of sensory stimulation is provided by members of the nuclear and extended families, leading to security in attachment and a capacity for separation and individuation. The young child's strivings for independence are taken care of as a built-in part of the tribes' traditional practices. Thus, one sees cherished infants and preschoolers with vitality, curiosity, and independence. These children made the author, a Headstart evaluation consultant in the Northwest, feel that they could face and alter the future according to their needs. In many cases where young parents were depressed or alcoholic, the author has seen members of the extended family take affected infants into their care. Clearly, the development of such infants and toddlers depended upon the human and economic abilities of the extended family to respond to the child's needs and to provide a responsible and responsive human environment.[2,10,35,36]

PROBLEMS IN DEVELOPMENT AND SECONDARY PREVENTION

Where family resources are strained by poverty and many children, a particular child's development may not be very rapid. Genetic and neonatal development disorders along with problems resulting from maternal deprivation test the capacity of parents to provide constant nurturance. Extended family may also find it difficult to help with ongoing care.[37-39]

Consistent caring, consistent expectations, and clear role models in the environment are especially critical to the survival of the child who experienced developmental delays resulting from a variety of causes.[39]

In many cases in the Headstart program, one could see that with increased attention and devotion of teachers and tribal aides, youngsters—some with early deprivation of maternal care or early developmental deviations—would improve markedly in personality. Progressively, they socialized more freely, learned better, and became delightful, vigorous, and curious young children who achieved most of the developmental goals of normal preschool children. Where such help was not available, withdrawal and hyperactive difficult home behavior was carried over to the school, with increased problems in learning. It is clear from Headstart and other such programs, that carefully designed preschools may prevent many behavioral and emotional problems in Native-American children.[40]

EARLY IDENTIFICATION AND TREATMENT OF DEVELOPMENTAL PROBLEMS

The use of good preschools, both to diagnose developmental problems and to program for them, is only now beginning to occur where Native-Americans are not too spread out and isolated.

One of the early stimulation programs the author recently visited among the Navajos was for developmentally delayed and retarded young children. It demonstrated the effectiveness of a dedicated staff and some very invested young parents. In this particular program, the children were responsive, looked less developmentally delayed, and were more ready to be involved in play and early learning through games than were other developmentally delayed children in other preschools. Preschool and early stimulation programs are essential for all young children (not only for those with developmental delays). But the creation of a core of early childhood stimulation and development specialists from Native-Americans for the reservations, pueblos, and urban Native-American infants is especially crucial.[41]

Critical needs in infancy and preschool years are to help with early identification of problems and for more precise programming for remediation. Child health and mental health professionals must be trained to become expert in these areas and to be more effective teachers. Thus, Native-American professionals and paraprofessionals can be taught to become more proficient in early identification and intervention.[42,43]

One way of reducing the need for preschool intervention is prenatal involvement of pregnant adolescent girls in group counseling and an

early stimulation practicum. Such efforts can ready them for participation in early stimulation programs with their own babies. Learning
with other young mothers, together with concerned professionals and
paraprofessionals from their own tribes, has proved effective in several
pilot projects.[44]

The school has a vital role in the development of Native-American
children, especially in transmission of cultural values and attitudes toward learning. Certainly, one of the very critical issues for the schoolage
child is that often *no one* tries to help make learning a creative and
interesting process of discovery and problem solving.[45]

ROLE OF ACADEMIC ACHIEVEMENT IN DEVELOPMENT AND SECONDARY PREVENTION

Although a minority of Indian children now attend boarding schools,
the impact of boarding schools on Indian children is serious and can be
remediated.

The author has had an opportunity to visit a number of boarding
schools for Native-American children. In each case, he had been told
contradictory stories. There were horror stories about how the schools
were unrelated to the tribes from which the children came; there were
stories of loneliness, degradation, and ill treatment of the children; stories of their failure to learn, of suicide attempts, of runaways, and so
on. The author also heard from parents, themselves products of the
boarding schools, about how the discipline, kindness, and opportunities
to learn had helped them, not to speak of the facts that they were fed,
clothed, and housed at a time when their families were destitute. The
author must admit, however, that, with only one exception, the tales of
horror were borne out as he observed large numbers of depressed,
anxious, and clearly symptomatic children. He also noted many unin-
volved, unconcerned, ignorant, and punitive adults, both Anglo and
Native-American.[46-48]

The author's concern with boarding school students is that these depressed, nonlearning youngsters must have been, at some point, some
of the curious, delightful children he had seen previously. Rather than
being afforded opportunities in their schoolage periods to become engrossed in learning, they became turned off, perhaps for the rest of their
lives. The interest and concern of parents (or their substitutes) with
learning and their encouragement and active support of the acquisition
of knowledge are critical to the child's desire to learn. Such encouragement and support did not exist in these boarding schools.[9,49-51]

In the one excellent boarding school, prevention of mental illness and positive support for mental health did occur in several ways. In each dormitory there were carefully selected, concerned young adults representing each of the tribes in the school. The teachers and counselors were alert to any signs of problems in living or learning. Most were young Native-Americans concerned with preserving their heritage and helping their students enjoy learning and become competent persons. They dealt with an everpresent special problem of Native-American children in learning situations, that of avoiding competition and being singled out as better (which is culturally frowned upon) by developing individualized learning goals. The modeling by these young adults, by their interest in learning and thirst for knowledge, was heartening to observers. Their individualized concern in working with students and actively seeking out any youngster who had problems, created a warm and alive learning atmosphere. This school model can be applied to the nonresidential schools on reservations, which often also do not stimulate their students to learn.[52]

PROBLEM-SOLVING LEARNING AN AID IN PREVENTION

Problem solving is a crucial issue in learning, which could be pioneered by Native-Americans since most Anglo teaching and learning ignores the question of how to teach problem solving.

In all survival cultures, the adults model the necessary problem solving for survival, be it hunting, fishing, or agriculture. For actual survival and the development of skills required to keep one's culture not only intact but progressing, learning problem solving and current survival are closely related. In the few cases where problem solving is encouraged through project learning, it meets resistance. Yet, becoming a problem-solving person is vital to mental health and prevention of a hopelessness and helplessness characteristic of depression and other mental illness.[19,53,54]

Educators and investigators concerned with cognitive development have noted the importance of involving children early in considering most aspects of education as an opportunity to learn how to think in problem-solving terms. This means being able to define a problem, gather data about it, and evaluate the findings or data in terms of solutions that may emerge with regard to that problem.[55] The use of collaborative projects as early as the third grade has been shown to encourage such thinking.[56] There is increasing data that, in Piagetian terms, environmental experience (that is, how and what learning has been encouraged at home and in school) will determine when, during the concrete operational developmental stage, the concepts of conservation will take place.[57] For some children the concepts of conservation are present by age 11 or 12, for some not until age 15 or 16.[58] One of the major concerns of developmentalists working with adolescents is that many adolescents never leave the concrete operational stage and move to formal operational thinking and understanding of abstract concepts such as those in science. Again these stage developments appear vulnerable to environmental and educational limitations. There is current interest in the possibility that learning to think in problem-solving terms early and continually may enhance the development of formal operational thinking. The ability to assess data, to think in problem-solving terms, and to be able to deal with abstract ideas seems to enhance the kinds of choices one makes in work and civic responsibilities and seems related to feelings of adequacy and competence.[58,59]

One tribe, after centuries of being moved from one reservation site to another, had a corn and alfalfa crop economy for many years. One year the eighth grade junior high school students, stimulated by their Native and Anglo teachers, took on as their project a review of what really were the best agricultural products for the local type of soil.

Visits to productive Anglo farms, soil analysis conducted by a reluctant county agent, and computer analysis done by a Native programmer at the local college, indicated that intensive truck farming was most likely to produce cash crops to supply a needed hotel market. Efforts by committees of students and teachers to present these findings to tribal elders met with rebuffs. It was clear that to change one's ways again was difficult to think about. A prent-student-teacher presentation at an open meeting, unheard of in this tribe, was able to disseminate the information. With such support, a pilot project was begun with land set aside by the tribal council and money obtained from the Department of Agriculture. The project was undertaken by concerned high school students and teachers. Since this meant a totally new approach, much more care than usual was needed in planting, weeding, and pest control. For some of these young people the project pointed to a way out of the adolescent dilemma of where to go after high school. Recent results are promising, but it takes time to alter the defensive ways of people who have been uprooted for hundreds of years, have continually readjusted, only to be uprooted again and again. The role of such activities in the life of involved adults and adolescents is clearly going to affect the mental health of the adolescents and their roles as effective and concerned adults and parents with their own children.[60]

Alaska Methodist University's efforts some years back to help develop Headstart teachers and aides from junior and senior high school students in local schools revealed how powerful such programs could be. A practical experience in helping one's own ethnic group in a preschool was coupled with child development seminars. As reported by the National Commission for Youth and from the author's own observations, this was an exciting project. It not only taught adolescents the skills of child care within a developmental framework, but it stimulated the students to raise questions about the problems of the children with whom they worked. They also wanted to understand the parents' problems. This led to exploration of their own past experiences. Such sharing, led by their own people who could be honest and open about their own feelings, also led to discussion of how they could avoid problems as parents. It led adolescents to consider pervasive alcoholism and drug addiction as signs of depression and giving up. They were also concerned with the reasons for so many adolescent pregnancies. Their discussions and readings helped them understand the psychological problems and needs that led to pregnancy and the resulting emotional difficulties for both the disturbed mother and child. Such open discussions among adolescents from different tribes were unheard of. The Eskimo and Aleut teachers, one male and one female, were remarkable people and had much to do with the success of the effort. Similar efforts elsewhere, using practical experience as a base for seminar learning and discussion, have occurred repeatedly in minority communities.[44] Real efforts of anticipatory guidance and problem solving occurred for some of these young people and resulted in their finding new goals and directions for living. How parents view their own futures and what they want for their children will alter the children's views of themselves and their sense of purpose in life. These alterations in view may be the most vital and powerful tools in prevention that we know.

PRIMARY PREVENTION FOR NATIVE-AMERICANS

The various Native-American communities and organizations and the government must find ways of helping adolescents whose parents are depressed and alcoholic to find new adult models in their communities, especially related to employment opportunities. Adolescents may then feel more effective as people and become more nurturant as parents.

In the few cases where organized efforts are being made to use work, both through light industries and service organizations, and a return to one's heritage as an antidote to depression, there have been strides. But for many young parents in many areas, there are still only few opportunities for such rehabilitation. Prevention of mental illness and emotional disturbances in the child may in large part depend on tribes and pueblos learning from every possible source. Parents' increased experiences with worthwhile work is one such source. Organized opportunities to learn about child development using child-rearing principles stated in their own heritage may be another means of favorably altering young parents' functioning.

CURRENT ISSUES

There are many problems currently facing the Native-American child, adolescent, and adult. The current problems of unemployment in both urban areas and in Indian communities breed serious depression, alcoholism and substance abuse, and suicide.[19,49] Adolescents who leave their homebase seeking better economic futures elsewhere, often fail in the cities and begin drug and alcohol use that continues when they return to their communities. There is a lack of adequate support systems for children, adolescents, and adults, especially in terms of health, mental health care, and prevention-focused education, both in their own communities and in urban centers where many Native-Americans come to live. We need to think more about secondary prevention, through early intervention programs, and tertiary prevention, through prompt and effective treatment for those psychiatric problems that come to health or mental health workers' attention.[61,62]

During the last year, as part of an Indian Health Service Outreach Team, the author has had some opportunity to view the role of program- and client-centered consultation to schools, health, and mental health settings, which might affect the mental health of their students or clients. He has worked with pediatricians at various sites to help them understand the opportunities in early identification and possible intervention in child abuse and other emotional problems. Case management strategies were discussed with mental health workers in the communities to help them to understand and apply a task-oriented crisis technique with families, aimed at fostering the development of both children and adults.[62-64]

It is clear that the professionals and paraprofessionals in many Native-American communities are eager to be more effective. They are eager to learn to serve in special education, Headstart, boarding school, or residential settings. Helping the indigenous mental health worker in the community, school, or hospital to refine his or her diagnostic and treatment skills through regular case reviews has proved to be most effective. These reviews need to be more frequent, with continuity of consultation and education by more mental health professionals, so that change in clients or students can be evaluated. It is clear from the author's work that the more such consultation occurs in the actual communities or schools where problems arise, the more effective it is. Often such meetings are held in centers distant from the communities to save consultant's time with reduced effectiveness.[63]

Currently, a pressing need exists for direct treatment of severely depressed or otherwise disturbed children and adolescents among Native Americans. We also need to learn how to involve their families. New program opportunities in secondary prevention and early intervention constantly occur. Recent opportunities include group discussions among girls at risk for suicide in one boarding school; a chance to provide program support and consultation to an early intervention program with clear goals and training for its workers in another site; and a pregnant adolescent child development program in another community. Without continued support and guidance from mental health specialists, these efforts are not likely to maintain their effectiveness. The problems, difficulties, and discouragements that beset all such programs can only be dealt with through a continued relationship between trained and experienced specialists and the community leaders involved in these activities.

CONCLUSIONS

The serious mental health problems in many Indian communities manifested by substance abuse, alcoholism, suicide, and so on, need to be examined from both an individual developmental and an epidemiologic point of view. The developmental problems related to depressed alcoholic parents affect children from infancy through adolescence. Epidemiologic issues of widespread alcoholism, glue sniffing and suicide are now being studied. It is clear from various preschool efforts and from the pilot projects cited that secondary prevention and early intervention are both possible and effective. There is a growing readiness in many Indian communities and settings to institute secondary prevention efforts. These efforts require sustained help and continuous consultation with trained mental health specialists.

The need for direct care of mentally ill, depressed, and suicidal children and adolescents is great. However, there is also a need for growing awareness in the Indian Health Service and Indian communities of the necessity to support and encourage early intervention and secondary prevention. Available means include early stimulation programs for infants with developmental problems, work in groups with pregnant adolescents, identification of adolescents at risk for suicide, and group and individual therapy to reduce the depression and helplessness that result from substance abuse. It is clear there are more and more opportunities for prevention. We need to be able to encourage and facilitate them.

REFERENCES

1. Erikson, E. H. (1963). *Childhood and Society*, 2nd ed. New York: W. W. Norton.
2. Leighton, D. and Kluckhohn, C. (1948). *Children of the People*. Cambridge: Harvard University Press.
3. Shore, J. H. (1975). American Indian suicide—fact and fantasy. *Psychiatry*, 38:86–91.
4. Levy, J. E. (1965). Navajo suicide. *Hum. Organ.*, 24:309–318.
5. Miller, S. I. and Schoenfeld, L. S. (1971). Suicide attempt patterns among the Navajo Indians. *International Journal of Social Psychiatry*, 17:189–193.
6. Swanson, D. W., Bratrude, A. P. and Brown, E. M. (1971). Alcohol abuse in a population of Indian children. *Disease of the Nervous System*, 32:835–842.
7. Westermeyer, J., Walker, D. and Benton, E. (1981). A review of some methods for investigating substance abuse epidemiology among American Indians and Alaska natives. *White Cloud Journal*, 2(2):13–21.
8. Report of the Third National Indian Child Conference: The Indian Family—Foundations for Future (May 17–21, 1981). Department of Health and Human Services, Indian Health Service, Office of Mental Health Programs, Albuquerque, NM.
9. Beiser, M. (1981). Mental health of American Indian and Alaska native children: Some epidemiologic perspectives. *White Cloud Journal*, 2(2):37–47.
10. Attneave, C. L (1979). The American Indian child. In *Basic Handbook of Child Psychiatry*, J. B. Noshpitz, ed. New York: Basic Books.
11. Beiser, M. (1972). Etiology of mental disorders: Socio-cultural aspects. In *Manual of Child Psychopathology*, B. Wolman, ed. New York: McGraw Hill.
12. Green, B. E., Sack, W. H. and Pambrun, A. (1981). A review of child psychiatric epidemiology with special reference to American Indian and Alaska native children. *White Cloud Journal*, 2(2):23–36.
13. Kempe, C. H. and Silver, H. K. (1959). The problem of parental criminal neglect and severe physical abuse of children. *American Journal of Diseases of Children*, 98:528.
14. Levy, J. E. and Kunitz, S. J. (1971). Indian reservations, anomie, and social pathologies. *Southwestern Journal of Anthropology*, 27:97–128.
15. Plowden Report (1966). Central Advisory Council for Education (England). *Children and Their Primary Schools*, Vol. 1. London: Her Majesty's Stationery Office.
16. Werner, O. and Fenton, J. (1973). Method and theory in ethnoscience and ethno-epistemology. In *A Handbook of Method in Cultural Anthropology*, R. Naroll and R. Cohen, eds.
17. Bryde, J. F. (1970). *The Indian Student: A Study of Scholastic Failure and Personality Conflict*. Vermillion: University of South Dakota Press.
18. Blos, P. (1967). Second individuation process of adolescence. *Psychoanalytic Study of the Child*, 22:162–186.

19. Berlin, I. N. (1980). Opportunities in adolescence to rectify developmental failures. In *Adolescent Psychiatry*, Vol. VIII, S. C. Feinstein, P. L. Giovacchini, J. G. Looney, A. Z. Schwartzberg, and A. D. Sorosky, eds. Chicago: University of Chicago Press, pp. 231–243.

20. Toews, J. (1980). Adolescent development issues in marital therapy. In *Adolescent Psychiatry*, Vol. VIII, S. C. Feinstein, P. L. Giovacchini, J. H. Looney, A. Z. Schwartzberg and A. D. Sorosky, eds. Chicago: University of Chicago Press, pp. 244–252.

21. Miller, D. (1980). Treatment of the seriously disturbed adolescent. In *Adolescent Psychiatry*, Vol. VIII, S. C. Feinstein, P. L. Giovacchini, J. G. Looney, A. Z. Schwartzberg, and A. D. Sorosky, eds. Chicago: University of Chicago Press, pp. 469–481.

22. Shore, J. H., Kinzie, J. D., Pattison, E. M. and Hampson, J. (1973). Psychiatric epidemiology of an Indian village. *Psychiatry*, 36:70–81.

23. Goldstein, J., Freud, A. and Solnit, A. J. (1973). *Beyond the Best Interests of the Child.* New York: Free Press.

24. Mindell, C. and Gurwitt, A. (1977). The placement of American Indian Children: The need for change. In *The Destruction of the American Indian Family*, S. Unger, ed. New York: Association on American Indian Affairs, pp. 61–66.

25. Berlin, I. N. (1978). Anglo adoption of Native-Americans: Repercussions in adolescence. *Journal of the American Academy of Child Psychiatry*, 17(2):387–388.

26. Kaufman, A. (1973). Gasoline sniffing among children in a Pueblo Indian village. *Pediatrics*, 51:1060–1064.

27. Nelson, I. (1977). Alcoholism in Zuni, New Mexico. *Preventive Medicine*, 6:152–166.

28. Shore, J. H. and Manson, S. M. (1981). Cross-cultural studies of depression among American Indians and Alaska natives. *White Cloud Journal*, 2(2):5–12.

29. Levy, J. E. and Kunitz, S. J. (1974). *Indian Drinking: Navajo Practices and Anglo-American Theories.* New York: Wiley.

30. Stratton, R., Zeiner, A. and Paredes, A. (1978). Tribal affiliations and prevalence of alcohol problems. *Journal of Studies on Alcohol*, 39:1166–1177.

31. Krause, R. F. and Buffler, P. A. (1979). Socioculture stress and the American Native in Alaska: An analysis of changing patterns of psychiatric illness and alcohol abuse among Alaska Natives. *Culture, Medicine and Psychiatry*, 3:111–151.

32. Johnson, D. L. and Johnson, C. A. (1965). Totally discouraged: A depressive syndrome of the Dakota Sioux. *Transcultural Psychiatric Research*, 1:141–143.

33. Jones, D. M. (1969). Child welfare problems in an Alaskan Native village. *Social Service Review*, 43:297–309.

34. Townsley, H. C. and Goldstein, G. S. (1977). One view of the etiology of depression in the American Indian. *Public Health Report*, 92(5):458–461.

35. Dennis, W. (1965). *The Hopi Child.* New York: Wiley.

36. Devereux, G. (1961). *Mohave Ethnopsychiatry.* Washington, DC: Smithsonian Institution Press.

37. McDermott, J. F. (1967). Social class and mental illness in children: The diagnosis of organicity and mental retardation. *Journal of American Child Psychiatry*, 6:309–320.

38. Shore, J. H. (1977). Psychiatric research issues with American Indians. In *Current Perspectives in Cultural Psychiatry*, E. F. Foulks, R. M. Wintrob, J. Westermeyer, and A. R. Favazza, eds. Jamaica, NY: Spectrum Publications, pp. 73–80.

39. Berlin, I. N. (1966). Consultation and special education. In *Prevention and Treatment of Mental Retardation*, I. Phillips, ed. New York: Basic Books, pp. 279–293.

40. Caldwell, B. M. and Richmond, J. B. (1968). The Children's Center in Syracuse, N.H. In *Early Child Care: The New Perspective*, L. L. Dittman, ed. New York: Atherton Press.

41. Caldwell, B. M. (1972). What does research tell us about day care? *Children Today*, 1:1.
42. Ablon, J., Metcalf, A. and Miller, D. (1967). *An Overview of Mental Health Problems of Indian Children*. Report to the Joint Commission on the Mental Health of Children.
43. Berlin, R. and Berlin, I. N. (1975). Parent's advocate role in education as primary prevention. In *Advocacy for Child Mental Health*, I. N. Berlin, ed. New York: Brunner/Mazel, pp. 145–157.
44. Kohler, M. (1971). The rights of children: An unexplored constituency. *Social Policy*, 1:36–43.
45. Mindell, C. and Maynard, E. (1967). Ambivalence towards education among Indian high school students. *Pine Ridge Research Bulletin*, No. 1, 26–31.
46. Hammerschlag, C., Alderfer, C. P. and Berg, D. (1973). Indian education: A human systems analysis. *American Journal of Psychiatry*, 130(10):1098–1102.
47. Krush, T. P., Bjork, J., Sindell, P. S. and Nelle, J. (1966). Some thoughts on the formation of personality disorder: Study of an Indian boarding school population. *American Journal of Psychiatry*, 122:868–876.
48. Ogden, M., Spector, M. I. and Hill, C. A. (1970). Suicides and homicides among Indians. *Public Health Reports*, 35(1):75–80.
49. Oetting, E. R. and Goldstein, G. S. (1978). *Drug Abuse among Indian Adolescents*. Report to N.I.D.A., Grant No. 2 RO1 DA01054, Ft. Collins, CO: Colorado State University.
50. Krush, T. P. and Bjork, J. (1965). Mental health factors in an Indian boarding school. *Mental Hygiene*, 49:94–103.
51. Kleinfeld, J. and Bloom, J. (1977). Boarding schools: Effects on the mental health of Eskimo adolescents. *American Journal of Psychiatry*, 134(4):441–471.
52. Goldstein, G. S. (1974). The model dormitory. *Psychiatric Annals*, 4:85–92.
53. Shure, M., Spivack, G. and Jaeger, M. (1971). Problem solving thinking and adjustment among disadvantaged preschool children. *Child Development*, 4:1791–1803.
54. Coche, E. and Douglas, A. (1977). Therapeutic effects of problem solving training and play reading groups. *Journal of Clinical Psychology*, 33:820–827.
55. Hollister, W. G. (1967). Concept of stress in education: A challenge to curriculum development. In *Behavioral Science Frontiers in Education*, E. M. Bower and W. G. Hollister, eds. New York: Wiley.
56. Berlin, I. N. (1981). *Problem Solving and Creativity: A Family School Collaboration*. Albuquerque, New Mexico: University of New Mexico Press, pp. 53–57.
57. Piaget, J. and Inhelder, B. (1969). *The Psychology of the Child*. New York: Basic Books.
58. Elkind, D. (1975). Recent research in cognitive development in adolescence. In *Adolescence in the Life Cycle*, S. E. Drogastin and C. H. Elder, Jr., eds. New York: Halstead, pp. 49–62.
59. Block, J. (1971). *Mastery Learning: Theory and Practice*. New York: Holt, Rinehart and Winston.
60. Kinsie, J. D. (1975). Personal communication, University of Oregon.
61. Leighton, A. (1971). Cosmos and the Gallup City Dump. In *Psychiatric Disorder and the Urban Environment*, B. H. Kaplan, ed. New York: Behavioral Publications.
62. Kinzie, J. D., Shore, J. H. and Pattison, E. M. (1972). Anatomy of psychiatric consultation to rural Indians. *Community Mental Health Journal*, 8:196–207.
63. Berlin, I. N. (1979). Mental health consultation to child serving agencies as therapeutic intervention. In *Basic Handbook of Child Psychiatry*, Vol. III, J. D. Noshpitz and S. I. Harrison, eds. New York: Basic Books, pp. 353–364.
64. Attneave, C. (1974). Medicine men and psychiatrists in the Indian Health Service. *Psychiatric Annals*, 4(1):49–55.

Part V

TEMPERAMENT STUDIES

The extensive temperament literature of previous years has encompassed studies of normal and deviant populations in various settings. However, only a few studies have considered the functional significance of the child's temperamental characteristics in the schoolroom, either with regard to the teacher's differential response to children with different temperamental traits, or to the influence of temperament, in interaction with other factors, on the child's adaptation to school and level of academic achievement. This year's selection of temperament studies does include several which provide a substantial basis for the systematic investigation of the relationship of the child's temperamental individuality to school functioning.

Keogh and her associates report the collection of questionnaire data from teachers in three preschools, involving a sample of over 300 three-to-six-year-old children, utilizing the NYLS 64-item Teacher Temperament Questionnaire. Factor analyses of the data yield three factors which appeared to have functional meaning within the school setting. From the factor loadings a psychometrically sound short form of the teacher questionnaire was developed, which appears practical as a research instrument.

Pullis and Cadwell report the use of this brief teacher questionnaire in a study relating the ratings from the three temperament factors to teachers' school performance estimates and classroom management decisions. Their findings emphasize the reliance of teachers on temperament information when making classroom management decisions. In fact, the teachers used information concerning their students' temperament characteristics more than any other type of information.

The paper by Greenberg and Field considers the question of whether handicapped infants' temperaments are perceived differently by teachers, mothers, and observers, and in different contexts. Their study reports the levels of interrater agreement among teachers, mothers, and observers, and compares the temperament ratings for the contrasting

335

groups of normal, developmentally delayed, Down Syndrome, cerebral palsied, and audiovisually handicapped infants. The methodological problems with regard to temperament questionnaire ratings of handicapped infants, as well as the implications of the findings, are highlighted in the discussion section.

The final paper by Weissbluth reports a significant correlation between infant sleep duration and temperament. The findings should be useful in counseling parents with respect to the sleep patterns in their infants.

21

A Short Form of the Teacher Temperament Questionnaire

Barbara K. Keogh

University of California, Los Angeles

Michael E. Pullis

University of Texas, Dallas

Joel Cadwell

Rutgers University

Renewed interest in temperament as an individual difference dimension of importance in children's behavior has led to reanalysis of both theoretical and methodological considerations relating to the construct. Temperament is now a topic of study from the perspectives of behavioral-genetics, developmental and clinical psychology, psychiatry, and pediatrics (Buss & Plomin, 1975; Carey, 1982; Goldsmith & Gottesman, 1981; Rothbart, 1981; Wilson, 1982; Wolkind & DeSalis, 1982). Measurement and conceptual issues have been pinpointed by Hubert, Wachs, Peters-Martin, and Gandour (1982). As noted in a recent review by Keogh and Pullis (1980), different theoretical orientations have provided somewhat different formulations on number, specificity, and stability of hypothesized temperament dimensions. Despite variations in specifics,

Keogh, Barbara K., Pullis, Michael E., and Cadwell, Joel. "A Short Form of the Teacher Temperament Questionnaire." *Journal of Educational Measurement*, 1982, Vol. 19, pp. 323–329. Copyright 1982, National Council on Measurement in Education, Washington, D.C.

This work was supported by Project REACH under contract #4-482130-25700-3 between the U.S. Office of Special Education and the University of California.

We wish to thank Alexander Thomas and Stella Chess for their continuing consultation and for their generosity in sharing ideas and information.

however, there is considerable agreement that significant and relatively enduring individual differences may be identified in children's behavioral styles, in the "how," not just the "how much," of their behavior.

The temperament formulation proposed by Thomas, Chess, and Birch (1968), and elaborated by Thomas and Chess (1977), seems particularly useful for the assessment of temperament variations in young children. Relying on their extensive clinical experience, these investigators defined nine dimensions of temperament: Activity Level, Adaptability, Approach/Withdrawal, Distractibility, Intensity, Persistence, Quality of Mood, Rhythmicity, and Threshold of Response. They also provided a system for assessing temperament in young children. Based on interview data collected as part of the New York Longitudinal Study (NYLS), Thomas and Chess (1977) developed a 72-item Parent Temperament Questionnaire (PTQ) and a 64-item Teacher Temperament Questionnaire (TTQ). In both questionnaires each temperament dimension is represented by eight items. (Rhythmicity items are not included in the Teacher Scale.) The items are worded to be appropriate for use by parents (PTQ) or by teachers (TTQ). Evidence from a number of different research groups (Billman & McDevitt, 1980; Carey, 1981; Maurer, 1980; Rutter, 1970) provides support for the Thomas and Chess dimensions and suggests that these stylistic differences, while situationally sensitive, have some stability across situations and over time.

Despite the appeal of the Thomas and Chess temperament constructs, measurement problems have limited research on clinical and educational applications. The original scaling work by Thomas et al. (1968) was carried out on a selected sample of children and families in New York City. Subsequent scale development by Carey and McDevitt (Carey, 1970; Carey & McDevitt, 1978; McDevitt & Carey, 1978) has focused on assessment of temperament within a clinical/pediatric context and has led to longer scales for use by parents. However, consideration of temperament within an educational context requires a scale which is psychometrically adequate yet practical for use by teachers. The present work was carried out with this goal. Focusing on the Thomas and Chess Teacher Temperament Questionnaire (TTQ), we have assessed reliabilities of items and dimensions, determined the extent of agreement among raters, identified the factor structure, and assessed the influence of sex and age of children on raters' perceptions. We have reduced the number of items in the original Questionnaire while maintaining its measurement properties. This article contains a summary of these analyses and identifies the items recommended for inclusion in a short form of the TTQ.

PSYCHOMETRIC ANALYSES OF THE TTQ

Initial work on the 64-item TTQ was based on data from 35 teachers in three preschools in the Los Angeles area. The sample consisted of over 300 three-to-six-year old children. The majority of children and teachers were Anglo, representing an SES range from low to upper middle class. All children were rated by at least two teachers. Initial analyses were performed at the item level. Following the Thomas and Chess (1977) instructions, the eight items comprising each dimension were weighted and summed, providing a single score for each of the eight dimensions. Correlation coefficients reflecting agreement between teachers' ratings were computed for dimension scores. Threshold of Response was the only dimension on which there was low agreement ($r = .19$). Correlations between the two teachers' ratings on the seven other dimensions ranged from .48 to .84 with an average correlation of .59. Rate-rerate correlations over a five-week period for a subset of teachers ranged from .69 to .88; the average value of r was .81. Internal consistency reliability coefficients for the eight dimensions ranged from .46 to .85. Unclear wording of items (e.g., double negatives, conditional statements with infrequent antecedents) reduced the internal consistency of some dimensions. In general, however, the reliability coefficients were moderately high although the dimensions tapping Mood and Distractibility were less reliable than others.

Separate factor analyses of the 64 items and of the eight dimensions yielded the same three-factor structure. The first factor was composed of the dimensions of Persistence, Distractibility, and Activity. We interpret this as a task related factor. Examination of the items loading on this factor confirmed this interpretation. The second factor, made up of Adaptability, Approach-Withdrawal, and positive Mood, appeared related to the child's flexibility, especially in social situations, as the specific items focused more on social interactions than on task behavior. The third factor, labeled Reactivity, was composed of dimensions of Intensity of Response and Threshold of Response; specific items concerned with the negative aspects of Mood also appeared in the factor. Although the factor analyses indicated that the eight dimensions of temperament were not factorially independent, the dimensions clustered in logical and interpretable ways. Further analyses were directed at determining possible influences of children's sex and age on teachers' ratings of temperament. In general, the ANOVA and *post hoc* comparisons confirmed past findings and intuitive notions concerning sex and age differences: boys were rated higher than girls in Activity, Intensity, and

Distractibility, but lower in Persistence; as age increased there was a general increase in Persistence accompanied by a decrease in Distractibility.

SHORT FORM OF THE TEACHER TEMPERAMENT QUESTIONNAIRE (TTQ)

Having established the three-factor structure of the Thomas and Chess TTQ and noting that all the items within a given dimension did not always load on the same factor, the original scale was revised by examining the factor loadings for the 64 items and retaining only those items with substantial weights. This process yielded a 23-item scale in which all eight dimensions were represented. In this form of the TTQ the teacher is asked to rate each item on a 6-point scale from "hardly ever" to "almost always." Psychometric properties of the scale were examined by Pullis (1979), who gathered data on over 300 children in kindergarten, first, and third grades. Pullis verified that the factor structure of the short form was consistent with that of the original 64-item scale, the 23 items clustering into three factors labelled Task Orientation, Personal-Social Flexibility, and Reactivity. When the items were grouped according to the factor structure and tested for internal consistency, alpha coefficients for the three factors were .94, .88, and .62, respectively. Examination of sex and grade differences yielded findings consistent with those of the psychometric analysis of the long form of the TTQ already discussed. Taken as a whole, Pullis' analyses supported the utility and feasibility of the 23 items as a research instrument. The 23 items and their factor loadings may be found in Table 1. The values in column 1 represent the preschool findings, those in column 2 the kindergarten, first and third grade findings (Pullis, 1979). Subsequent work with samples of preschool and elementary school regular and special education children (Keogh, 1982, in press; Keogh & Kornblau, 1982) has confirmed that there is substantial agreement between teachers' ratings of the same children and that there are identifiable correlates of the temperament ratings.

Taken as a whole, results of the psychometric analyses of the Teacher Temperament Questionnaire suggest that the 23-item short form is a reliable technique for assessing teachers' perceptions of children's temperament. The two forms are factorially consistent; the factors have demonstrated internal consistency; agreement among raters is acceptably high; and the scores are consistent with expectancies for age and sex of children. On a practical level teachers are able to use the scales efficiently and quickly. While the educational applications of the tem-

Table 1

Selected TTQ Items and Factor Loadings
for Preschool and Kindergarten, Grades 1 & 3 Samples

Item	Thomas & Chess TTQ Item Number	Factor	Pre-School	K, 1, & 3*
Child seems to have difficulty sitting still, may wriggle a lot or get out of seat.	1	I	.84	.80
If child's activity is interrupted, he/she tries to go back to the activity.	5	I	.73	.84
Child is easily drawn away from his/her work by noises, something outside the window, another child's whispering, etc.	9	I	.84	.86
Child can continue at the same activity for an hour.	31	I	.66	.87
Child is able to sit quietly for a reasonable amount of time (as compared to classmates).	34	I	.86	.88
Child cannot be distracted when he/she is working (seems able to concentrate in the midst of bedlam).	36	I	.78	.62
If other children are talking or making noise while teacher is explaining a lesson, this child remains attentive to the teacher.	44	I	.83	.84
Child starts an activity and does not finish it.	48	I	.74	.73
Child sits still when a story is being told or read.	64	I	.76	.77
When with other children, this child seems to be having a good time.	2	II	.49	.62
Child will initially avoid new games and activities, preferring to sit on the side and watch.	10	II	.63	.86
Child enjoys going on errands for the teacher.	14	II	.65	.60

Table 1 (continued)

Item	Thomas & Chess TTQ Item Number	Factor	Pre-School	K, 1, & 3*
If initially hesitant about entering into new games and activities, child gets over this quickly.	15	II	.72	.69
Child takes a long time to become comfortable in a new physical location (e.g., different classroom, new seat, etc.).	25	II	.48	.67
Child will show little or no reaction when another child takes his/her toy or possession away.	27	II	.38	.19
Child plunges into new activities and situations without hesitation.	30	II	.74	.65
Child takes a long time to become comfortable in a new situation.	40	II	.57	.72
Child is bashful when meeting new children.	47	II	.55	.79
When playing with other children, this child argues with them.	29	III	.29	.32
Child is sensitive to temperature and likely to comment on classroom being hot or cold.	39	III	.41	.37
Child overreacts (becomes very upset) in a stressful situation.	43	III	.52	.69
When child can't have or do something he/she wants, child becomes annoyed or upset.	56	III	.53	.60
Child is highly sensitive to changes in the brightness or dimness of light.	57	III	.44	.43

*From the work of M. Pullis, 1979.

perament scales require further study, the short form of the TTQ appears useful as a research instrument.

REFERENCES

Billman, J. and McDevitt, S. C. (1980). Convergence of parent and observer ratings of temperament with observations of peer interaction in nursery school. *Child Development*, 51:395–400.

Buss, A. H. and Plomin, R. A. (1975). *Temperament Theory of Personality Development*. New York: Wiley.

Carey, W. B. (1970). A simplified method for measuring infant temperament. *Journal of Pediatrics*, 77(2):188–194.

Carey, W. B. (1981). The importance of temperament-environment interaction for child level and development. In *The Uncommon Child*, M. Lewis and R. L. Rosenblum, eds. New York: Plenum.

Carey, W. B. (1982). Clinical use of temperament in pediatrics. In *Temperamental, Differences in Infants and Young Children*, M. Rutter, R. Porter and G. M. Collins, eds. London: Ciba Foundation.

Carey, W. B. and McDevitt, S. C. (1978). Revision of the Infant Temperament Questionnaire. *Pediatrics*, 61:735–739.

Goldsmith, H. H. and Gottesman, I. I. (1981). Origins of variation in behavioral style: A longitudinal study of temperament in young twins. *Child Development*, 52(1):91–103.

Hubert, N. C., Wachs, T. D., Peters-Martin, P. and Gandour, M. J. (1982). The study of early temperament: Measurement and conceptual issues. *Child Development*, 55:571–600.

Keogh, B. K. (1982). Children's temperament and teachers' decisions. In *Temperamental Differences in Infants and Young Children*, M. Rutter, R. Porter and G. M. Collins, eds. London: The Ciba Foundation.

Keogh, B. K. (In press). Individual differences in temperament: A contributor to the personal-social and educational competence of learning disabled children. In *Current Topics in Learning Disabilities*, J. D. McKinney and L. Feagens, eds. Norwood, NJ: Ablex Publishing Corp.

Keogh, B. K. and Kornblau, B. S. (1982). Children's temperament and teachers' perceptions of teachability. Report in preparation, UCLA.

Keogh, B. K. and Pullis, M. E. (1980). Temperament influences on the development of exceptional children. In *Advances in Special Education*, Vol. 1, B. K. Keogh, ed. Greenwich, CT: JAI Press.

Maurer, R., Cardoret, R. J. and Cain, C. (1980). Cluster analysis of childhood temperament data on adoptees. *American Journal of Orthopsychiatry*, 51:522–534.

McDevitt, S. C. and Carey, W. B. (1978). The measurement f temperament in 3–7 year old children. *Journal of Child Psychology and Psychiatry*, 19:245–253.

Pullis, M. E. (1982). An investigation of the relationship between children's temperament and school adjustment. Unpublished doctoral dissertation, University of California, Los Angeles.

Rothbart, M. K. (1981). Measurement of temperament in infancy. *Child Development*, 52(2):569–578.

Rutter, M. (1970). Psychological development: Predictions from infancy. *Journal of Child Psychology and Psychiatry*, 11:49–62.

Thomas, A. and Chess, S. (1977). *Temperament and Development*. New York: Brunner/Mazel, Inc.

Thomas, A., Chess, S. and Birch, H. G. (1968). *Temperament and Behavior Disorders in Children*. New York: New York University Press.

Wilson, R. (1982). Intrinsic determinants of temperament. In *Temperamental Differences in Infants and Young Children*, M. Rutter, R. Porter and G. M. Collins, eds. London: Ciba Foundation.

Wolkind, S. N. and Desalis, W. (In press). Infant temperament, maternal mental state and child behavioral problems. In *Temperamental Differences in Infants and Young Children*, M. Rutter, R. Porter and G. M. Collins, eds. London: Ciba Foundation.

PART V: TEMPERAMENT STUDIES

22

The Influence of Children's Temperament Characteristics on Teachers' Decision Strategies

Michael Pullis

University of Texas at Dallas

Joel Cadwell

Rutgers University

Thirteen primary level teachers provided information on 321 students concerning the children's temperament characteristics, school performance estimates, and classroom management decisions. Factor analysis of the temperament measures yielded three independent factors: Task Orientation, Adaptability, and Reactivity. These factors replicate earlier findings with a similar instrument and meld with other research on teachers' behavioral ratings. The most important finding to emerge concerned the strong and consistent relationship between the students' temperament characteristics and teachers' classroom decisions. Multiple regression analyses indicated that most of the teachers used Task Orientation information across classroom management decision-making situations.

Pullis, Michael and Cadwell, Joel., "The Influence of Children's Temperament Characteristics on Teachers' Decision Strategies." *American Educational Research Journal*, 1982, Vol. 19, No. 2, pp. 165–181. Copyright 1982, American Educational Research Association, Washington, D.C.

This research was supported, in part, by a grant from the Bureau of Education for the Handicapped, United States Office of Education, and Project REACH of the University of California, Los Angeles. The gracious cooperation of the DuQuoin, Illinois Unified School District is acknowledged.

Research on children's performance in school has historically focused on intellectual factors. While obviously important to the understanding of children's success or failure in school, emphasis on intellectual constructs (usually some measure of potential, knowledge, or skill) may well have resulted in less vigorous investigation of other sources of developmental variation (Keogh & Pullis, 1980). For example, Thomas and Chess (1977) contend that most research has focused either on the content of achievement or on the underlying motivation of academic performance, but has failed to consider the stylistic aspects of achievement-related behaviors (i.e., *how* children approach, avoid, interact, and respond to school tasks). Using a similar argument, several investigators have criticized the almost total reliance on cognitive measures as predictors of academic achievement and have advocated the inclusion of affective measures in the prediction equation (Kohn, 1977; McKinney et al., 1975; Perry, Guidubaldi, & Kehle, 1979). Although each author argues for a relationship between school performance and nonintellective characteristics, the mechanism through which these factors might influence school performance has never been systematically investigated. In an attempt to specify this process, the present study examined how children's temperament characteristics are related to teachers' classroom decisions.

Though there are several different theoretical conceptualizations dealing with nonintellective characteristics of children, the approach of Thomas and Chess (1977) was chosen because of its emphasis on the influence of children's temperament on their interactions with adults. Defining temperament as within-person stylistic characteristics that reflect general response tendencies in learning and social situations, Thomas and Chess have identified nine dimensions of temperament: Activity Level, Rhythmicity, Approach/Withdrawal, Adaptability, Intensity of Response, Threshold of Responsiveness, Quality of Mood, Distractibility, and Attention Span and Persistence. Using these temperament dimensions, they developed a transactional model of parent-child interaction. According to this model, the child is seen as having a relatively stable behavioral style or temperament, which is reflected in his or her behavior. The parents, on the other hand, have some flexibility in their response to the child's behavior. For instance, the parents can avoid explosive tantrums from their overly persistent child by recognizing when the child is engrossed in a task and not interrupting until his or her attention has waned. It is the cumulative stress resulting from a mismatch between the child's behavioral style and the parents' reactions that produces behavioral disorders. Moreover, Thomas, Chess, and

Birch (1968) have demonstrated that the problems associated with the "lack of fit" between child characteristics and parenting strategies can be attenuated when parents understand their child's temperament and respond appropriately.

Thomas and Chess have attempted to extend their work with parents to the classroom by assuming that temperament might have the same influence on teacher-student relationships as it does with parent-child interactions. They hypothesized that the temperament characteristics of children, in combination with teacher strategies and the structure of the classroom, might have powerful effects on school performance. For example, Stella Chess (1966), using a clinical case study approach, described several instances where changes in teachers' reactions to problem behaviors resulted in improved adaptation by the difficult student. Gordon and Thomas (1967), studying the relationship between teachers' perceptions of student temperament and their estimates of student intelligence, found that teachers' estimates of their students' ability were influenced significantly by the students' temperament. In particular, teachers were more likely to underestimate the intelligence of children who did not readily approach new situations and who were somewhat slow in adapting. Gordon and Thomas suggested that these inaccuracies in teachers' estimates may affect school performance because the teachers' expectations do not correspond to the actual capabilities of the children.

Other researchers using this temperament framework, have also demonstrated a relationship between temperament and adaptation to school. Carey, Fox, and McDevitt (1977) found that infants with extreme temperament ratings tended to have a more difficult adjustment to early school demands. Lambert and Windmiller (1977) reported that parents' retrospective ratings of their child's temperament were related to the child's current membership in groups considered educationally at risk. Hall and Keogh (1977) documented a relationship between temperament and ratings of educational competence and educational risk. Interviews with teachers revealed that certain temperament patterns covaried with sex and intellectual ability in the determination of risk. Still others have reported modest correlations between temperament ratings and school performance measures such as achievement test scores and social interaction ratings (See Keogh & Pullis, 1980 for a comprehensive review).

These studies provide tentative support for an association between temperament and school performance, yet they fail to reveal the mechanism through which variations in temperament affect school performance. According to the transactional model, it is the teacher's response to a child's relatively stable behavioral style that is important. For example, a child who is reluctant to approach group learning activities may become disruptive or withdrawn when the teacher demands immediate participation, but may slowly join the group when the teacher recognizes the child's temperament and responds to accommodate it.

As an initial step to the analysis of this transactional model the present study was designed to determine teachers' sensitivity to individual differences in children's temperament in specific classroom decision-making situations. Teachers were asked to rate their students' temperaments and make several classroom management and placement decisions. In addition, teacher ratings of traditional student attributes were obtained. Using a policy-capturing or regression-modeling approach (Shavelson, Cadwell, & Izu, 1977; Shulman & Elstein, 1975), the teachers' decision strategies were "captured" by regressing the decisions onto the student characteristics. If the teacher focused on particular student characteristics when making decisions, then measures of those characteristics will be related significantly to the decisions and the regression equation will document this relationship. If the temperament characteristics of children influence teachers' decisions, then temperament may indeed be an important factor mediating classroom interactions and school performance.

METHODS

Subjects

The subjects were 321 elementary school children from a small school district in Illinois. The students were predominantly white (96%); the remainder were black. These students came from families whose socioeconomic status ranged from lower class to upper middle class, with a majority of the families classified as lower middle to middle class. The sample contained a larger proportion of boys (N = 177) than girls (N = 144): 74-kindergarten, 145-first grade, and 102-third grade.

Information on the students was provided by 13 primary-level teachers. All teachers participating in the study were female: 12 were white and 1 was black. The teachers' experience averaged 11.1 years; the range was from 5 to 33 years. The teachers had undergraduate degrees in either elementary education or early childhood education. All of the teachers had additional hours of graduate work in compliance with requirements for continuing education. Six teachers held Master's degrees and two more were working toward advanced degrees.

Materials and Procedure

All student information was collected using teacher ratings. The teachers were asked to complete a three-part questionnaire for each student in their classroom. Teachers completed the questionnaires on their own time, reporting that it took from 2 to 5 hours to provide information on all of their students.

Teacher estimates of student aptitudes.—In the first part of the questionnaire, teachers were asked to rate each child in their class on five areas of classroom functioning or behavior: (1) intelligence or general ability, (2) motivation during classroom activities, (3) social interaction skills, (4) academic performance, and (5) working up to potential. The response to each of the items was a single value within a 6 point Likert scale, where low ratings reflected poor performance and high ratings indicated outstanding performance or capacity.

Temperament ratings.—The second part of the questionnaire required teachers to make 23 temperament ratings on each student. Each item described a child's behavior in a classroom setting. The teacher responded on a 6-point Likert scale by indicating the frequency with which the particular behavior occurred (1 = hardly ever to 6 = almost always). The 23 items were selected from the original 64-item Teacher Temperament Questionnaire (Thomas & Chess, 1977) on the basis of an exploratory factor analysis (Keogh et al., 1979). This factor analysis showed that only three factors were needed to account for most of the common variance among the original temperament items. Using these results, the items with the highest loadings on each factor were chosen.

Classroom management and placement decisions.—In the last section of the questionnaire, teachers were provided with brief descriptions of five classroom situations and asked to indicate the frequency with which they had to monitor each child's behavior in each situation. Responses were made on the same 6-point Likert scale used for rating temperament. The situations were chosen because they are common occurrences in primary grade classrooms and because individual differences in behavioral style might influence teachers' strategies for dealing with these events. The five classroom situations were (1) independent seatwork, (2) small-group activity where students are required to share materials, (3) transition from one academic activity to another, (4) transition from outside activity to classroom activity, and (5) free play activity in class in lieu of recess. In addition, teachers also made placement recommendations for the following school year ranging from full-time special education to regular promotion.

RESULTS

The data analysis was conducted in two phases. First, the measurement properties of the temperament questionnaire were investigated. This phase included a factor analysis of the 23 temperament items and an examination of the correlations between the teachers' ratings of temperament and their ratings of more traditional student aptitudes (ability, motivation, social skills, etc.). Second, the teachers' decision strategies were studied by regressing the classroom management and placement decisions on the teachers' ratings of student aptitude and temperament. The regression coefficients from this analysis indicated the contribution of each student characteristic to the teachers' decisions.

All analyses were performed using only teacher ratings. Since each teacher rated several students, it was assumed that data concerning individual students rated by the same teacher would not be independent. Because such dependencies violate the assumptions underlying factor analysis, correlation, and regression procedures, these analyses were conducted with deviation scores calculated by subtracting the teachers' mean rating over students from each individual student's score (Cronbach, 1976). Thus, when the data across different teachers were used, the pooled within-teacher correlation or variance-covariance matrix was analyzed.

Measurement Properties of the Temperament Questionnaire

The teacher ratings of behavioral style were factor analyzed to determine if the eight original dimensions proposed by Thomas et al. (1963) could be distinguished or if the dimensions were so highly interrelated that only the three higher order factors reported by Keogh et al. (1979) could be identified. An exploratory factor analysis of the 23 temperament items extracted three common factors accounting for 60 percent of the variance. These factors were subjected to a varimax rotation resulting in the three independent temperament factors presented in Table I.

The findings were essentially identical to those from Keogh et al. (1979). The first factor, Task Orientation, contained items from the dimensions of Activity Level, Persistence, and Distractibility. These items reflect the student's ability to remain seated during work activities, to

Table 1

Factor Loading of Temperament Items (Pooled Within Teacher)

Item No.	Dimension	Factor 1 Task Orientation	Factor 2 Adaptability	Factor 3 Reactivity
1.	Activity	.799	−.116	.190
2.	Persistence	.824	.186	.029
3.	Distractibility	.8599	.032	.114
4.	Appr./Withdrawal	−.072	.856	−.150
5.	Adaptablilty	.025	693	−.044
6.	Positive Mood	.133	.623	.176
7.	Threshold	−.044	−.166	.369
8.	Intensity	.035	−.188	.032
9.	Activity	.887	−.038	.078
10.	Persistence	.868	.122	.020
11.	Distractibility	.619	−.044	.009
12.	Appr./Withdrawal	.449	.647	.006
13.	Adaptability	.265	.672	.146
14.	Negative Mood	.465	−.078	.432
15.	Threshold	−.031	−.093	.437
16.	Intensity	.205	.266	.692
17.	Activity	.771	−.006	.160
18.	Persistence	.731	.262	−.002
19.	Distractibility	.834	.066	.064
20.	Appr./Withdrawal	−.154	.789	−.126
21.	Adaptability	.106	.718	.103
22.	Negative Mood	.363	.127	.710
23.	Positive Mood	.016	.599	−.114

Note All items recoded so that a higher score indicates a more positive response. A copy of the questionnaire is available upon request from the first author.

persist on tasks until completion, and to not be distracted. Items from the dimensions of Approach/Withdrawal, Adaptability, and Positive Mood loaded on the second factor, labeled Adaptability. Students scoring high on this subscale tend to react positively to new stimuli, easily modify their behavior in response to routine changes, and respond positively during social interactions. The last factor, Reactivity, included items from the dimensions of Threshold of Response, Intensity, and Negative Mood. This last factor refers to a student's tendency to overreact to stressful situations and become overly upset when frustrated. Given the replication of the Keogh et al. (1979) findings, the 23 items were subdivided so that items with the highest loadings were grouped together to form nonoverlapping subscales. The score on each subscale was calculated as the mean rating on the items forming the subscale.

To assess the internal consistency reliability of the subscales, coefficient alpha was computed. The following reliabilities were obtained: Task

Orientation (.943), Adaptability (.883), and Reactivity (.689). The reliability for Reactivity was computed after deleting Item 8 from the subscale. The item contained awkward wording, which teachers found to be confusing.

To determine the relationship between the temperament ratings and the ratings of the other student attributes, the correlations between the three temperament subscales and the five estimates of student aptitudes were computed (see Table II). First, the intercorrelations among the temperament subscales should be noted. Of the three temperament measures, only Task Orientation and Reactivity were moderately correlated. Adaptability was relatively independent of the other two temperament subscales. These relationships could have been predicted from the results of the factor analysis. A few of the items with high factor pattern coefficients on Reactivity also had moderate loadings on Task Orientation. Since factor scores were not calculated, it is to be expected that the subscales would be correlated to some degree.

Although Task Orientation and Reactivity were not independent, the subscales did not have the same patterns of correlation with the other teacher estimates. For example, teachers' ratings of Task Orientation were highly related to their ratings of motivation, academic performance, and potential. These correlations tend to support the original interpretation of this factor. Moreover, Task Orientation does not appear to be merely another measure of ability, since it has a somewhat lower correlation with the ability estimate. Reactivity, on the other hand, was significantly related to only one estimate, students' social interaction skills. While Task Orientation and Reactivity were moderately correlated, their differential patterns of relationship to the other teacher estimates

Table II
Correlations Among the Student Characteristics (Pooled Within Teacher)

	Task Orientation	Adaptability	Reactivity	Ability	Motivation	Soc. S.	Academic	Potential
Task Orientation	1.000							
Adaptability	.200	1.000						
Reactivity	.406*	.103	1.000					
Ability Est.	.527*	.358*	.124	1.000				
Motivation	.714*	.447*	.199	.511*	1.000			
Social Skills	.418*	.608*	.319*	.443*	.602*	1.000		
Academic Per.	.708*	.442*	.197	.745*	.766*	.594*	1.000	
Potential	.632*	.333*	.173	.446*	.719*	.463*	.763*	1.000
Mean	3.81	4.79	5.05	4.03	4.12	4.32	4.03	3.53
Standard Deviation	1.36	1.01	0.86	1.12	1.12	1.06	1.27	0.97

*$p < .05$

provided evidence that the subscales were measuring different aspects of temperament.

Teacher Decision Making

The study was designed to investigate how teachers utilize temperament information in making classroom management and placement decisions. By regressing the teachers' decision on the measures of student characteristics, the contribution of each characteristic to the decision can be assessed. The regression procedure, however, requires some degree of independence among the student variables in order to unambiguously separate the effects of the different measures or ratings. As was indicated in Table II, the teacher estimates of student characteristics were not independent. Although the degree of intercorrelation does not rule out a regression analysis using all the student variables, the following strategy was chosen. First, based on logical and substantive considerations, a priori models of teacher decision making were specified. For each decision, the a priori model contained those student variables believed to be important for that decision. The temperament subscales were included in all of these models. Second, regression analyses were then performed with *all* teacher ratings in the equation. This step tested if any student information, not in the a priori model, ought to be included in the decision. The a priori models were supported by the data with only one additional estimate, motivation, found significant in the models for Individual Seatwork and Placement decisions.

Once the set of student characteristics had been determined, the regression analysis for each decision model was performed using the data from all the teachers. Since it was hypothesized that teachers might employ different decision strategies, the interactions between teachers and each student characteristic were formed and tested. These interactions were constructed by adding to the regression equation 12 dummy variables representing the 13 teachers and creating the product terms between the dummy variables and the teacher estimates. In each of the decision models significant teacher-by-student estimate interactions were found, indicating that teachers were using different strategies when making the decisions. Therefore, the data from each teacher were analyzed separately for each decision, and the results are reported in Tables III-VIII.

Most of the decisions concerned the frequency with which the teacher had to monitor each student in different school situations because of the possibility of inappropriate or disruptive behavior. The various settings were chosen to provide a broad sampling of situations where student temperament characteristics might influence teachers' decisions.

The first decision asked the teachers to estimate how frequently they had to monitor each child when the class was working individually at their seats on academic tasks. Table III contains the regression coefficients for each teacher. Task Orientation appears to be the most important piece of information in the teachers' decisions. The negative sign of the coefficients means that the higher the Task Orientation rating of a student, the less need there was for monitoring. Eight of the 13 teachers in the study were sensitive to the Task Orientation of their students. Five teachers used no other information in reaching their decision. If Task Orientation information was not used, then either the teachers used some combination of the other student characteristics or the teachers' decisions were not related to any of the student estimates. It should be noted that Task Orientation was not merely serving as a proxy for ability, since the ability estimate was also in the regression equation. Finally, one finding contrasting the decision strategies of teachers at different grade levels should be mentioned. All third-grade teachers used Task Orientation information. Although this tendency for third-grade teachers to rely on Task Orientation will also be found in other decisions, the sample sizes and small differences between grades limits the generalizability of this finding.

Table III

Decision Model for Individual Seatwork

	Teacher	Mean Rating	Regression Weights for Independent Variables				
			Ability Estimate	Task Orientation	Adaptability	Reactivity	Motivation Estimate
Kindergarten	1	3.08	−0.45	−0.47*	0.26	−0.35	−0.50*
	2	1.83	−0.13	−0.43	0.10	−0.25	−0.24
	3	2.24	0.02	−0.83*	−0.46	0.41	−0.44
First Grade	4	2.57	0.03	−1.16*	0.43	−0.48	0.28
	5	2.65	0.20	−0.94*	0.16	−0.06	−0.21
	6	1.88	0.09	−0.37	−0.01	−0.34	−0.62*
	7	2.84	0.73*	−0.58	−1.38*	0.51	−0.79
	8	2.42	−0.67*	−0.19	0.17	0.49	−0.77*
	9	2.36	−0.16	−0.56	−0.07	−.034	−0.12
Third Grade	10	3.35	0.25	−0.82*	−0.31*	−0.37	−0.28
	11	2.31	0.22	−1.32*	0.21	0.08	0.20
	12	2.88	0.19	−1.59*	−0.14	0.67*	−0.04
	13	3.15	0.31	−1.14*	0.04	−0.10	−0.22

*$p < .05$

Table IV

Decision Model for Group Activity

	Teacher	Mean Rating	Regression Weights for Independent Variables				
			Ability Es-timate	Task Ori-entation	Adaptabil-ity	Reactivity	Social Es-timate
Kindergarten	1	2.88	− 0.33	− 0.54*	0.80*	− 0.30	− 0.91*
	2	1.88	0.25	− 0.72*	0.85*	− 0.35	− 0.76
	3	1.40	0.53*	− 0.32*	0.16	− 1.09	− 0.56*
First Grade	4	1.87	− 0.13	− 0.75*	0.15	− 0.46	0.30
	5	2.57	0.03	− 0.82*	0.35	− 0.76*	− 0.22
	6	1.92	0.26	− 0.67*	0.48	− 0.29	− 0.61
	7	2.64	0.40	− 1.08*	− 0.40	0.19	− 0.05
	8	1.33	0.25	0.08	0.01	− 0.38	0.04
	9	2.04	0.24	− 0.40	− 0.01	− 0.10	− 0.11
Third Grade	10	3.35	0.45*	− 1.45*	− 0.27	− 9.64	0.18
	11	2.00	0.34	− 1.01*	0.32	− 0.05	− 0.42
	12	2.38	− 0.65*	− 0.58*	0.34	− 0.29	0.36
	13	2.81	0.29	− 1.03*	− 0.22	− 0.30	0.16

$p < .05$

For the second decision, teachers estimated how often they had to monitor their students when the class was engaged in small-group activities. As shown in Table IV, eleven of the teachers relied on the Task Orientation information. The regression coefficients were again negative, indicating that task oriented students needed less monitoring. The two teachers who did not use Task Orientation information did not appear to be responding to any of the student characteristics. While grade level differences are only suggestive, the kindergarten teachers seemed to be particularly sensitive to the Adaptability and social skills information. It may be that kindergarten children find it more difficult to work in small groups where they are required to share materials. However, the coefficients for Adaptability are positive, suggesting that the more adaptable child requires more monitoring. Such a finding is interpretable if one assumes that the highly adaptable student "over-responds" in group settings, and, thus, requires the attention of the teacher in order to allow the other students to complete their own work.

Table V contains the regression coefficients for each teacher on the third decision, a rating of monitoring frequency during the transition from one academic assignment to another. Again, most (nine) of the teachers were responsive to the Task Orientation information. The other teachers did not appear to be using any of the student characteristics. Some teachers did respond to other student estimates, but no common

Table V
Decision Model for Academic Transition

	Teacher	Mean Rating	Regression Weights for Independent Variables				
			Ability Es-timate	Task Ori-entation	Adaptabil-ity	Reactivity	Motivation Estimate
Kindergarten	1	3.08	−0.54	−0.55*	0.95*	−0.69*	−0.16
	2	1.63	−0.39	−0.14	−0.27	−0.02	
	3	1.76	0.48*	−0.66*	−0.28	−0.65	−0.19
First Grade	4	1.57	−0.28	−0.37	−0.51	−0.44	0.36
	5	2.87	0.06	−1.23*	0.08	−0.19	0.05
	6	1.92	0.21	−0.85	−0.29	0.23	−0.16
	7	2.68	0.22	−0.76*	0.51	0.30	−1.29*
	8	2.25	−0.31	−0.80*	−0.20	0.30	−0.17
	9	2.00	−0.11	−0.45*	0.05	0.15	−0.40
Third Grade	10	3.19	−0.03	−0.57*	0.24	−0.39	−0.48*
	11	2.54	0.34	−1.50*	0.02	−0.15	0.45
	12	2.25	−0.08	−1.03*	0.05	−0.13	0.03
	13	2.42	0.32	−1.04*	−0.03	0.01	−0.14

*$p < .05$

decision strategy emerged. Finally, examining possible grade differences in strategies, all third grade teachers had significant Task Orientation regression coefficients. Moreover, except for one teacher, Task Orientation was the only information the third grade teachers used.

The fourth decision required teachers to make the same estimate of monitoring frequency, but changed the setting so that students were now returning from an outside activity and preparing to work at their seats. The pattern of results in Table VI was consistent with the findings from earlier decisions. Ten of the 13 teachers utilized Task Orientation information. The third-grade teachers totally relied on Task Orientation and nothing else. The kindergarten and first-grade teachers, however, tended to pay more attention to the other temperament information. In fact, nonacademic transition was the first decision in which Reactivity entered the teachers' decision models. Looking at the regression coefficients, Task Orientation had its usual negative weights demonstrating that the more task oriented child required less monitoring. The weights for Reactivity were also negative, showing that students likely to overreact in stressful situations or when frustrated required closer supervision. On the other hand, Adaptability tended to be given a positive weight indicating, as found earlier for the small-group activity, extremely adaptable students needing more monitoring. This finding was observed only for

Table VI
Decision Model for Nonacademic Transition

	Teacher	Mean Rating	Regression Weights for Independent Variables			
			Task Orientation	Adaptability	Reactivity	Social Estimate
Kindergarten	1	3.40	−0.71*	0.78*	−0.48	−0.49
	2	1.79	−0.38	0.44	−0.81*	−0.37
	3	1.64	−0.17	0.87*	−1.48*	−0.87*
First Grade	4	1.70	−0.32*	0.31	−0.93*	−0.72*
	5	2.91	−1.02*	0.72*	−1.25*	0.10
	6	2.16	−0.74*	0.25	−0.25	−0.22
	7	2.44	−1.11*	0.54	−0.01	0.39
	8	1.25	−0.11	−0.48*	−0.89*	0.00
	9	1.64	−0.24	0.22	−0.84	−0.32
Third Grade	10	2.96	−0.99*	0.15	−0.43	−0.16
	11	2.42	−1.22*	0.55	−0.18	0.04
	12	3.00	−1.19*	0.43	−0.28	0.25
	13	2.50	−0.94*	0.16	−0.26	−0.14

*$p < .05$

teachers of the younger children (especially kindergarten). Recalling that the Adaptability subscale has a strong social interaction component, a possible interpretation of this finding is that the extremely adaptable child may have a difficult time in the transition from the playground (a social setting) to classroom seatwork (a setting where social interaction is inappropriate). In addition, two of the teachers took into consideration the social skills of the children by indicating that they would monitor children with good social interaction skills less frequently.

Table VII reveals that the results for the fifth decision, frequency of monitoring during free play activity in the classroom, were similar to those from the nonacademic transition decision. Again, the Task Orientation coefficients were significant for 10 of the 13 teachers (including all third-grade teachers); Adaptability was positively related to the need for monitoring (particularly for kindergarten children); there was a negative relationship between Reactivity and monitoring frequency; and a few teachers took into account the children's social interaction skills by rating the students with appropriate social skills as less likely to require monitoring.

The last decision, the placement recommendation, was the most difficult to model given the available student information. As can be seen from Table VIII, almost half of the teachers had no significant coeffi-

Table VII
Decision Model for Free Play

	Teacher	Mean Rating	Regression Weights for Independent Variables			
			Task Orientation	Adaptability	Reactivity	Social Estimate
Kindergarten	1	3.28	−0.49*	0.70*	−0.50	−0.92*
	2	2.08	−0.48*	0.55	−0.27	−0.33*
	3	1.68	−0.13	0.82*	−1.87*	−0.82*
First Grade	4	2.00	−0.79*	0.40	−0.46	−0.04
	5	3.35	−0.19	0.38	−1.44*	−0.30
	6	2.08	−0.57*	0.48	−0.36	−0.61*
	7	2.32	−1.03*	0.85*	−0.53*	0.15
	8	1.29	−0.62*	−0.10	0.21	0.28
	9	2.20	−0.19	0.29	−0.34	−0.29
Third Grade	10	3.15	−0.96*	0.37	−0.44	−0.40
	11	1.73	−0.59*	0.94*	−0.18	−0.72
	12	2.63	−0.67*	0.42	−0.63	−0.43
	13	2.96	−0.81*	0.68	−0.01	0.15

*$p < .05$

Table VIII
Decision Model for Placement Recommendations

	Teacher	Mean Rating	Regression Weights for Independent Variables					
			Ability Estimate	Task Orientation	Academic Estimate	Adaptability	Reactivity	Motivation Estimate
Kindergarten	1	3.72	0.15	0.12	0.08	−0.00	−0.01	−0.04
	2	3.67	0.01	0.31	0.15	0.11	−0.17	−0.15
	3	3.80	−0.07	0.03	0.29*	0.47*	−0.27	−0.03
First Grade	4	3.70	0.33*	0.10	−0.31	−0.01	−0.15	0.32
	5	3.65	−0.14	0.08	0.38*	−0.07	0.17	−0.02
	6	3.44	0.41*	−0.15	0.21	−0.06	0.43*	−0.03
	7	3.84	−0.02	0.17	0.17	−0.09	−0.04	−0.06
	8	3.58	0.20	−0.00	0.31	0.09	−0.27	−0.05
	9	3.60	0.05	−0.09	0.53*	0.12	0.16	−0.11
Third Grade	10	3.62	0.13	−0.03	0.27	−0.09	0.14	0.06
	11	3.77	0.29*	0.10	−0.11	0.21	−0.24*	−0.20
	12	3.67	0.47*	0.07	0.08	0.06	0.00	−0.21
	13	3.73	0.21	0.01	0.12	0.03	0.10	−0.04

*$p < .05$

cients. The failure to capture these teachers' decision strategies may have resulted from the lack of variability in placement decisions with teachers recommending regular promotion or promotion with some academic assistance for 95 percent of the students. The seven teachers who had at least one significant regression weight tended to use the ability or academic performance estimate but not both. This mutually exclusive relationship between the ability and academic performance estimates may have been due to their high intercorrelations. The temperament information was used sparingly and then only in combination with the ability or academic performance estimates. It appears that teachers whose placement decisions could be modeled were relying on the child's ability or academic performance when making their decisions.

DISCUSSION

The most important finding to emerge was the teachers' reliance on temperament consistently entered the regression equation even when controlling for ratings of ability, motivation, and social interaction skills. In fact, the teachers used information concerning their students' temperament characteristics more than any other type of information. This was the case both in terms of the number of teachers that used the temperament information, as well as the magnitude of the regression weights. Of the three temperament factors, teachers were particularly sensitive to their students' Task Orientation characteristics. The consistency with which Task Orientation was used by many of the teachers across all of the classroom decision-making situations was not anticipated. It was thought that this dimension would be important only in the academic situations. Nevertheless, it appeared that students with positive task orientation were viewed as needing less supervision across all classroom settings. The finding that the temperament variables were not related to the placement recommendation can be explained by the lack of variability in the teachers' recommendations. In addition, this decision, unlike the others, was not addressed to specific classroom interaction situations.

While the temperament information was used quite often and across classroom situations, general statements concerning teachers' strategies must be qualified, as all teachers did not use the same decision policy. In particular, there were at least two grade-related trends. First, in situations involving children interacting in groups (Group Activity, Nonacademic Transition, and Free Play), the kindergarten teachers were more likely to use Adaptability information in forming their decisions.

Unexpectedly, these coefficients were positive, suggesting that more adaptable children required more monitoring. While seemingly unintuitive, other investigators have reported similar findings. Both Carey, Fox, and McDevitt (1977) and Thomas and Chess (1977) have found that extremely adaptable children were often rated by their teachers as having difficulties adjusting during the first years of school. This somewhat paradoxical finding that adaptable children have adjustment problems is a consequence, in part, of our definition of Adaptability. An examination of the Adaptability subscale reveals a strong social component (recall the high correlation between teachers' estimates of social interaction skills and Adaptability). Perhaps some of the younger children were overly sensitive to social demands and, therefore, were not goal-directed within the group situations.

The other grade-related trend concerned the third-grade teachers' use of Task Orientation. In every classroom situation, all third-grade teachers relied on Task Orientation as the primary source of information for their decisions. During the debriefing period, these teachers revealed that a major concern was their students' ability to make the trasition to the fourth grade where they would be expected to function independently. This concern may have been reflected in their emphasis on Task Orientation.

In addition to the findings concerning teachers' decision processes, the study provided some insight into the structure of the nonintellective domain. Although the temperament questionnaire was originally constructed to measure eight different dimensions, the factor analysis yielded only three relatively independent factors. Moreover, similar constructs have been identified in other studies of teachers' behavioral ratings (Kohn, 1977; Peterson, 1961; Schaefer, 1971). Kohn, for example, found three factors for teacher ratings of elementary school behavior which he called Interest-Participation versus Apathy-Withdrawal, Cooperation-Compliance versus Anger-Defiance, and Task Orientation. Obviously, the Task Orientation factors from Kohn's and our studies measure similar constructs. What is not obvious from the names of the other factors is that Interest-Participation is similar to Adaptability and Anger-Defiance resembles Reactivity. This convergence of findings from several different studies supports the validity of the present temperament instrument and suggests that teachers tend to use three dimensions to span the nonintellective domain.

Before concluding this discussion, some limits to the generalizability of the current study should be noted. First, children's temperament was assessed using teacher ratings. No attempt was made to obtain "objective" measures of temperament, since the transactional model holds that it is teachers' perceptions that are crucial. Although one would be surprised if there were no relationship between teachers' ratings and children's actual behavior, the nature of this relationship is beyond the scope of this investigation. Second, because teachers were asked to respond to hypothetical classroom situations, any inferences as to what teachers might do while actually teaching must be made solely on logical grounds. We can generalize only to the extent that the situations were realistic, and the teachers were aware of their actual monitoring practices. Lastly, given that all of the data were generated by teachers, a final question might be raised about the validity of the findings. Was the observed relationship between children's temperament and teachers' management decisions an artifact of the data generation process? That is, would one not expect to find such a relationship between any two sets of teachers' ratings. If only temperament information had been requested and entered into the regression equations, then the relationship might be due to the kind of general halo-effect one often finds among ratings by the same person. However, teachers also estimated their students' ability, motivation, social interaction competence, academic performance, and potential. The effect of children's temperament on teachers' decisions was found controlling for these more traditional measures of children's characteristics. The fact that all the data were teacher ratings cannot account for the teachers' reliance on temperament.

The present study was intended as an initial step in studying the transactional model proposed by Thomas and Chess. The next phase would include the observation of actual classroom interactions. Such an approach might reveal more precisely how teachers respond to students' behavioral style and if a mismatch results in stress and continued problems. If the transactional model is correct, then intervention might consist of in-service training aimed at increasing teachers' awareness of their students' behavioral style and their strategies for responding to students' behavior. As a preliminary test of the feasibility of such an intervention program, an informal debriefing session was conducted as part of the present study. The teachers responded quite positively, indicating that this may be a promising approach for enhancing teachers' sensitivity to the nonintellective characteristics of their students and their strategies for accommodating such characteristics.

REFERENCES

Carey, W., Fox, M. and McDevitt, S. (1977). Temperament as a factor in early school adjustment. *Pediatrics*, 60:621–624.

Chess, S. (1968). Temperament and learning of school children. *American Journal of Public Health*, 58(2):2231–2239.

Cronbach, L. (1976). *Research on Classrooms and Schools; Formulation of Questions, Design and Analysis*. Occasional Paper of the Stanford Evaluation Consortium, Stanford University.

Gordon, E. and Thomas, A. (1967). Children's behavioral style and teachers' appraisal of their intelligence. *Journal of School Psychology*, 5(4):292–300.

Hall, R. and Keogh, B. (1977). Qualitative characteristics of educationally high-risk children. *Learning Disabilities Quarterly*, 1(2):62–69.

Keogh, B. and Pullis, M. (1980). Temperament influences on the development of exceptional children. In *Advances in Special Education*,. B. K. Keogh, ed. Greenwich, Conn.: JAI Press.

Keogh, B., Pullis, M., Cadwell, J. and Burstein, N. (1979). *Studies of Temperament in Young Children: Measurements Considerations*. Project REACH report. University of California, Los Angeles.

Kohn, M. (1977). *Social Competence, Symptoms and Underachievement in Childhood: A Longitudinal Perspective*. Washington, D.C.: V. H. Winston & Sons.

Lambert, N. and Windmiller, M. (1977). An exploratory study of temperament traits in a population of children at risk. *Journal of Special Education*, 11(1):37–47.

McKinney, J., Mason, J., Perkerson, K. and Clifford, M. (1975). Relationship between classroom behavior and academic achievement. *Journal of Educational Psychology*, 67:198–203.

Perry, J., Guidubaldi, J. and Kehle, T. (1979). Kindergarten competencies as predictors of third-grade classroom behavior and achievement. *Journal of Educational Psychology*, 71:443–450.

Peterson, D. R. (1961). Behavior problems of middle childhood. *Journal of Consulting Psychology*, 25:205–209.

Schaefer, E. S. (1971). Development of hierarchical, configurational models for parent and child behavior. In *Minnesota Symposium on Child Psychology*, Vol. 5., J. P. Hill, ed. Minneapolis: University of Minnesota Press.

Shavelson, R. J., Cadwell, J. and Izu, T. (1977). Teachers' sensitivity to the reliability of information in making pedagogical decisions. *American Educational Research Journal*, 14:83–97.

Shulman, L. and Elstein, A. (1975). Studies of problem solving, judgment, and decision making: Implications for educational research. In *Review of Research in Education*, F. N. Kerlinger, ed. Itasca, Ill.: F. E. Peacock.

Thomas, A. and Chess, S. (1977). *Temperament and Development*. New York: Brunner/Mazel Publishers.

Thomas, A., Chess, S. and Birch, H. (1968). *Temperament and Behavior Disorders*. New York: New York University Press.

Thomas, A., Chess, S., Birch, H., Hertzig, M. and Korn, S. (1963). *Behavioral Individuality in Early Childhood*. New York: New York University Press.

PART V: TEMPERAMENT STUDIES

23

Temperament Ratings of Handicapped Infants During Classroom, Mother, and Teacher Interactions

Reena Greenberg and Tiffany Field

Mailman Center for Child Development
University of Miami Medical School

This study investigated whether handicapped infants' temperaments are perceived differently by teachers, mothers, and observers and in different contexts. The temperament of 55 normal and same-developmental age, developmentally delayed, Down syndrome, cerebral palsied, and audio-visually handicapped infants was assessed by the infants' mothers, teachers, and an independent observer using the Carey Infant Temperament Questionnaire. In addition, using a rating scale adapted from that questionnaire, observers rated the temperament of these infants during classroom play interactions and during dyadic play interactions with the infants' mothers and teachers. Although interrater agreement coefficients were moderately high, mothers tended to rate their infants' temperament as being less difficult than did the observers who, in turn, assigned less-difficult ratings

Reprinted with permission from the *Journal of Pediatric Psychology*, 1982, Vol. 7, No. 4, 387–405.

We would like to thank the infants, mothers, and teachers who participated in this study. Further thanks go to Norma Hanna, Jo Anne Dickinson, Laurel Allan, and Sherilyn Stoller for assistance with data collection. This research was presented at the biennial meeting of the Society for Research in Child Development, Boston, April 1981, and was supported by grant 90CW605(1) from the Administration for Children, Youth, and Families.

363

than teachers. Normal, developmentally delayed, and Down syndrome infants received less-difficult ratings than cerebral palsied and audio-visually handicapped infants on most of the temperament dimensions rated during classroom play. The interaction context also appeared to affect temperament ratings, with more-difficult ratings assigned during classroom play than during the dyadic interactions.

Infant temperament may be affected by a handicapping condition and the associated frustrations felt by the infant. Temperament assessments, typically made by parents or teachers, my be affected by the frustrations felt by parents and teachers in dealing with these infants. Accordingly, they may differ from the perceptions of an observer who is not taking care of the infant. Teachers' and parents' perceptions of handicapped infants may also be colored by stereotypes associated with different handicapping conditions, for example, that Down syndrome infants are less intense and cerebral palsied infants are more intense than normal infants. In addition, the temperament of a handicapped infant may vary across situations such as a classroom or a one-to-one dyadic play situation.

The purpose of this study was to tap parents', teachers', and independent observers' assessments of the temperament of normal infants and infants experiencing different handicapping conditions. Comparisons were made between the temperament of normal, developmentally delayed, Down syndrome, cerebral palsied, and perceptually handicapped infants during free play in their classrooms and dyadic interactions with their mothers and teachers. Thus, three variables were investigated, the person making the assessment (mother, teacher, or independent observer), the condition of the infant (normal, developmentally delayed, Down syndrome, cerebral palsied, or perceptually handicapped), and the situation (classroom or group play vs. dyadic floor play interactions with the infant's mother or teacher).

METHOD

Subjects

The subjects were 43 handicapped infants including developmentally delayed, Down syndrome, cerebral palsied, and audiovisually impaired infants with deafness or blindness as well as 12 normal infants. The normal infants averaged 9 months of age (range 4–14 months). The handicapped infants averaged 22 months chronological age (range 7–35 months) and 10 months developmental age (range 3–24 months). Thus,

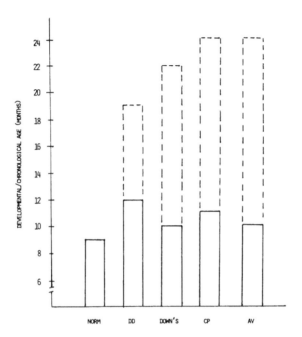

Fig. 1. a. Developmental ages (solid lines) of normal (NORM) and chronological ages (broken line) of developmentally delayed (DD), Down syndrome, cerebral palsied (CP), and audiovisually handicapped (AV) infants ($F < 1$ for developmental age, $F(4, 50) = 2.83$, $p < .05$ for chronological age).

all infants were equivalent in developmental age (see Figure 1). The amount of developmental delay as assessed by the inverse of the ratio of developmental age to chronological age ranged from 1% to 90% with the developmentally delayed infants averaging a 32% delay, the Down syndrome 52%, cerebral palsied infants 56%, and the audiovisually impaired a 58% delay (see Figure 2). The developmentally delayed infants were significantly less delayed than the handicapped infants.

The infants attended an all-day nursery school which included one normal nursery and three handicapped nursery classes. The handicapped nursery classes served 16 infants with varying handicaps. The infants were assigned to a particular nursery according to severity of handicapping condition or developmental delay, with one nursery serving minimally delayed, another moderately delayed, and a third severely delayed infants.

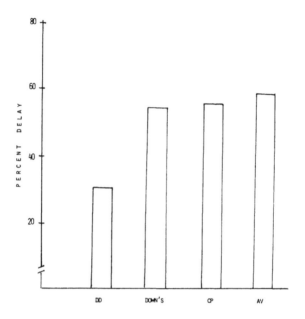

Fig. 2. Percentage developmental delay of developmentally delayed (DD), Down syndrome, cerebral palsied (CP), and audiovisually handicapped (AV) infants ($F < 1$).

Procedure

The infants were rated by their mothers, two teachers, and an independent observer on the Carey Infant Temperament Questionnaire (Carey, 1970). We used the original version rather than the revised version of this scale (Carey & McDevitt, 1978) because the lesser educated mothers of our sample noted that the shorter questionnaire with fewer choices (three instead of six choices) was easier for them to complete. Although many of the handicapped infants were toddler age, the Toddler Temperament Scale designed by the same authors was not given because these handicapped toddlers were developmentally comparable to infants, and the normal comparison group also comprised infants.

Following the first semester of nursery school, the infants' mothers and teachers were requested to complete the Infant Temperament Questionnaire (ITQ). Independent observers also completed the questionnaire for the infants they had observed during classroom free play over this 3-month period. During this period the children were observed in their four separate classrooms for 3 hours per week by four different trained observers. Prior to their observation series the observers were given a listing of all the questionnaire items which comprise each temperament dimension. During the observations they rated each infant on a three-point scale adapted from the "mothers' general impressions of infants' temperament" summary sheet of the Infant Temperament Questionnaire. The only dimension which the coders determined a priori that they could not rate based on their classroom observations was the rhythmicity dimension. Their ratings for each of the dimensions for each observation session were then averaged over the course of the semester. These ratings for each dimension comprised the classroom interaction ratings.

For the dyadic interactions with mothers and teachers, each infant was videotaped in a 10-minute floor play observation which occurred in a small playroom and for which toys were provided. These dyadic interactions were rated in the same manner that the classroom observations were rated. Thus there were four sets of questionnaire ratings (mother, teacher, assistant teacher, and observer) and three sets of interaction temperament ratings based on the dyadic interactions with mother and teacher and classroom free play interactions.

RESULTS

Interrater Agreement

A correlational analysis was conducted to determine the interrater concordance or agreement on the infant temperament questionnaire and on the interaction ratings. As can be seen in Table I, the interrater concordance coefficients were moderate. The coefficients of concordance for the teacher ratings on the questionnaire were significant at least at the $p < .05$ level on all dimensions except intensity and persistence. Coefficients of concordance for mother/teacher ratings (head teachers' ratings being used for this analysis) were significant for rhythmicity, adaptability, intensity, and mood. For teacher-observer ratings, significant values emerged for all dimensions except intensity. Interrater agreement on a greater number of dimensions by teachers and teachers-observers than teachers and mothers may have related to the fact that teachers and observers rate the child in the same environment (the classroom). Although a child's temperament may differ at home and school, mothers and teachers may have different expectations and different base lines for comparisons. In a study on temperament in normal infants,

Table I. Concordance Coefficients for Infant Temperament Questionnaire Ratings by Different Raters

Temperament dimension	Raters[a]		
	T_1T_2	T_1M	T_1OB
Activity	.48	.08[b]	.41
Rhythmicity	.79	.78	—
Adaptability	.58	.45	.38
Approach	.32	.21[b]	.38
Threshold	.50	.07[b]	.44
Intensity	.01[b]	.42	.18[b]
Mood	.26	.33	.38
Distractibility	.40	.05[b]	.48
Persistence	.12[b]	.19[b]	.34
Summary	.85	.84	.83

[a]Teachers (T_1), assistant teachers (T_2), mothers (M), and observers (OB).
[b]r values nonsignificant, $p > .05$.

toddlers, and preschool children, we also noted more frequent concordance between teachers than between parents and teachers (Field & Greenberg, in press).

Table II lists correlation coefficients for the classroom and dyadic interaction ratings. Correlation coefficients were significant for all dimensions in the case of classroom and teacher interaction ratings, for all but the approach dimension in the case of classroom and mother interaction ratings, and for all dimensions of dyadic interactions with mothers and teachers. Thus, in addition to the interrater agreement across most of the dimensions of the questionnaire, there appeared to

Table II. Correlation Coefficients for Temperament Ratings Based on Observations of Classroom Interactions with Mothers and Teachers

Interaction ratings	Interaction situation		
	Class-Teacher	Class-Mother	Mother-Teacher
Activity	.32	.52	.86
Rhythmicity	—	—	—
Adaptability	.69	.84	.67
Approach	.36	.19[b]	.10[b]
Threshold	.35	.52	.42
Intensity	.52	.77	.60
Mood	.56	.78	.10[a]
Distractibility	.31	.67	.50
Persistence	.63	.90	.70

[a]r values nonsignificant, $p > .05$.

be some stability of infant temperament across the classroom, teacher, and parent interaction situations, suggesting stability in the infants' temperament across these situations, or stability in the raters' perceptions of the infants' temperament, or both.

No comparisons were made between temperament questionnaire and interaction temperament ratings because of the different nature of the rating tasks and scales that were used.

Infant Temperament and Questionnaire Ratings

A 5 (group) × 3 (rater) MANOVA followed by univariate analyses of variance were performed on the nine temperament dimensions and summary ratings on the ITQ. A significant main effect for group or infant handicapping condition and post hoc comparisons of these suggested that normal (NORM) and Down (DOWN) infants were rated as having less difficult temperaments than the developmentally delayed (DD) infants who in turn were rated as less difficult than the cerebral palsied (CP) and perceptually handicapped or audiovisually (AV) impaired infants (see Figure 3a). A main effect for rater (Figure 3b) suggested that mothers rated infants' temperament as less difficult than the observers who in turn rated infants as less difficult than the teachers had rated them.

Classroom and Dyadic Interaction Ratings

MANOVA and univariate analyses were performed on the nine temperament dimension ratings for classroom play. Results are presented in Figures 4a–4h as follows: (4a) the observer assigned less difficult classroom ratings for the activity dimension to normal and developmentally delayed infants (lower ratings being "easy") than Down infants, who in turn received easier ratings than the CP or audiovisually impaired infants. This finding was not surprising since infants with the latter condition, a motor handicap, blindness, or deafness were noticeably less active in all situations than their less handicapped peers, although all infants tended to be low to medium on activity level; (4b) on the adaptability dimension the Down infants were rated as more adaptable than all other infants. This finding provides some support for the stereotype that Down infants are generally accepting of novel situations and changes in routine and are generally pleasant and friendly. However, it should be noted that all infants' rating fell within the range of generally adaptable to variable on this dimension; (4c) on the approach dimension the

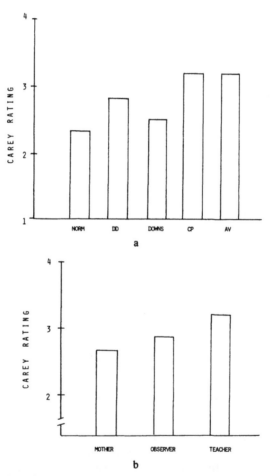

Fig. 3. a. Summary ratings on Infants Temperament Questionnaire for normal (NORM), developmentally delayed (DD), Down syndrome, cerebral palsied (CP), and audiovisually handicapped (AV) infants ($F(4, 48) = 4.11, p < .01$). Ratings range from 1 (easy) to 4 (difficult). b. Summary ratings on Infant Temperament Questionnaire by mothers, observers, and teachers ($F(2, 48) = 3.61, p < .05$).

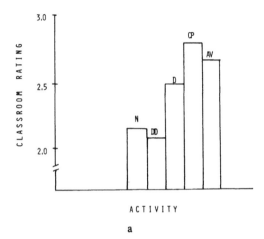

a

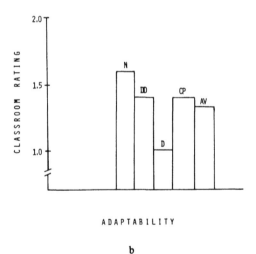

b

Fig. 4. Classroom temperament ratings for normal (N), developmentally delayed (DD), Down syndrome (D), cerebral palsied (CP), and audio-visually handicapped (AV) infants. Ratings range from 1 to 3. a. Activity ($F(4, 50) = 3.48, p < .05$); b. adaptability ($F(4, 50) = 2.71, p < .05$); c. approach ($F(4, 50) = 6.13, p < .001$); d. threshold ($F(4, 50) = 4.09, p < .01$); e. intensity ($F(4, 50) = 5.85, p < .001$); f. mood ($F(4, 50) = 2.67, p < .05$); g. distractibility ($F(4, 50) = 7.01, p < .001$); h. persistence ($F(4, 50) = 7.01, p < .001$);

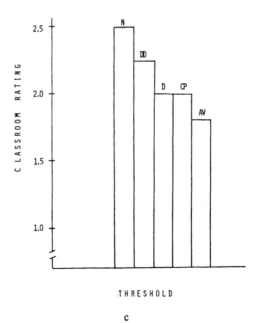

c

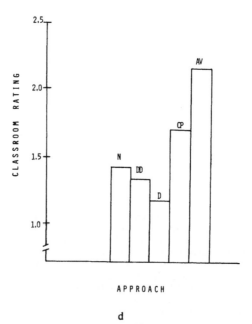

d

Fig. 4. Continued.

normal, developmentally delayed, and Down syndrome infants were more accepting and responsive to new people, places, and toys than the CP or audiovisually impaired infants. Their easy ratings on this dimension as well as for the activity dimension may simply relate to their greater mobility, gross and fine motor skills; (4d) on the threshold dimension the normal and developmentally delayed infants were noted to have lower thresholds to sensory stimulation or were responsive to lesser quantities of stimulation than the Down syndrome, CP, or AV-impaired infants (a higher rating being considered less difficult). The handicapped infants appeared to react similarly to different people and were only reactive to moderate amounts of stimulation. This finding is consistent at least with Cicchetti and Sroufe's (1978) finding that more stimulation is required, for example, to elicit laughter in the Down syndrome infant; (4e) on the intensity dimension the intensity of responses for normal infants was greater than those of the handicapped infants, for example, to hunger, new food, diaper changes, baths, sounds, strangers, and familiar people. The intensity of responses among handicapped infants, by contrast, was generally variable to mild; (4f) on the mood dimension most of the infants were generally positive to variable, although more frequent positive affect was noted among the normal and developmentally delayed than the other groups of infants. The Down syndrome, CP, and blind-deaf infants might be more appropriately described as generally having neutral or flat affect; (4g) on the distractibility dimension the normal and developmentally delayed infants were more readily distracted from ongoing behavior, e.g., crying, by sounds, toys, or people than were the sensory handicapped infants. The Down syndrome infants were more readily distracted (distractibility used here as a positive quality) than any of the other groups of infants except the normal infants. This finding may be inconsistent with that of Cicchetti and Sroufe (1978), who reported that once a crying response, for example, was elicited from a Down syndrome infant, the examiner might have considerable difficulty "turning him off" or "distracting him" from an ongoing behavior like crying; (4h) on the persistence dimension the normal and developmentally delayed infants were noted to attend to and maintain activities such as toy play, play with self and pees for more sustained periods than the other groups of infants. The handicapped infants, because of more delayed motor and cognitive development, may have difficulty sustaining activities over which they have less control.

Analyses of variance were also conducted for temperament ratings across the interaction contexts (classroom, dyadic teacher, and dyadic mother interactions). As can be seen in Figure 5a and 5b, ratings were

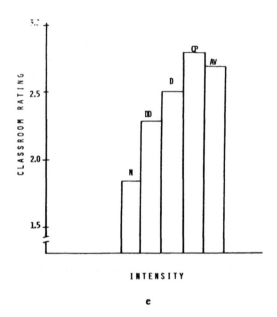

e

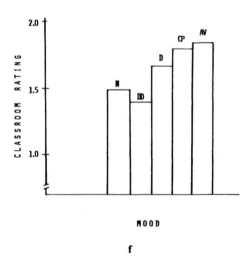

f

Fig. 4. Continued.

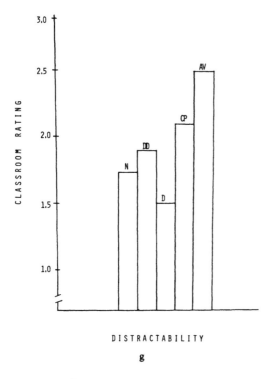

DISTRACTABILITY

g

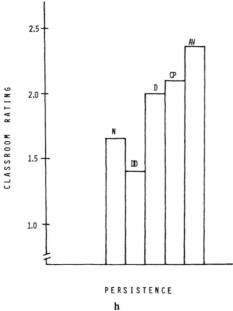

PERSISTENCE

h

Fig. 4. Continued.

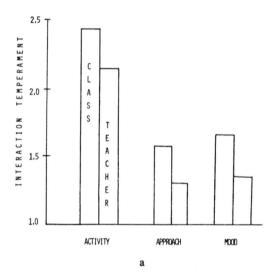

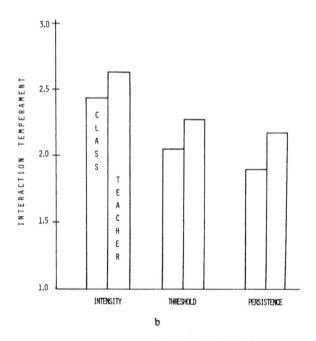

Fig. 5. Classroom and teacher dyadic interaction ratings: a. activity ($F(2, 52) = 5.31, p < .01$); approach ($F(2, 52) = 6.19, p < .005$); and mood ($F(2, 52) = 8.45, p < .001$); b. intensity ($F(2, 52) = 3.71, p < .05$); threshold ($F(2, 52) = 4.11, p < .05$); and presistence ($F(2, 52) = 3.94, p < .05$).

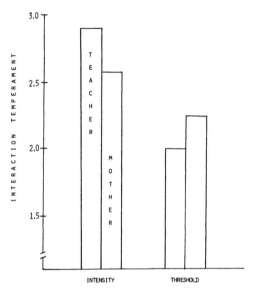

Fig. 6. Teacher and mother dyadic interaction ratings for intensity $(F(2, 52) = 3.37, p < .05)$ and threshold $(F(2, 52) = 423, p < .05)$.

easier for the dyadic interactions with the teacher than classroom ratings on several of the temperament dimensions, including activity, approach, mood, intensity, and threshold. The only dimension for which classroom ratings were easier was the persistence dimension. While persistence is one of the most valid dimensions in predicting later problem-solving ability in the classroom as reported by Carey, Fox, and McDevitt (1977), the easy rating for persistence in the classroom in this study may have been confounded by the distractions of the dyadic floor play interaction situations such as novel toys. Only two of the dimensions, adaptability and distractibility, were not differentially affected by group and dyadic situations.

Temperament was also rated easier in the infants' dyadic interactions with their mothers than in the classroom. Ratings in the two dyadic situations (i.e., the mother and teacher interactions) did not differ except on the intensity dimension which was rated as less difficult during interactions with teachers and on the threshold dimension on which the infants received easier ratings during interactions with their mothers (see Figure 6).

While the dyadic interactions with teacher and mother appeared to facilitate rating on activity, approach, mood, intensity, and threshold

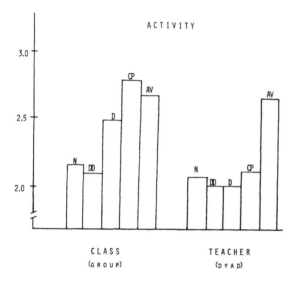

a

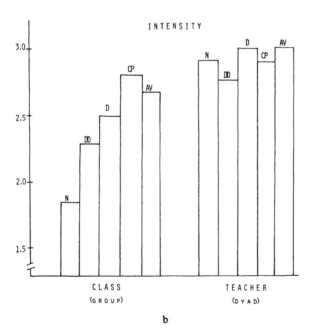

b

Fig. 7. Classroom and teacher interaction ratings for which there were significant group by context interaction effects and for which specific groups received better ratings during dyadic teacher than classroom situations: a. activity ($F(8, 46) = 3.71$, $p < .005$), b. intensity ($F(8, 46) = 4.23$, $p < .001$).

dimensions, interaction effects between interaction situation and infant condition suggested that only some of the infants benefited from the dyadic interaction. For example, on the activity dimension (see Figure 7a), only the temperament of Down syndrome and CP infants improved in the dyadic interaction. And on the intensity dimension (see Figure 7b), only the temperament of normal, developmentally delayed, and Down syndrome infants improved in the dyadic interaction.

DISCUSSION

The developmentally delayed children were ambulatory; they related to each other and to the teacher; they played, and displayed different emotions. For them, the classroom situation was enriching. Their temperament, even though reflecting individual differences, was fairly positive. Most of these children seemed happy, smiled appropriately, and remained entertained either by the teachers or themselves.

The children who fell in the middle range, those with moderate physical and mental handicaps, but who were not severely disabled, exhibited more mood swings, did not entertain themselves as readily, needed more supervision and individual attention from the teacher, and were more "cranky." They set the tone for the classroom. When they cried the others tended to cry; if they were content, the whole classroom seemed peaceful. Unfortunately, happy expressions were rare with this group.

Finally, the severely handicapped children seemed to go from one extreme to another. They were either passive and unresponsive or they were crying. Smiles were totally missing. These children required either no attention or total attention from the teachers, and such attention was generally focused on making them comfortable.

Drawing on knowledge of a child's classroom behavior and skills, the teachers were able to direct the child's activity during their dyadic interactions and show the child's performance capabilities "in the best light." The absence of other children combined with the pristine laboratory environment and the teacher's undivided attention may have helped to promote less difficult temperament. Mothers (when filmed played with their children) appeared to be less directive with them than the teachers in that situation. In contrast with teachers, who usually managed to elicit better task performance, the presence of the mothers seemed to promote more affective behavior.

The Carey Temperament Scales were developed to tap the temperament of normal children. The use of these scales with a handicapped population poses certain problems. Although the categories (activity, regularity, adaptability, approach, intensity, threshold, mood, distractibility, and persistence) are appropriate for both normal and handicapped populations, they need to be redefined to include more aspects of handicapped behavior. The range of scoring needs to be wider in order to tap those behaviors that differentiate handicapped children from normal children.

The recurrent problem within most of the categories was the lack of a dimension which considers passivity and neutral or flat affect. The question arises as to how flat affect is to be coded. There is a need for a "neutral" dimension—one which would reflect the lack of any given activity or response.

When rating handicapped children on temperament a basis for comparison must be determined. Should handicapped temperament be compared to that of a normal population, thereby assessing how different the two populations are? Should each child's temperament be compared to other children in his or her class, thereby assessing "temperament by disorder"? Should a handicapped child's temperament be compared with his or her own self on a day-to-day basis, thereby assessing temperament which may be situationally specific?

Many of the behaviors and modes of responding were not covered in our three-point rating scale based on the ITQ. Examination of each category reveals the following considerations:

Threshold and activity dimensions appeared to be the most clear-cut. They were easy to define and apply to the handicapped group with no specific problems.

The question that arises with the adaptability dimension is how to rate passive behavior. The behaviors that are rated as a 1 (adaptable) are very different within the handicapped population. Some children remain motionless and accept anything that is done or given to them, and therefore are considered adaptable. Other children are actively involved in the process of adapting; they accept and reject changes with a certain amount of effort, yet they too are considered adaptable. These two sets of behavior are markedly different, but because the rating is the same, there was no way to differentiate in what way the child was adapting.

Many of the same problems come into play for the approach dimension. Once again, the question is how should "no reaction" be coded? Does a child reject a toy because s/he does not have the motor control to reach for it? An item is needed that conveys neither approach nor withdrawal. If a child neither accepts nor rejects a new situation, it cannot be coded as variable. An entire mode of responding is omitted.

Although intensity is a dimension which focuses on both intensity and passivity, a middle item is needed. If a child is not intense or mild but reacts "in between," then a moderate score would be more appropriate than variable. The term *variable* speaks to a changing mode of behavior, while the term *moderate* refers to a behavior between intense and mild.

The mood dimension offers two choices and does not include a rating for "no mood." Many times the handicapped infant was not positive, variable, or negative—it was simply flat. Flatness refers to moods devoid of positiveness or negativity, suggesting a neutral response is necessary.

Similar problems were evident for the distractibility and persistence dimensions. This rating system does not include total passivity, which would affect ratings on the distractibility and persistence dimensions. Some children were not easily distracted when focused on a game or toy and therefore were rated a 3 (not distractible). Other children did nothing, yet were not distractible, so they also were assigned a rating of 3. These behaviors need to be differentiated. Is "staring off into space" considered a persistent behavior when the child appears to be amused and persistently may reject efforts to distract him or her? In general, then, it would appear that for future ratings of handicapped infants, we should include ratings that reflect passivity, lack of active play, flat affect, and neutral responses.

In addition to these limitations, the methodological problems of this study cannot be ignored. Generalizability of these findings may be limited by small sample size and the extent to which these children were representative of these handicapping conditions. Also, the infants' mean developmental age was 2 months beyond the 8 month upper limit for the standardized ITQ. Finally, differences between groups were based on global impressions of the temperament dimensions rather than the itemized ratings. Nonetheless, these findings tentatively suggest differences between infants and differences between infants experiencing different handicapping conditions. In addition they suggest that a dyadic play context may facilitate easier temperament. Finally, because there was moderate interrater agreement between teachers, mothers might be a useful addition to the clinical records of handicapped children.

REFERENCES

Carey, W. B. (1970). A simplified method for measuring infant temperament. *Journal of Pediatrics*, 77:188–194.
Carey, W. B., Fox, M. and McDevitt, S. (1977). Temperament as a factor in early school adjustment. *Pediatrics*, 60:621–624.
Carey, W. B. and McDevitt, S. C. (1978). Revision of the infant temperament questionnaire. *Pediatrics*, 61:735–739.
Cicchetti, D. and Sroufe, L. A. (1978). An organizational view of affect: Illustration from

the study of Down's syndrome infants. In *The Development of Affect*, Vol. 1, M. Lewis and L. A. Rosenblum, eds. New York: Plenum Press.

Field, T. and Greenberg, R. (1982). Temperament ratings by parents and teachers of infants, toddlers, and preschool children. *Child Development*, 53:160–163.

24

Sleep Duration and Infant Temperament

Marc Weissbluth

Children's Memorial Hospital, Chicago

Individual temperament and mental and physical health may be interrelated in infants as well as adults.[1-3] In adults, mental and physical health status appears to be related to sleep duration.[4,5] In fact, recent studies in adults suggest that short sleep durations are related to increased morbidity.[6] Additionally, among adults and older children,[7] environmental and social factors influence sleep duration. In contrast to sleep duration in adults, sleep duration in infancy seems determined primarily by neurologic maturation[8-10] and, perhaps to a lesser degree, by infant temperament.[11] This prospective study was conducted to determine the relationship between sleep duration and infant temperament.

METHODS

The two criteria for inclusion in the study were that the patients were under the age of 8 months at the time of the first office visit and that they were brought to the author's private general practice office for well-child care. No infant referred to the author for any suspected problems was included in the study. The study population consisted of 60 consecutive infants (26 boys) meeting the entry criteria. The parents were

Reprinted with permission from *The Journal of Pediatrics*, 1982, Vol. 99, No. 5, 817–819. Copyright 1982 by The C. V. Mosby Company.

The author wishes to thank Yvonne Shy for secretarial assistance and Rosemary Egan, Janet Reis, and Daniel Garside for assistance in data analysis and for their critical reviews.

predominantly white and middle to upper class. The median age of the infants at the first examination was 21 days; 88% of the infants were first examined before the age of 2 months.

The author gave The Carey Infant Temperament Questionnaire (revised 1977)[12] with a stamped self-addressed envelope to each family when the infant was at least 4 months of age. At this visit, the author conducted a standardized interview with the mother to determine the duration of evening and day sleep. All 60 questionnaires were returned and scored by the author. Infant temperament diagnoses were assigned using the published values and criteria of the Infant Temperament Questionnaire (revised 1977).

To determine whether individual temperament characteristics were interrelated or related to sleep duration, Pearson product moment correlations were performed for the nine infant temperament characteristics (activity, rhythmicity, approach/withdrawal, adaptability, intensity, mood, persistence, distractibility, threshold) and day sleep, night sleep, and total sleep duration. The large number of computations performed in this analysis might produce, by chance alone, high correlations which are clinically meaningless. Therefore, statistical significance was conservatively defined as $P < 0.01$. To determine the effect of infant temperament diagnoses on sleep, Student t tests (two-tailed) were performed for easy versus difficult infant temperament diagnoses and easy plus intermediate low versus difficult plus intermediate high infant temperament diagnoses. Four infants diagnosed as slow to warm-up were not included in these comparisons. Statistical significance in these analyses was defined as $P < 0.01$.

RESULTS

Correlations Between Temperament Characteristics and Sleep Duration

Four of the five infant temperament characteristics (mood, adaptability, rhythmicity, and approach/withdrawal), which are used to establish temperament diagnoses of "easy" or "difficult," were highly negatively correlated with total sleep duration (Table). High ratings in these four characteristics describe negative mood, slow adaptation, irregularity, and withdrawal. Intensity, the fifth temperament characteristic used to determine an infant temperament diagnosis, was not correlated with day, night, or total sleep duration. Mood rating was the temperament characteristic which had the highest correlation with total sleep duration. Mood ratings were correlated with persistence ratings ($r = 0.3502, P$

Table. Sleep duration and temperament characteristics

	N	Day sleep	Night sleep	Total sleep
Correlation coefficients				
Infant temperament characteristic	60			
Mood		-0.3223†	-0.4377‡	-0.5406‡
Adaptability		ns	-0.3951‡	-0.3623†
Rhythmicity		ns	ns	-0.3396†
Approach/withdrawal		ns	-0.3452†	-0.3380†
Persistence		-0.4274‡	ns	-0.3050*
Sleep durations (mean hours ± 1SD)				
Diagnostic clusters				
Easy	20	3.7 ± 1.3^{ns}	11.7 ± 1.1‡	15.3 ± 1.6‡
Difficult	8	2.7 ± 1.5	9.6 ± 1.9	12.3 ± 1.5
Easy and intermediate low	36	3.6 ± 1.2^{ns}	11.4 ± 1.4*	15.0 ± 1.8‡
Difficult and intermediate high	20	2.8 ± 1.2	10.2 ± 1.7	13.1 ± 1.8

ns = No significant difference.
*$P < 0.01$.
†$P < 0.005$.
‡$P < 0.001$.

< 0.005). A high persistence rating describes low persistence or short attention span. Persistence ratings were not correlated with any other temperament characteristic. However, persistence rating was the temperament characteristic which had the highest correlation with day sleep duration. Only the temperament characteristics shown in the Table were significantly correlated with day, night, or total sleep duration. Correlation coefficients between mood, intensity, adaptability, and approach/withdrawal were all significant (r = 0.3316 to 0.7695, $P < 0.005$ to $P < 0.001$). No significant correlations were observed between night sleep and day sleep duration.

Student t Tests for Paired Comparisons

Easy versus difficult infant temperament diagnosis. By definition, easy infants compared to difficult infants were positive in mood, mild, very adaptable, approaching, and rhythmical (all $P < 0.001$). Additionally, easy children were less active ($P < 0.05$), more distractible ($P < 0.005$), and had higher sensory threshold ($P < 0.001$) than in difficult children. Persistence was the only infant temperament characteristic rating which was similar in easy and difficult children. Differences in sleep duration between easy and difficult infants are shown in the Table.

Easy plus intermediate low versus difficult plus intermediate high infant temperament diagnosis. Statistically significant results, similar to the preceding paired comparison, were observed in this paired comparison with the exception that ratings for activity as well as for persistence were similar for the two groups (Table).

DISCUSSION

This study suggests a general relationship between infant sleep duration and temperament. Temperamental differences among babies were described by Thomas and associates[11,13] and an easy method of measuring these differences was introduced by Carey.[14] Thomas noted statistical interrelations between the traits of mood, intensity, adaptability, and approach/withdrawal; these traits clustered together during the infant's first five years. In this study also, strong interrelationships among these four traits appeared. Withdrawing, negative in mood, slowly adaptable, and intense infants in Thomas' study also were rated in that study as irregular, and were diagnosed as having difficult temperaments. Infants with easy temperaments had opposite characteristics. In Thomas' study, four additional temperament characteristics were described: persistence, activity, distractibility, and threshold; only persistence and activity at age one year had no intercorrelations with any other temperament characteristic. Similarly, in this study, only persistence and activity ratings were similar among the different diagnostic groups.

Total sleep duration was highly correlated with four of the five temperament characteristics used to diagnose easy/difficult temperaments. Difficult children slept about two hours less each night and one hour less each day than the easy children did. Whereas night sleep duration was most highly correlated with mood ratings, day sleep duration was most highly correlated with persistence ratings. Brief day sleep duration was associated with high persistence ratings or short attention span. Knowledge of these relationships should be helpful in counselling parents with respect to the sleep patterns in their infants.

REFERENCES

1. Betz, B. J. and Thomas, C. B. (1979). Individual temperament as a predictor of health or premature disease. *John Hopkins Medical Journal*, 144:81.
2. Vaillant, G. E. (1979). Natural history of male psychologic health: Effects of mental health on physical health. *New England Journal of Medicine*, 301:1249.
3. Carey, W. B. (1972). Clinical applications of infant temperament measurements. *Journal of Pediatrics*, 81:823.
4. Breslow, L. and Enstrom, J. E. (1980). Persistence of health habits and their relationship to mortality. *Preventive Medicine*, 9:469.
5. Association of Sleep Disorders Centers. (1979). Diagnostic classification of sleep and arousal disorders, prepared by The Sleep Disorders Classification Committee, H. P. Roffwarg, Chairman. *Sleep*, 2:1–137.
6. Palmer, C. D., Harrison, G. A. and Hirons, R. W. (1980). Sleep patterns and life styles in Oxfordshire village. *J. Biosoc. Sci.*, 12:437.
7. Ragins, N. and Schachter, J. (1971). A study of sleep behavior in two-year old children. *Journal of the American Academy of Child Psychiatry*, 10:464.
8. Parmelee, A. H., Wenner, W. H. and Schulz, H. R. (1964). Infant sleep patterns; From birth to 16 weeks of age. *Journal of Pediatrics*, 65:576.
9. Holmes, G. L., Logan, W. J., Kirkpatrick, B. V., and Meyer, E. C. (1979). Central nervous system maturation in the stressed premature. *Annals of Neurology*, 6:518.
10. Stern, E., Parmelee, A. H. and Harris, M. A. (1973). Sleep state periodicity in prematures and young infants. *Dev. Psychobiol.*, 6:357.
11. Thomas, A., Chess, A. and Birch, H. G. (1968). *Temperament and Behavior Disorders in Children*. New York: New York University Press.
12. Carey, W. B. and McDevitt, S. C. (1978). Revision of the infant temperament questionnaire. *Pediatrics*, 61:735.
13. Thomas, A., Chess, S., Birch, H. G., Hertzig, M. E. and Korn S. (1963). *Behavioral Individuality in Early Childhood*. New York: New York University Press.
14. Carey, W. B. (1970). A simplified method for measuring infant temperament. *Journal of Pediatrics*, 77:188.

Part VI

CLINICAL ISSUES

The range of topics included in this section emphasizes anew, as in the past few years, the scope of the clinical issues which are engaging the serious attention of researchers and clinicians.

The paper by Rapoport and Ismond presents an authoritative review of the current status of research in pediatric psychopharmacology, neurodiagnostic techniques, and psychogenetics. This review will provide the clinician with a much needed framework for the evaluation of the complex research studies in these fields. The authors emphasize that the research to date, as exciting and promising as many of the findings are, has as yet had little influence upon practice, nor is there yet the likelihood of immediate practical benefit. They emphasize that, clinically, the discovery of a trait marker with high specificity would be the major biological breakthrough for child psychiatry. They are optimistic about the future of biological research, but emphasize, most appropriately, the responsibility of clinicians to utilize our available knowledge in the psychosocial area for effective preventive and therapeutic actions.

The deleterious effect of chronic malnutrition on the psychological development of children has been documented in a number of studies in recent years. Severe pre- and early postnatal caloric deficits have been shown to hinder significantly neuronal cell division and size. A number of studies have exposed the damaging behavioral consequences of prolonged childhood malnutrition. The paper by Barrett and his co-workers report a systematic controlled study of the effects of early caloric supplementation in young children with chronic malnutrition on social and emotional functioning at school age. The results indicated the importance of adequate energy intake in infancy for later social-emotional development. These findings are of special importance at this time, when the federal government is engaged in cutting back the highly important programs of food supplementation for needy children.

Each solution brings new problems, and the advances in oncology which are saving or prolonging the lives of childhood cancer victims are

389

no exception to this truth. As Brunnquell and Hall point out in their sensitive clinical review of this issue, the child is faced with the task of coping with a life-threatening disease, and also with the strange and distressing effects of the treatment measures. The authors explore the issues of separation and loss, control and competence, the restriction of mobility and activity, the effects of isolation, and the sequelae of treatment, as well as fear of disfigurement, interpersonal issues, and family issues, with appropriate clinical vignettes throughout. They offer many valuable therapeutic suggestions, but emphasize that no quick or easy solutions exist.

In a similar vein, Ravenscroft's paper provides a broad dynamic view of the psychological effects of acute physical trauma for a child or adolescent. The consequences for patient and family are detailed, and principles for effective medical, surgical, and ward team management are outlined. The paper offers useful guidelines for the clinician in the treatment of the fears, denials, and other defense mechanisms of both child and family.

Systematic clinical studies of somnambulism in children have been conspicuous by their absence, and Klackenberg's paper fills this gap. His report goes beyond a prevalence study to a consideration of the correlation with a number of behavioral variables. The findings indicate that the alarm so frequently induced in parents by this dramatic symptom may in fact not be justified by the relatively benign nature of the psychopathology it reflects.

PART VI: CLINICAL ISSUES

25

Biological Research in Child Psychiatry: The Interplay of Theory and Investigation

Judith L. Rapoport and Deborah R. Ismond

Unit on Child Mental Illness, National Institute of Mental Health, Bethesda, Maryland

Three areas of biological research are reviewed for child psychiatry: pediatric psychopharmacology, neurodiagnostic techniques, and psychogenetics. Eventually these areas of research may help refine diagnosis, predict treatments and give hints as to etiology. At present however such research is in early stages and this review suggests important new areas for clinicians to follow.

This paper makes predictions about the embryonic field of Biological Research in Child Psychiatry, and speculations about the effects on clinical practice. This is an ambitious task, undertaken in the spirit of generating interest and discussion, and for which somewhat arbitrary selection of topics is made.

Biological research in psychiatry has a variety of aims. Goals include: refining diagnosis, predicting treatment response, prognosticating, and (ideally) providing state and trait markers, and suggesting and/or identifying etiology. Time will judge the degree to which any of these goals

Reprinted with permission from the *Journal of the American Academy of Child Psychiatry*, 1982, Vol. 21, No. 6, 543–548. Copyright 1982 by the American Academy of Child Psychiatry.

Dr. Rapoport is Chief, Unit on Childhood Mental Illness. Ms. Ismond is a psychologist in the Unit.

are met. In these preliminary stages, I have a more limited (if this paper can be called limited!) approach.

Discussion is structured around three areas: pediatric psychopharmacology; genetics; and neuropsychological research, particularly the use of newer neuroradiological diagnostic techniques. I will review the current ideas, effects on practice (if any) and new areas for future research.

PEDIATRIC PSYCHOPHARMACOLOGY

The easiest area to discuss is pediatric psychopharmacology. The advent of two major textbooks for child psychiatrists in the last 5 years (Wiener 1977, Werry 1978) has had a clear impact on training programs and Board standards in Child Psychiatry and has legitimized what had been a growing area of treatment and training over the past 15 years.

An extraordinary expansion of information and practice has occurred with respect to pediatric psychopharmacology extending to other disciplines (pediatrics, neurology) and to general psychiatry. Not surprisingly, the advent of effective (at least short-term) treatments has led to increased interest in Hyperkinesis/Attention Deficit Disorder as well as in Tourettes Syndrome, earlier recognition of these disorders and much exciting research on the role of neurotransmitters.

The phenomenon of tardive dyskinesias and cognitive impairment in retarded children given phenothiazines has become common knowledge to child psychiatric trainees, and the option to use of tricyclics for enuresis, school phobia and possibly childhood depression can be discussed intelligently by most practitioners although styles vary widely. The psychopharmacologists' double-blind techniques, and preoccupation with rating scales has influenced much non-pharmacological research in child psychopathology, so that techniques are now more like those used in the related area of child development.

There are also areas of failure for pediatric psychopharmacology. In spite of some excellent studies, there are no agents that have been shown to affect core symptoms of autism, mental retardation or learning disabilities, and drug treatment of these populations remains of primary research interest. Here we have a clear example where knowledge changed practice and focused interest on biological factors in psychopathology.

One is tempted to speculate on areas likely to become "hot" in the future. Future questions deal with prophylactic treatment and modification of behavior. Recent basic work has provided exciting ideas about the use of neuroleptics in altering early CNS development. Usually such effects are considered as toxic and undesirable. It has been shown that neuroleptics which have the ability to block dopamine may interfere with dopamine receptor development (Friedhoff and Rosengarten, 1979). Haloperidol, a potent neuroleptic, when administered to rats prenatally, significantly reduces the number of specific dopamine binding sites in the brain. On the other hand, administration of haloperidol immediately postpartum, via mother's milk, produced an *increase* in the number of binding sites. This deficit persists, in the rat, into adulthood and has a behavioral correlate. Dopamine is believed to play a role in symptom expression in psychosis, in regulation of mood and emotional expression, and in attentional phenomena. A pilot study is currently underway at New York University to determine if preliminary evidence may be found linking fetal exposure to neuroleptics with disturbances in certain aspects of behavioral function and, speculatively, if the risk for development of schizophrenia is altered in the offspring of schizophrenic women who were treated with neuroleptics throughout their pregnancy.

Other studies of "prenatal neuropsychopharmacology" deal with effects of drugs of abuse, and I would like to cite some pertinent alcohol research, with possible clinical correlates. Recent studies of behavioral effects of alcohol in *adult* rats (Taylor et al., in press) indicate that exposure of rats to alcohol *in utero* alters their tolerance to alcohol as adults. (*Post natal* maternal alcohol effects have, of course, also been well documented [Broadhurst, 1978]). In addition, other animal studies show that offspring exposed to ethanol either *in utero* or during lactation have greater ethanol preferences later as adults in addition to impaired learning and hyperactivity (Rosett, 1979). These basic studies take on particular importance in the light of exciting new data on the inheritance of alcohol abuse among adopted daughters of alcoholic biological mothers compared to other daughters (Bohman et al., 1981). In this study, there was a threefold excess of alcohol abuses among adopted daughters of alcoholic mothers, and a lesser effect in daughters of alcoholic fathers. In view of the large amount of unexplained variance in genetic studies attempting prediction of both alcohol abuse and alcohol dependence in adult human populations, these basic studies have important implications for the new and exciting area of psychiatric-genetic epidemiology. It might, for example, be that subtle but specific patterns of maternal drinking predispose offspring as adults to abuse even if parents are not themselves identified abusers.

More basic developmental issues are addressed by animal studies of biological correlates of the interaction between the developing animal and its environment. Extensive work, for example, has documented the contribution of sensory stimulation to development of normal CNS function, and more specific recent work shown the exquisite sensitivity of some enzyme systems involved in growth to even hourly maternal stimulation (Shanberg and Kuhn, 1980). Such investigations open up a new basic area of developmental psychopharmacology.

NEURODIAGNOSTIC TECHNIQUES AND BIOLOGICAL CHILD PSYCHIATRY

Emergent neurodiagnostic techniques are viewed with enthusiasm by biologically oriented psychiatry. For example, at one time the clinical EEG was explored as a possible basis for psychiatric diagnosis schema and the correlated average evoked responses with clinical state are an offshoot of such advances. The so called, neurological "soft signs" were another addition to the "biological correlates" research approach.

Computerized brain tomography has proved invaluable to pediatric neurology for early diagnosis of tuberous sclerosis, and the classification and evaluation of some childhood epilepsies (Bachman et al., 1977). This new system has also been applied to neuropsychiatric disorders and although all the studies are very recent, the results are intriguing. I shall briefly review new studies in three areas: autism, "MBD" and dyslexia.

Four studies have reported CT scan findings in subjects with autistic symptoms. These are reviewed in Table I.

None of these studies are ideal; however, all indicate that there are some (not all) subjects with autism having abnormal scans, particularly left side lesions. The methodology is still primitive, however, and the precise measurements and differentiation from controls as well as the difficulty and ethical issues involved in obtaining truly normal control groups are all problems to be considered. The reports of Hier et al. (1979), Damascio et al., (1980), Campbell et al. (1980) and Caparulo et al. (1981) all indicate a variety of abnormalities that seem to be associated with autism, though methodology varied widely between studies both as to patient selection, use of controls and method of reading the scans. It is promising that positive results are being obtained and it is hoped that future refinements will include such elegant standardized measurements as used in schizophrenia research by Weinberger and colleagues (1980).

Five studies (one repeated from the first group) have addressed various aspects of Minimal Brain Dysfunction and more specifically, dyslexia and speech and language delay. These are summarized in Table II. As seen, three studies with populations described as "Minimal Brain Dysfunction" or Attention Deficit Disorder (Bergström and Bille, 1978,

Table I
CT Scans in Pediatric Neuropsychiatric Syndromes
Infant Autism

Author	n	Age	Findings	Comment
Hier et al., 1979	16 autistic 44 retarded 100 neurological	7-27	Reversed posterior cerebral asymmetry 57% autistic 23% retarded 25% neurological	Suggests specificity of asymmetry in relation to language development
Damascio et al., 1980	17	4-31	Clear lesions – 3 cases	1) 50% of scans were normal 2) Patients included with head abnormalities and neurological abnormalities
Campbell et al., 1982	45 autistic 19 controls 9 nonfocal seizures 4 headaches 3 spinal cord tumor 2 head trauma 1 intoxication, cause unknown	2½-7½ 3-9	11 autistics showed ventricular enlargement (5 mildly prominent ventricles); remaining autistics and all controls were judged normal	1) Data presentation not clear 2) Controls used best of all CT studies
Caparulo et al., 1981	22 autistic 17 Pervasive Developmental Disorder nonautistic type 16 Speech & Language Developmental Disorder 14 Attention and Learning Disorder 16 Tourettes			18% autistic 59% Developmental Disorder 43% Language Disorder 24% Attention Deficit Disorder 37% Tourettes Syndrome 1) 20 (24%) of 85 patients marked had abnormal scans; 37% had "any" abnormality

Table II
CT Scans in Pediatric Patients With Behavioral and Cognitive Disabilities

Author	n	Age	Findings	Comment
Dyslexia Hier et al., 1978	24	14-47	1) 10 patients have reversal, i.e., R>L posterior parieto-occipital region. 2) patients with reversal have lower verbal IQ than other 14	3.2 = expected frequency. $P<01$
Speech Delay Hier & Rosenberger, 1980	30	8-22	2 cases abnormal with 1 temporal focal lesion. Lesion included: bilateral or unilateral dilation of lateral ventricles (12). Third ventricle 1 wide fissure or cyst 2.	1) mental retardation & cerebral palsy ruled out 2) Abnormalities in 1 moderate and 1 severe speech delay patient
"Minimal Brain Dysfunction" Bergström & Bille, 1978	46	4-15	15 (32.6%) had cerebral atrophy, asymmetry or an anomaly	1) pneumoencephalogram controls
Thompson et. al., 1980	44	11 yrs (mean) ± 3.43	2 (5%) had abnormality: a) gliosis in right occipital region b) agenesis of the corpus callosum	1) no control data reported 2) no measurements of asymmetry etc. reported
Caparulo et. al., 1981	14	"LD" + ADD	4 (25%) abnormal ventricular dilation	1) no precise blind control measurements, scans read "clinically"

Thompson et al., 1980, and Caparulo et al., 1981) suggest that there may be anatomical abnormalities in patients with Attention Deficit Disorder. Two reports say that at least 25% may have a variety of abnormalities including cerebral dilation and asymmetry, while one study is essentially negative.

Two other papers deal with the specific disabilities of dyslexia and speech delay. As a group, dyslexics tend to have reversed posterior parieto-occipital diameters (i.e., right is greater than left) and the patients who show this reversal are likely to be the ones with the lowest verbal IQ (Hier et al., 1978). The same research group has also reported that two of 30 patients with speech delay had focal left temporal lesions which could be diagnosed only by CT scan; patients with lesions could not be distinguished clinically from the rest of the sample (Hier and Rosenberger, 1980). Here too, methodology of measurement and of obtaining control data varies and the comments made with respect to the studies of autism also apply. However, this is a promising, possibly important neurological measure.

This clinical neurodiagnostic research has already had some influence on practice and certainly on research. Our ongoing work at the NIMH routinely includes CT scans in studies of Attention Deficit Disorder, Obsessive Compulsive Disorder, and Adult Autism and we are in the process of obtaining satisfactory scans of control populations. It is unlikely that research groups will carry out CT scans on normal volunteers. Radiation exposure is comparable to that for a routine skull series; however, the concern about radiation precludes this approach and alternate populations, such as children with first seizures, headaches, etc., whose scans are likely to be normal will most likely be used. The neuroradiological field has other techniques of equal interest and potential. Measurements of regional cerebral blood flow suggest that changes in flow are related to altered patterns of regional cerebral neuronal activity (Hagberg and Ingvar, 1976). The adaptation of ^{18}F Fluorodeoxyglucose method for measurement of local cerebral glucose utilization in man, also called positron emission tomography (PETT scan) (Reivich et al., 1979), enables visualization of deeper brain structures. The measures of physiological activity may detect subtle changes in function where structural alteration is lacking. The amount of radiation exposure, with current techniques, is unacceptable for research purposes with pediatric groups. However, radiation exposure is likely to be reduced in the near future through the use of other isotopes. Studies with adult psychiatric patients and controls are underway at a variety of centers, on populations of schizophrenic, Tourettes and normal-aged groups. Eventually, childhood disorders will be studied; for the moment studies of adults with autism, dyslexia and Tourettes Disease will be of great interest to child psychiatry and, with modifications of the technique, repeated scans on the same patient during different states and/or during different activities will greatly enhance the information that can be obtained. An even newer technique, Nuclear Magnetic Resonance (NMR) is being evaluated for clinical and basic work (Brownell et al., 1982). When placed in a strong magnetic field, the magnetism of the atomic nucleii result in the alignment of most of the nuclei with the external field. Nucleii of different energy are separated in their orientation within the field. The introduction of radio waves with resulting effect on the orientation of nucleii provides an index of the molecules' identity.

This new technique may provide superior anatomic diagnosis, superior in resolution to that of the CT scan, and avoiding the use of X-ray and/or contrast media. Images may also be available in any cross-sectional plane.

Most exciting, however, may be the ability of NMR to reflect metabolic state, providing some metabolic information about brain function through measurement of nuclear ion density, high energy phosphate bonds, or water flow. Predictably, localization by other means from neurological examination to extensive neuropsychological testing, will be expanded in connection with these research approaches. A new golden age for pediatric neuropsychological research is upon us!

GENETIC RESEARCH IN PSYCHIATRY

Genetic research goals are to refine diagnosis, predict outcome and treatment response, and ideally provide trait markers. In the field of mental retardation, properly a field assigned at least in part to child psychiatry, our major advance has come with the recognition of chromosomal abnormality of Downs Syndrome which accounts for one-third of all cases of mental retardation (Bagadia et al., 1979). With amniocentesis for all pregnancies over 40, abortions could prevent one-third of all Downs syndrome cases or one-ninth of mental retardation as it exists in the western world.

In schizophrenia and depression, genetic counseling might conceivably be of value for some individual families, but only 4% of patients suffering from schizophrenia have a clear family history. In half the parents of schizophrenic children, the first psychotic episode appears after the child or children are born. Most important, there are no clear biological markers for vulnerability.

Similarly, the genetic basis of depression is nowhere near the point where decisions to marry or have children can be based on knowledge of one's own or spouses's hereditability of the disorder. Retrospectively, however, there is evidence that the *well spouse* of the bipolar proband would have wished for such council (Targum and Gershon, 1980). There are some data that offspring of the parents with unipolar depression have at least a 40% likelihood of having the disorder (Nurnberger and Gershon, in press).

Another benefit of genetic research, particularly from adoption strategies, would be evidence of phenocopy effects on major disorders. This has clearly not been found for schizophrenia. However, there is some evidence for this with respect to depression. First, the high rate of same sex transmission of depression broadly defined is not compatible with genetic models and suggests social-environmental effects (see Nurnberg and Gershon discussion of Weissman studies).

Similarly, a phenocopy of depression seems to be demonstrated in the adoption alcoholism studies of Goodwin et al. (1977). In that study, daughters of alcoholics had a higher rate of depression if raised by their biological parents, but not if they were adopted away at birth.

A major advance in genetic research would be if trait markers could be the identification of a biological marker which would identify trait, that is, which could be found in individuals at risk for a disorder when they were in the well state. In depression, for example, the altered excretion patterns of cortisol and the dexamethasone suppression test revert to normal when the patient recovers from depression.

One finding of major interest as a potential marker for vulnerability to affective illness has been reported by Gershon et al. (1979). This is REM sleep induction in response to arecoline. This response is significantly quicker in patients in remission, and off medication, than in normal controls. Currently, normal twins and relatives of patients who show the response are being tested in order to see if this marker predicts vulnerability to affective disorder.

Such a finding, of a biological trait marker for any major disease, would be a major breakthrough for primary prevention. We had hoped that the association of minor physical anomalies with hyperactive and inattentive behaviors in boys could be such a finding. However, this association is neither powerful nor specific (Rapoport and Ferguson, 1981). A newborn screening of 1,000 newborns then followed to age three showed only weak prediction of hyperactivity and speech delay. While statistically significant, the measure was, itself, not clinically useful.

None of the behavioral syndromes in children of normal intelligence has yet had an appropriate marker identified. If the Gershon finding with respect to REM indication were to hold up, a study of offspring of depressed patients having this response would be a major interest. Another putative marker, that of elevated acedaldehyde in offspring of alcoholics not themselves alcoholic, has been reported (Shuckit, 1979). If such a finding is replicated, similar identification of high risk individuals with prospective follow-up should be carried out.

DISCUSSION

Enthusiasm for biological research stems from the reproducibility of measures, and from the nature of its concepts which are understood by the biomedical community at large. Some of this research has added credibility in a field where authority and dogma have at times taken the place of factual information. However, with the exception of a few applications, particularly psychopharmacological, there is yet little influence upon practice or even the likelihood of immediate practical benefit from biological research. Even the most promising measures appear to have both low specificity and low sensitivity, thus limiting clinical application. This has been reviewed in detail for one syndrome (hyperkinesis) and if one applies the standards of general medicine, then none of the biological measures even approach clinical significance (Rapoport and Ferguson, 1981).

Our studies with minor physical anomalies and childhood behavior disorders, for example, while providing some interesting support for a biological influence on behavior, have not yielded specific subgroups or predicted treatment or outcome.

Clinically, the discovery of a trait marker with high specificity would be the major biological breakthrough for child psychiatry. As noted above, this has not yet occurred. Catecholamines and other neurotransmitters have been omitted from this discussion, as none of these measures has, as yet, shown either specificity or strength of association to meet any of the goals outlined above.

If a major biological breakthrough does not occur, primary prevention can still be approached through social-environmental support discussed elsewhere in this panel. A final caveat: We have reason to be optimistic about the advances in biological research, particularly in view of some current pharmacological treatment trials. This review is not intended to lull clinicians into waiting for "biological breakthroughs." The tools are already available for effective psychological treatments. There is sufficient knowledge of epidemiological risk, psychosocial strategies and preventive psychiatry for rational, focused, preventive action, even in the absence of such advances.

REFERENCES

Bachman, D., Hodges, F. and Freeman, J. (1977). Computerized axial tomography in neurologic disorders of children. *Pediatrics*, 59:352–363.

Bagadia, V., Eisenberg, L., Olutawura, M., Rafaelsen, O. and Vartanian, F. (1979). Knowledge and technology needed for further development of mental health program. *Neuropsychobiology*, 5:332–339.

Bergstrom, K. and Bille, B. (1978). Computed tomography of the brain in children with minimal brain damage: A preliminary study. *Neuropediatrie*, 9:378–384.

Bohman, M., Sigvardsson, S. and Cloninger, R. (1981). Maternal inheritance of alcohol abuse. *Archives of General Psychiatry*, 38:965–969.

Broadhurst, P. L. (1978). In *Drugs and the Inheritance of Behavior*. New York: Plenum Press, pp. 135–139.

Brownell, G. L., Budinger, T., Lauterbur, P. and McGeer, P. (1982). Positron tomography and nuclear magnetic resonance imaging. *Science*, 215:619–626.

Campbell, M., Rosenbloom, S., Perry, R., George, A., Krichoff, I., Anderson, L., Small, A. and Jennings, S. (1981). Computerized axial tomographic scans in young autistic children. Presented at Annual Meeting of the American Psychiatric Association, New Orleans, May, 1981.

Caparulo, B., Cohen, D., Rothman, S., Young, G., Katz, N., Shaywitz, S. and Shaywitz, B. (1981). Computed tomographic brain scanning in children with developmental neuropsychiatric disorders. *Journal of the American Academy of Child Psychiatry*, 20:338–357.

Damascio, H., Maurer, R. and Damascio, A. (1980). Computerized tomographic scan findings in patients with autistic behavior. *Archives of Neurology*, 37:504–510.

Eisenberg, L. (1974). Primary prevention and early detection in mental illness. *Bulletin of the New York Academy of Medicine*, 51:118–129.

Friedhoff, A. J. and Rosengarten, H. (1979). Enduring changes in dopamine receptor cells of pups from drug administration to pregnant and nursing rats. *Science*, 203:1133–1135.

Gershon, E. and Hamovit, J. (1979). Genetic methods and preventive psychiatry. *Progress in Neuropsychopharmacology*, 3:565–573.

Gershon, E., Nurnberger, J., Siraram, N. and Gillin, C. (1979). In *Neuropsychopharmacology*, B. Saletu, ed. New York: Pergamon Press.

Goodwin, D., Schulsinger, F., Knop, J., Mednick, S. and Guze, S. (1977). *Archives of General Psychiatry*, 34:1005–1009.

Hagberg, B. and Ingvar, D. H. (1976). Cognitive reduction in presenile dementia related to regional abnormalities of the cerebral blood flow. *British Journal of Psychiatry*, 128:209–222.

Hier, D., LeMay, M. and Rosenberger, P. (1979). Autism and unfavorable left-right asymmetries of the brain. *Journal of Autism and Developmental Disorders*, 9:153–159.

Hier, D., LeMay, M., Rosenburger, P. and Perlo, V. (1978). Developmental dyslexia. *Archives of Neurology*, 35:90–92.

Hier, D. and Rosenberger, P. (1980). Focal left temporal lobe lesions and delayed speech. *Developmental and Behavioral Pediatrics*, 1:54–57.

Nurnberger, J. and Gershon, E. (In press). Genetics of Affective Disorders. To be published in *Depression and Antidepressants: Implications for Cause and Treatment*, E. Friedman, ed. New York: Raven Press.

Rapoport, J. and Ferguson, B. (1981). Evidence for biological validity of the hyperactive child syndrome. *Developmental Medicine and Child Neurology*, 23:667–682.

Reivich, M., Kuhl, D., Wolf, A., Greenberg, J., Phelps, M., Ido, T., Casella, V., Fowler, J., Hoffman, E., Aloni, A., Sam, P. and Sokoloff, L. (1979). The [18]Flouride oxyglucose method for the measurement of local cerebral glucose utilization in man. *Circ. Res.,* 44:127–137.

Rosett, H. (1979). Clinical pharmacology of the fetal alcohol syndrome. In *Biochemistry and Pharmacology of Ethanol,* Vol. 2, E. Majchrowicz and E. Noble, eds. New York: Plenum Press, pp. 485–509.

Shanberg, S. and Kuhn, C. (1980). Maternal deprivation: An animal model of psychosocial dwarfism. In *Enzymes and Neurotransmitters in Mental Disease,* E. Usdin, T. Sourks and M. Youdim, eds. New York: John Wiley and Sons, pp. 373–393.

Shuckit, M. and Rayses, V. (1979). Ethanol ingestion: Differences in blood-acetaldehyde concentration relatives of alcoholics and controls. *Science,* 203:54–55.

Taylor, A., Liu, S., Randolph, B., Branch, B. and Kokka, W. (1981). Fetal exposure to ethanol alters drug sensitivity in adult rats. *Alcoholism: Clinical and Experimental Research,* in press.

Thompson, J., Ross, R. and Horwitz, S. (1980). Computed axial tomography and minimal brain dysfunction. *Journal of Learning Disabilities,* 13:334–337.

Weinberger, D., Bigelow, L., Kleinman, J., Klein, E., Rosenblatt, J. and Wyatt, R. (1980). Cerebral ventricular enlargement in chronic schizophrenia. *Archives of General Psychiatry,* 37:11–13.

Werry, J. (1978). *Pediatric Psychopharmacology: The Use of Behavior Modifying Ways in Children.* New York: Brunner/Mazel.

Weiner, J. (1977). *Psychopharmacology in Childhood and Adolescence.* New York: Basic Books.

26

Chronic Malnutrition and Child Behavior: Effects of Early Caloric Supplementation on Social and Emotional Functioning at School Age

David E. Barrett and Marian Radke-Yarrow

National Institute of Mental Health, Bethesda, Maryland

Robert E. Klein

Institute of Nutrition of Central America and Panama, Guatemala City, Guatemala

The effects of chronic malnutrition on child behavior were examined by determining the relationships between prenatal and postnatal caloric supplementation and social–emotional functioning at school age in chronically malnourished, rural Guatemalan children. Subjects were 138 children, ages 6 to 8, who had participated in the Institute of Nutrition of Central America and Panama Longitudinal Study. Independent variables were measures of maternal caloric supplementation during pregnancy, child caloric supplementation from birth to 2 years, and child caloric supplementation from age 2 to 4. Dependent measures were assessments of social interaction and affect, obtained by observing children in small-group activities with peers, and cognitive tests. High caloric supplementation from birth to 2 years predicted high levels of social involvement, both happy and angry affect, and moderate activity level at school age. Low supplementation was associated with passivity, dependency on adults, and anxious behavior. These relationships were significant when socioeconomic status and maternal supplementation were controlled. Cognitive measures were not strongly predicted by supplement intake. Results indicate the importance of adequate energy intake in infancy for later social–emotional development.

Chronic malnutrition characterizes much of the world's child population. The effects of severe malnutrition on the structural integrity of the organism are well documented. Impairment of defenses against disease (Neumann, Jelliffe, & Jelliffe, 1978), reduced neural cell growth (Dyson & Jones, 1976), and delayed neural maturation (Dobbing, 1964) are all associated with nutritional deficit in early life. Chronic undernutrition has been associated with reduced stature, head circumference, and physical development (Livingston, Calloway, MacGregor, Fischer, & Hastings, 1975; Underwood et al., 1967).

Less well understood are the behavioral consequences of malnutrition, particularly mild-to-moderate undernutrition. Whereas there is documentation of lasting impairments in cognitive processes in children who experienced severe malnutrition in infancy (MacLaren, Yaktin, Kanawati, Sabbagh, & Kadi, 1973; Monckeberg, 1968), the relations between mild-to-moderate malnutrition and later cognitive dysfunction are not strong (see Pollitt & Thomson, 1977, for a review). Further, research has not made clear whether empirical relations between degree of nutritional deficit in early life and later cognitive outcomes remain significant when other important socioeconomic variables (e.g., conditions of housing, stimulation in the home) are controlled (Lloyd-Still, 1976).

Particularly important is the fact that very little is known about the effects of chronic malnutrition on children's later social behaviors and emotional characteristics. Few human studies have examined relationships between measures of nutritional deficit in early life and later social and emotional behavior. However, the few studies that have done so raise provocative issues and suggest that social–emotional well-being may be particularly vulnerable to the effects of early malnutrition.

The studies that have been done in this area have focused on infancy, comparing the behavioral characteristics of infants with a history of undernutrition (including prenatal nutritional deficit) with those of better nourished infants. From the research a consistent pattern of behavioral characteristics of malnourished infants appears, including impaired attentional processes (Lester, 1975); reduced social responsiveness (Brazelton, Tronick, Lechtig, Lasky, & Klein, 1977; Mora et al., 1979); heightened irritability and inability to tolerate frustration (Mora et al., 1979); and low activity level, reduced independence, and diminished affect (Chavez & Martinez, 1979). Lester (1979) suggested that such effects may occur within a synergistic system where the malnourished infant is less successful at engaging caretakers in interaction and, in turn, is responded to less often and with less sensitivity, resulting in a failure to develop normal patterns of social interaction. If so, we should expect that insufficient nutrition early in life would be associated with poor interpersonal skills and general lack of social responsiveness in later childhood. Thus, the recent research on malnourished human infants provides a theoretical rationale for an investigation of the effects of malnutrition on social–emotional functioning in childhood.

Another, and perhaps even more compelling, theoretical basis for this study is derived from the large amount of research on the behavioral characteristics of severely malnourished animals. Experimentally malnourished animals are characterized by apathy, passivity, and inability to sustain attention (Strobel & Zimmrman, 1971). They show reduced exploration and curiosity (Frankova, 1973), fearful avoidance of new stimuli (Strobel & Zimmerman, 1972), and a failure to respond normally to social initiations from other animals. All of these characteristics would appear to indicate a "functional avoidance" and a "functional deprivation" (Barnes, 1976) of new situations and stimuli. Other characteristics of severely malnourished animals are nonpurposive behavior (Frankova & Barnes, 1968), excitability (Barnes, Moore & Pond, 1970), and unpredictable aggression (Platt & Stewart, 1968).

Thus, although we can not extrapolate directly from animals to humans, the above findings from the animal research link malnutrition to important functional disorders. Lack of social responsiveness, emotionality, avoidance of new stimuli, and poor behavioral organization comprise a critical complex of behaviors which, if characteristic of malnourished children, are likely to be associated with impaired emotional responding and poor interpersonal skills. As previously indicated, the studies on malnourished human infants suggest that this may be the case: Undernourished infants show reduced responsiveness to persons, lack of initiative, and heightened irritability relative to better nourished peers. Such characteristics, if they continue to mark the course of early social development, may be expected to impair the quality of the infant's early social interactions and thereby inhibit the development of social competencies and positive emotional characteristics in childhood.

In the present article, the behavioral implications of chronic malnutrition in school-age children are investigated. The article addresses this issue by analyzing relationships between the adequacy of prenatal and postnatal nutrition and later social–emotional behavior. On the basis of the theoretical formulation presented above, we hypothesized that children who experienced greater nutritional deficit in the early years of development would, at school age, show impaired social–emotional functioning relative to children whose nutrition was more adequate. In addition, relationships between prenatal and postnatal nutrition and cognitive development at school age were examined in order to bring further light to the issue of the vulnerability of cognitive functions to chronic nutritional insult. In view of the cited research indicating attentional impairments in malnourished infants, we hypothesized that these cognitive measures tapping primarily attentional processes would be most clearly related to undernutrition.

METHOD

Children in the present study had been participants in the Institute of Nutrition of Central America and Panama (INCAP) Longitudinal Study (1969–1977; Klein, 1979). In that study an attempt was made to establish causal relations between chronic undernutrition and physical and cognitive development. The method used was to provide nutritional supplements to an endemically malnourished population and to examine the relationship between amount of supplement intake and later development. The INCAP investigators (Engle, Irwin, Klein, Yarbrough, & Townsend, 1979; Klein 1979) consistently found that supplement caloric intake was the best predictor of physical growth and cognitive development up to the preschool years, relative to other nutritional (e.g., diet calories or protein) and social–environmental variables. Therefore, in the present study supplemental caloric measures were the primary indices of nutritional history; these were used as independent variables to predict behavior at school age. Dependent measures were assessments of social interaction and affect, obtained by observing children in small-group activities with peers, and cognitive tests. Nonnutritional social–environmental factors were controlled.

Subjects

Subjects were 78 boys and 60 girls from the villages of Santo Domingo, Conocaste, and San Juan in the county of El Progresso, Guatemala. Children were between the ages of 6 years 1 month and 8 years 3 months at the time of the data collection. Villages were represented in the study in approximate proportion to village size: There were 60 subjects from

Santo Domingo, 54 from Conocaste, and 24 from San Juan. These three agricultural communities are located 30–60 kilometers northeast of Guatemala City. The adult literacy rate is approximately 50%. The study population has been identified as chronically malnourished: 80% to 85% of preschool-age children were classified as at least mildly to moderately undernourished in INCAP's baseline survey according to Gomez et al.'s (1956) criterion of weight for age.

In selecting the samples an attempt was made to ensure adequate variability in nutritional history. Therefore, supplemental caloric intake of mother and child was used as a selection variable. On the basis of INCAP's longitudinal data, all children in the villages were assigned to "good," "average," or "poor" classifications with respect to caloric supplementation of the mother during pregnancy and of the child from birth to 4 years.[1] Because height for age has often been used as an index of degree of nutritional deprivation (Brozek, 1979), children were also classified as "tall" (third or fourth quartile) or "short" (first or second quartile). The sample was then selected so that (a) there would be approximately equal numbers of well-supplemented and poorly supplemented children and equal numbers of tall and short children, and (b) within villages, the characteristics of the sample with respect to supplementation history and height would reflect the village population. The final sample of 138 children included 56 with good supplementation, 29 with average supplementation, and 53 with poor supplementation. Sixty-eight children were tall, 70 were short.

Nutritional Assessments

Estimates of mean energy and protein intake based on dietary surveys carried out at the beginning of the INCAP Longitudinal Study (1969) showed that at all ages, mean daily energy intakes for the study popu-

---

[1]Children were assigned scores of 1 to 3 for mother caloric supplementation history and scores of 1 to 5 for child caloric supplementation history. For mother supplementation history, scores were assigned as follows: 1 = less than 5,000 supplemental calories during pregnancy; 2 = 5,000–20,000 supplemental calories during pregnancy; 3 = more than 20,000 supplemental calories during pregnancy. For child supplementation, scores were based on the percentage of 3-month periods in which the child was poorly supplemented (less than 5,000 calories) or well-supplemented (more than 10,000 calories). Ratings were as follows: 1 = poorly supplemented in more than three fourths of the periods; 2 = poorly supplemented in more than one half of the periods; 3 = poorly supplemented in less than one half of the periods, but not well supplemented in more than one half of the periods; 4 = well supplemented in more than one half of the periods; 5 = well supplemented in more than three fourths of the periods. Combinations of mother and child supplement ratings were used to classify children as good, poor, or average in supplementation.

lation were substantially below estimated daily requirements. For example, 4-year-old children in 1969 received about 80 kcal/kg/day, compared with estimated needs of 96–99 kcal/kg/day (World Health Organization, Note 1). Daily protein intake was at or above both required and safe levels.

From a physiological standpoint, this energy deficit means that children were likely to burn protein to satisfy energy needs, thus threatening the available store of body protein. The hypothesized effect of supplemental calories would be to spare body protein by providing adequate nutrients for energy needs. Thus, low supplemental caloric intake, in a supplemented population, would represent relative energy deficit and risk for retarded growth and development.

Empirical evidence supports this interpretation. In the present population, maternal caloric intake was related to placental weight (Lechtig, Yarbrough, Delgado, Klein, & Behar, 1975) and birthweight (Lechtig, Yarbrough, Delgado, Habicht, Martorell, & Klein, 1975). Our data show that caloric supplementation prior to the age of 2 years predicted height at age 4 ($r = .39$, $p < .005$, and $r = .33$, $p < .05$, for boys and girls, respectively) and also at present age ($r = .33$, $p < .005$, and $r = .27$, $p < .05$, for boys and girls, respectively). Further, Martorell, Lechtig, Yarbrough, Delgado, and Klein (1976) reviewed the studies on the effects of protein and/or caloric supplementation on postnatal physical growth in developing countries. They concluded that in the experiments reviewed, protein-calorie supplementation was causally related to physical growth. The relative importance of proteins versus calories depended on which nutrient was limiting in the home diet. When calories but not protein were limiting, calories alone seemed to improve growth rates. Thus, on both theoretical and emprical grounds, level of caloric supplement intake appears to be an appropriate index of nutritional status for our study population.

INCAP Longitudinal Design: Relation to the Present Study

To infer that supplementation is related to later behavior, one must rule out alternative explanatory variables relating to intake or outcome, that is, individual differences (e.g., in social class and circumstances, motivational characteristics, etc.) that might covary with both supplement intake and later behavior and, in our population, village differences that might be related to level of supplementation and behavior. Although INCAP investigators have not identified any personality or socioeconomic variables that were correlated with supplement intake (Engle et al., 1979), the villages themselves did differ in mean supplemental caloric intake. This was by virtue of the original INCAP Longitudinal Study design, which is described in detail below. Thus, the possibility that supplement effects might be confounded with village differences had to be considered. Further, the possibility that supplementation might differentially affect children in the different villages required attention.

In the INCAP Longitudinal Study, the investigators wished to determine the relative effectiveness of a protein-calorie supplement and a calorie-only supplement in promoting physical growth and cognitive development. Four study villages that had been matched on a number of social–environmental and epidemiological characteristics (see Klein, 1979) were selected to be studied. Two villages were provided the protein–calorie supplement, the other two villages received the calorie-only supplement. The protein-calorie supplement (*atole*) consisted of a vegetable protein mixture, dry skim milk, and sugar, whereas the calorie-only supplement (*fresco*) contained only sugar and flavoring. One cup (180 ml) of protein–calorie supplement contained 11.5 g of protein and 163 kcal. One cup of calorie-only supplement contained 59 kcal. Both preparations included essential vitamins and minerals that were thought to be limiting in the diets of the study populations.[2] Because the protein–calorie supplement contained approximately three times the calories of the calorie-only supplement, proportionately more children in the protein–calorie villages had good supplementation histories than those in the calorie-only villages.[3]

When the present study began in 1979, one of the villages in the study had received the calorie-only supplement, and two villages had received the protein–calorie supplement.[4] Since the villages differed in supplemental caloric intake, it was necessary to ensure that any relationships between caloric intake and later behavior were not specific to type of village (atole or fresco). Further, it was necessary to determine whether

---

[2]Each supplement contained the following vitamins and minerals: ascorbic acid (4.0 mg/cup), thiamine (1.1 mg/cup), riboflavin (1.5 mg/cup), niacin (18.5 mg/cup), vitamin A (1.2 mg/cup), iron (5.0–5.4 mg/cup), and fluoride (.2 mg/cup).

[3]Village means for mothers' daily supplemental calories ranged from 65 kcal per day (Santo Domingo) to 111 kcal per day (Conocaste). Means for children for the period of birth to 2 years ranged from 8 kcal per day (Santo Domingo) to 108 kcal per day (Conocaste). For children ages 2 to 4, means ranged from 103 kcal per day (Santo Domingo) to 325 kcal per day (San Juan).

[4]Due to financial constraints, observations could be made in only three of the four villages that had participated in the longitudinal study. We chose not to make observations in Espiritu Santu, one of the two smaller villages and the one farthest from INCAP in Guatemala City.

different villages might respond differently to caloric intervention due to preexisting village differences that had not been adequately controlled by the original matching procedure. The current analysis was designed to take into account these interpretive issues.

In the INCAP Longitudinal Study, supplements were administered at central food stations in each village. Attendance was voluntary. Daily supplemental caloric intake was recorded (kcal/kg/day) for all women during pregnancy and for all children under 7 years of age. For the present analysis, three variables were constructed from these data: total supplemental caloric intake of the mother during pregnancy, total supplemental caloric intake of the child from birth to 2 years, and total supplemental caloric intake of the child from 2 to 4 years. These variables were used as predictor variables in regression analyses (controlling for socioeconomic variables) to predict the behavioral measures.

All present analyses were conducted across villages and within each of the two largest villages, one of which had been given a protein–calorie supplement. Thus, we could determine whether the effects of caloric supplementation were specific to and/or different for particular villages.

Social Environment Index

To represent individual differences in living conditions, INCAP's standardized measure of socioeconomic status (SES) was used (Klein, 1979). This SES measure is a composite of three ratings of family living conditions: house quality (condition of roof, walls, kitchen, bedroom, dining room); parents' clothing (mother's and father's use of modern clothing, including sweaters and shoes); and mother's report of family teaching and stimulation of preschool children.

Behavior Assessments

Children were observed in social interactions in six-person groups. In addition, each child was tested on a psychological battery. The children were brought to a central location in the village for the observations and tests. Assessments took place within a 2-day period. There were approximately 5 hours of small-group observations per child, 2½ hours on each of the two mornings. Afternoons were used for individual testing. There were three observer/testers.

Group observations. In each six-person group children were of the same sex, were within 1 year in age, were of varied statures, and had different supplementation histories. Male and female groups were observed alternately in each village. In each of the two small-group sessions, children were observed in approximately nine different situations. The situations were joined together so that they comprised a smoothly running sequence of gamelike activities. The paradigm was adapted from Yarrow, Scott, and Waxler (1973). Situations included free play in a novel environment, group problem-solving tasks, construction activities (e.g., clay), competitive games, and impulse-control situations.

An ongoing record of each child's behavior was obtained using a standard time-sampling procedure. Across the variety of activities, each child was observed for a series of 2-min periods (divided into 30-sec intervals). Behaviors were coded in five classes: interaction with peers, contact with adults, behavior with the physical environment, level of activity, and emotions. Specific coding categories are shown in Table 1. Each child was observed for approximately 25 2-minute intervals. Each child's score for a particular category is the mean frequency of that behavior per 2-minute interval.

Each observer was generally assigned to two children per activity, observing each of them in alternating 2-minute periods until the end of the activity. For certain predesignated reliability assessments, each observer was assigned to three children so that matching observational records could be obtained. These data were analyzed for observer agreement using the intraclass correlation (Bartko, 1966). The unit of measurement in these analyses was the 2-minute observation; thus all scores entered by a particular observer were scores of 0 (no instances of the behavior in the 2-minute observation period) to 4 (four instances of the behavior). Intraclass correlation coefficients are reported in Table 1.[5]

Individual tests. After each morning session, and after a break for lunch (there were also snack breaks during each morning session), three children from the group came back to the testing center for individual testing. Cognitive tests, standarized by INCAP for use in the villages, were Verbal Inferences, Memory for Objects, Digit Span, Concept Identification, Hidden Figures, and Block Design. Also administered were the Bender-Gestalt Test and a test for the ability to follow directions after a period of delay. Those tests assumed to measure attentional capacities were Digit Span, Hidden Figures, the test of persistence and

---

[5]As Table 1 shows, six categories had intraclass correlations of .00. These were due to low frequencies of occurrence in the reliability sample. Reliability data from our parallel study in the United States (Barrett, Yarrow, Ziegler, & Livingston, Note 2; see also the section on instrument development) showed high interobserver agreement for five of the six categories: seeks physical contact (intraclass $r = .81$), imaginative play ($r = .81$), sad ($r = .94$), loses control, cries ($r = .86$), and destruction with materials ($r = .96$). Only physical play-alone had a zero-level intraclass correlation (.00) in that study. Therefore, with the exception of physical play-alone, all of the categories were retained in the present analysis.

Table 1
*Behaviors Coded on Time-Sampling Basis
in Small-Group Activities*

Behavior	Reliability
Interaction with peers	
Friendly interaction	.89*
Helps, shares, comforts	.24*
Physical aggression	.50*
Verbal aggression	1.00*
Rough and tumble play	.81*
Intrudes, interferes	.79*
Dominates, asserts self	.81*
Seeks help	.68*
Submissive	.65*
Defends self	.72*
Positive response to bid	.88*
Negative response to bid	.95*
No interaction	.90*
Contact with adults	
Seeks attention	.59*
Seeks physical contact	00
No interaction	.63*
Behavior with environment	
Involved in group activity	.88*
Plays with materials	.89*
Destructive with materials	.00
Wanders	.95*
Physical play alone	.00
Imaginative play	.00
Distracted by outside events	.84*
Only watching	.92*
Inactive	.79*
Level of activity	
Low	.67*
Moderate	.70*
High	.72*
Very high	.74*
Emotion	
Happy, laughs, smiles	.84*
Anxious	.85*
Angry, hostile	.53*
Sad	.00
Loses control	.00
No emotion shown	.79*

Note. Reliabilities are estimated by intraclass correlation coefficients. See Footnote 5 for a note on the interpretation of zero-level intraclass correlations.
* $p < .001$.

distractibility, and the task of following directions. In our analysis we also included scores on a cognitive composite consisting of the average of the child's standard scores on the INCAP tests.

Reliability estimates for cognitive and persistence measures were made in the INCAP Longitudinal Study. Test-retest correlation coefficients or coefficients of internal consistency were obtained: Verbal Inferences = .87 (test-retest); Persistence = .97 (test-retest); Hidden Figures = .81 (test-retest); Digit Span = .65 (test-retest); Memory for Objects = .69 and .72 (internal consistency for males and females, respectively); Concept Identification = .72 and .45 (internal consistency for males and females); Block Design = .83 and .54 (internal consistency for males and females).

Instrument Development

Methods and instruments were developed in the United States for a parallel study on the effects of malnutrition on children's behavior. The United States study was carried out in San Diego, California, concurrently with the present study, by Barrett, Yarrow, Ziegler, and Livingston (Note 2).

For the Guatemala research, the instruments developed in the San Diego study were translated from English to Spanish, and procedures were revised so that they were appropriate for the ability levels and expectations of children in Guatemala. Observers were trained by the first author for a period of 12 weeks. The observers were three women with extensive experience testing children from the villages in the INCAP study.

Data Analysis

For each dependent variable of interest, multiple regression analyses were carried out to examine the individual and cumulative predictive ability of the supplementation variables. The first analysis was conducted across villages. Socioeconomic status was entered into the equation, followed by supplemental calories of the mother during pregnancy, supplemental calories of the child from birth to 2 years and supplemental calories of the child from ages 2 to 4. The analyses thus addressed these questions: (a) How well can we predict individual differences on the dependent variable on the basis of prenatal supplementation, having controlled for home environment? (b) How much of the variance in the dependent measure can we account for on the basis of supplementation during infancy, having accounted for the effects of SES and maternal supplementation? (c) How much further can we account for variance in the dependent variable, if we now include a measure of supplementation in the child's third and fourth years? It should be noted that the same analyses also allowed us to determine which of the supplementation measures was the best predictor of the outcome measure, controlling for SES (see Nie, Hull, Jenkins, Steinbrenner, & Bent, 1975, pp. 358–359).

Within-village analyses. The same analyses were conducted within each of the two larger villages, one a protein–calorie village and the other a calorie-only village. These analyses allowed us to see whether any relationships between supplement intake and behavior were specific to village.

Within-village analyses were important for several reasons: (a) The villages differed in presence/absence of protein supplementation. Were relationships between caloric supplementation and behavior dependent on whether the supplement was protein-rich or protein-free? (b) Both supplemental caloric levels and home-diet caloric levels were significantly higher in the large protein–calorie village than in the calorie-only village over the course of the INCAP Longitudinal Study. Were relationships between calorie supplementation and behavior dependent on absolute level of energy intake? (c) The villages differed on several objective measures of quality of home and social environment. Although the villages had originally been matched on a number of general SES indices and demographic characteristics (e.g., means of livelihood, home diet), analyses based on more recent data show that the villages differed significantly on such variables as value of producer durables, access to water supply, modernity of cooking facilities, and number of rooms in the house. Further, the general atmosphere of the villages differed. For example, San Juan, the smaller, protein–calorie village, was shady and cool, physically attractive, and well cared for. Conocaste, the large protein–calorie village, was, in contrast, extremely hot and depressing, with a harsher, browner landscape, and with little physical beauty. Certainly such qualitative differences might affect the persons living in these environments. Thus, it was important to see whether relationships between nutritional history and later behavior were similar for the different villages.

Supplementary Analyses

Two further analyses were performed. Multiple regression analyses were carried out within sexes to determine whether supplementation effects generalized. Also, correlational analyses were performed to examine relationships between height, weight, and behavior.

RESULTS

Results of the multiple regression analyses for the prediction of social–emotional outcomes across villages are presented in detail in Table 2. Table 3 summarizes results of multiple regression analyses across and within villages. In the tables, dependent variables significantly associated with one or more independent variables are presented. Because of the clarity of the theoretical framework in which we have hypothesized empirical relations, results are reported for significance levels at or below .10. Attendance to marginally significant associations helps to trace out the relationships within the hypothesized network of variables. Results of the supplementary analyses for within-sex supplementation effects and relations between height, weight, and behavior are presented in summary form.

Social–Emotional Measures

Table 2 gives results for the multiple regression analysis for the prediction of social and emotional characteristics across villages. For each dependent variable the table shows the simple correlation of the variable with the SES composite and, at each succeeding step of the analysis, the resulting multiple correlations, beta weights, and F values for the increment in the squared multiple correlation, due to the entry of the last-entered variable. The results are reported up to and including the last independent variable that significantly increases the value of the squared multiple correlation.

Three variables were significantly predicted by SES alone. There were negative correlations between SES and only watching other children, and between SES and no activity (sum of only watching and inactive), and a positive correlation with happy affect. The first supplementation variable representing mother supplementation (MS) during pregnancy significantly increased the variance accounted for in the first two of these measures. Better maternally supplemented children (controlling for SES) were less often only watching and less often showed no activity than did poorly supplemented children. Children of better supplemented mothers more often requested help from a peer.

The addition of the variable representing child supplementation from birth to 2 years (CS1) significantly increased the multiple correlation for

Table 2
Multiple Regression Analysis for Prediction of Social–Emotional Variables

Dependent variables	Step 1		Step 2			Step 3					Step 4					
	r	R	β_{SES}	β_{MS}	F_{MS}	R	β_{SES}	β_{MS}	β_{CS_1}	F_{CS_1}	R	β_{SES}	β_{MS}	β_{CS_1}	β_{CS_2}	F_{CS_2}
1. Helps	.06	.07	−.06	.01	.01	.18	−.03	.12	−.21*	3.64*						
2. Seeks help from peer	.07	.25**	.10	.24***	7.45***	.29**	.07	.14	.18*	2.89*						
3. Defends self	.06	.12	.07	.11	1.50	.13	.07	.09	.04	.10	.22	.09	.07	−.17	.28**	4.12**
4. Negative to bid from peer	.08	.08	.07	−.03	.14	.17	.10	.07	−.18*	2.79*						
5. No interaction with adult	−.09	.10	−.08	.05	.31	.18	−.12	−.05	.18*	2.81*						
6. Involved in group activity	.12	.20*	.15	.16*	3.03*	.27**	.10	.03	.23**	4.66**						
7. Only watching	−.21**	.32***	−.24**	−.25**	6.57**											
8. No activity	−.22**	.27***	−.24***	−.17*	3.53*											
9. Moderate activity level	.07	.13	.09	.11	1.53	.24*	.00	−.02	.24**	4.82**						
10. Very high activity level	.09	.10	.09	.06	.37	.19	.06	−.05	.19*	3.11*						
11. Happy	.15*	.19*	.17*	.13	1.94	.29**	.12	−.02	.26**	5.88***						
12. Angry	.04	.10	.05	.10	1.10	.24*	.01	−.05	.27**	6.19***						
13. Anxious	−.12	.15	−.13	−.09	.90	.27**	−.08	.07	−.28**	6.74***						

Note. SES = socioeconomic status; MS = mother supplementation; CS_1 = child supplementation; CS_2 = child supplementation from birth to 2 years; CS_3 = child supplementation, 2–4 years. Predictor variables for the steps are as follows: Step 1, SES; Step 2, SES and MS; Step 3, SES, MS, CS_1; Step 4, SES, MS, CS_1, CS_2. Significance levels for r indicate significance of regression equation with 1, 122 degrees of freedom; for R, $df = k$, $124 - (k - 1)$. k is the number of variables in the analysis. F values represent increase in R^2 associated with the entry of the last variable in the equation. β values show standardized regression coefficients with all variables in the equation at a given step in the equation. Results are reported up to and including the final step in the equation where a last-entered variable makes a significant increase in R^2.
*$p < .10$. **$p < .05$. ***$p < .01$.

Table 3: *Summary of Multiple Regression Analyses*

Predictor variable	Across villages				Calorie-only village				Protein–calorie village			
	SES	MS	CS1	CS2	SES	MS	CS1	CS2	SES	MS	CS1	CS2
Friendly	.10	.12	-.00	-.08	.02	.19	.05	.50**	.23	.20	.09	-.25
Helps	-.07	.01	-.21*	.00	-.19	.22*	-.30**	.06	.15	-.18	-.38*	.11
Intrudes	.11	.01	.08	-.10	.21	-.15	.09	.29	.15	.10	.40*	-.10
Seeks help	.07	.24**	.18*	.06	-.02	-.00	.16	.26	.12	.43***	.03	.03
Defends self	.06	.11	.04	.28***	.20	.14	.21	.41**	.05	.14	.15	.14
Negative to bid	.08	-.03	-.18**	.02	.16	.02	-.07	-.01	.01	.11	.19	.08
No interaction (peer)	-.13	-.10	.06	.06	-.12	-.18	.02	-.41**	-.22	-.22	-.11	.26
Seeks contact with adult	.09	.05	-.12	.07	.15	.15	.33**	-.04	.00^b	.00^b	.00^b	.00^b
No interaction (adult)	-.09	.05	.18*	.07	-.08	.05	.14	.19	-.12	-.08	-.18	.04
Involved in group activity	.12	.16*	.23**	.04	.08	.12	.10	.22	.18	.30**	-.31	-.23
Plays with materials	.15*	.06	.05	.17	.19	-.02	.04	.44**	.22	.09	.17	.15
Imaginative play	-.05	-.04	-.08	.08	.07	-.02	.08	.36*	-.20	-.03	-.28	-.22
Only watching	-.21**	-.25**	.02	.08	-.07	-.39**	.23	-.21	-.33**	-.31**	.09	.16
No activity (environment)	-.22**	-.17*	-.01	-.08	-.17	-.11	.02	-.55***	-.32**	-.34**	.13	.09
Low activity level	-.09	-.12	.04	.02	.06	-.18	-.02	-.35*	-.32**	-.23	.03	.13
Moderate activity level	.07	.11	.24**	-.02	-.02	.06	.17	.20	.13	.11	.06	-.15
Very high activity level	.09	.06	.19*	.06	.31**	.10	-.01	.14	.12	.18	-.16	-.29
Happy	.15*	.13	.26**	-.00	.11	.15	.36**	.32*	.23*	.17	.16	-.22
Anxious	-.12	-.09	-.28**	-.06	-.12	.00	-.26*	-.10	-.19	-.06	.02	.20
Angry	.04	.10	.27**	.17	.08	.05	.07	.23	.06	.02	.37*	.22
Persistence	.03	.06	.01	.32**	.13	.06	-.10	.44**	.07	.12	.11	.40**
Distraction	-.18**	-.14	-.01	-.09	-.26*	-.13	-.12	-.10	-.09	-.18	.06	.01
Following Directions	.00	-.02	.02	.34**	-.01	.21	.04	.30	-.16	-.06	.13	.35*
Hidden Figures	.11	.17*	-.13	-.02	.29**	.36***	-.26*	.44**	-.07	.13	.28	-.03
Digit Span	.19**	.02	.02	.14	.15	.06	.07	.16	.16	-.05	-.04	.12
Block Design	.16*	.03	.03	-.13	.22*	.01	-.03	.41**	.13	.04	.14	-.17
Concept Identification	.23**	-.00	-.04	.00	.19	.11	.09	.21	.26*	-.18	.20	-.02
Bender Gestalt^c	-.13	-.08	.06	-.07	-.16	-.14	-.00	-.34*	-.11	-.08	.11	-.04
Cognitive Composite	.19**	.06	.01	.08	.22*	.15	-.11	.44**	-.19	-.03	.23	.04

Note. Entries in the table are standardized partial regression coefficients (beta weights). Each shows the weight given a particular independent variable in predicting the criterion at the step at which it was entered into the equation. Significance levels indicate the significance of the increase in R^2 due to the entry of the independent variable. SES = socioeconomic status; MS = mother supplementation; CS1 = child supplementation from birth to 2 years; CS2 = child supplementation, 2–4 years. [a] MS had the strongest association with helps at Step 3 (β = .36, $p < .05$). CS1 acted as a supressor variable. [b] Regression statistics were not computed due to insufficient variability in the criterion variable. [c] High scores on the Bender Gestalt indicate poor performance.
* $p < .10$. ** $p < .05$. *** $p < .01$.

10 variables. High caloric supplementation during this period was positively associated with seeks help from peer, involved in group activity, moderate activity level, happy affect, and angry expression (better supplemented children showed anger more often). High supplementation was negatively related to anxious expression, and to negative response to bid for help from peer. There was also a marginal negative relationship with helps peer, and a marginal positive association with very high activity level. Better supplemented children interacted less frequently with an adult observer.

The fourth variable in the equation, representing child supplementation from 2 to 4 years (CS2) significantly increased the prediction of only one measure—defends self—and assumed a positive beta weight in the equation.

Considered together, the findings indicate that maternal caloric supplementation during pregnancy and child caloric supplementation during the first 2 years were related to high levels of social responsiveness, interaction with the environment, activity level, and expression of affect—both positive (happy) and negative (angry)—at school age.

Individual Tests

As shown in Table 3, SES was positively correlated with Digit Span ($r = 19, p < .05$), Concept Identification ($r = .23, p < .05$), Block Design ($r = .16, p < .10$), and Cognitive Composite ($r = .19, p < .05$). SES was negatively related to amount of time distracted by attractive toys during work on the impossible puzzle ($r = -.18, p < .05$). None of the supplementation variables significantly improved the prediction of these measures. MS significantly improved prediction of Hidden Figures performance, $F(1, 121) = 3.56, p < .10$, with better maternally supplemented children scoring higher. CS1 did not significantly improve prediction of any measures. CS2 improved the prediction of Persistence on the impossible puzzle, $F(1, 119) = 5.29, p < .05$, and on the Following Directions test, $F(1, 119) = 4.92, p < .05$. The variable CS2 was weighted positively in both analyses.

In summary, SES but not the supplementation variables predicted overall cognitive performance; higher SES children performed better than lower SES children. Of the supplementation measures, only one—supplementation from 2 to 4 years—significantly improved the prediction of more than one dependent measure, and this occurred on tests that primarily tapped attentional characteristics (i.e., Persistence and Following Directions).

Within-Village Analyses

Social–emotional measures. The within-village analyses generally supported the findings from the overall analyses. Caloric supplementation during pregnancy and early childhood was predictive of social involvement, interest in the physical environment, affect, and activity level. Results are summarized in Table 3. In Conocaste, the large village given the protein–calorie supplement, MS was associated with low rates of only watching, $F(1, 43) = 5.10$, $p < .05$, and no activity, $F(1, 43) = 6.05$, $p < .05$, and high rates of involved in group activity, $F(1, 43) = 4.41$, $p < .05$, and seeks help from peer, $F(1, 43) = 9.75$, $p < .01$, with SES in the equation. CS1 increased the squared multiple correlation for angry, $F(1, 42) = 3.20$, $p < .10$, and for helps peer, $F(1, 42) = 3.51$, $p < .10$, with better supplemented children showing more anger and less helping than less well-supplemented children. There were, in addition, substantial though nonsignificant positive associations between CS1 and happy affect and defends self. These results are consistent with those of the across-villages analyses. Similarly, in Santo Domingo, the village given the calorie-only supplement, several of the relationships identified in the across-villages analyses were replicated. MS significantly improved prediction of only watching, $F(1, 53) = 5.46$, $p < .05$, assuming a negative beta weight. CS1 significantly increased squared multiple correlation values for happy affect, $F(1, 52) = 5.73$, $p < .05$, and anxious expression, $F(1, 52) = 2.91$, $p < .10$, with beta weights positive and negative, respectively. CS2 significantly improved prediction of defends self, $F(1, 51) = 4.82$, $p < .05$.

However, in each village there were marginally significant relationships between supplementation variables and behavior measures that were not predicted or suggested by the overall analyses. In Conocaste, the protein–calorie village, the addition of CS1 to the equation improved the prediction of intrudes (i.e., takes materials from peer), with a positive beta weight for CS1, $F(1, 42) = 3.84$, $p < .10$. Also, there was a positive though not significant relationship between CS1 and negative response to bid for help from peer. In Santo Domingo, the calorie-only village, there were several unexpected findings. First, child caloric supplementation from 2 to 4 years, rather than the maternal or infancy supplementation measures, was the most consistent predictor of the social–emotional measures. With the other predictor variables in the equation, CS2 was significantly associated with high rates of friendly interaction, $F(1, 51) = 7.01$, $p < .05$, plays with materials, $F(1, 51) = 5.20$, $p < .05$, imaginative play, $F(1, 51) = 3.40$, $p < .10$, and happy affect, $F(1, 51)$

$= 2.99, p < .10$, and with low rates of no interaction with peers, $F(1, 51)$ $= 4.51, p < .05$, no activity, $F(1, 51) = 8.96, p < .01$, and low activity level, $F(1, 51) = 3.26, p < .10$. Second, child supplementation from birth to 2 years (CS1) was positively associated with seeks physical contact from adult, $F(1, 52) = 4.87, p < .05$, a finding that seems inconsistent with the general finding that early caloric supplementation is related to less attention-seeking from adults. Third, there was a significant supplement effect for helps peer: Mother supplementation (MS) was the most important predictor and was weighted positively, $F(1, 52) = 5.92, p < .05$.

To summarize, whereas the within-village findings supported the general interpretation that early caloric supplementation is related to later levels of social responsiveness, affect, and activity, there was a tendency for supplement effects to be specific to the more prosocial, affiliative behaviors in Santo Domingo, the village given the calorie-only supplement, and to intrusive, aggressive behaviors in Conocaste, the village given the protein–calorie supplement. Further, in Santo Domingo, supplementation *after* infancy (i.e., ages 2–4) was a more important predictor of social–emotional functioning at school age than was maternal supplementation during pregnancy or child supplementation during the first 2 years.

Individual test scores. The results of the within-village analyses were generally consistent with the across-village analyses, indicating that caloric supplementation had significant effects on attentional characteristics. Results are summarized in Table 3. In both villages, CS2 was significantly associated with high scores on Persistence on the impossible puzzle, $F(1, 41) = 4.62, p < .05$, for Conocaste and $F(1, 51) = 5.26, p < .05$, for Santo Domingo. In Conocaste, the protein–calorie village, CS2 was also associated with high scores on the Following Directions test, $F(1, 41) = 3.43, p < .10$. In Santo Domingo, the calorie-only village, MS and CS2 were associated with Hidden Figures performance, $F(1, 53) = 8.34, p < .01$, for MS and $F(1, 51) = 7.02, p < .05$, for CS2. However, results also indicated that in the less well-supplemented village, Santo Domingo, caloric supplementation had significant effects on performance on more strictly cognitive measures. In this village, child caloric supplementation from ages 2–4 (CS2) was related to performance on Block Design, $F(1, 51) = 4.51, p < .05$, Bender-Gestalt, $F(1, 51) = 2.92, p < .10$, and Cognitive Composite, $F(1, 51) = 5.44, p < .05$.

Supplementary Analyses

Supplementation effects within sex groups. Multiple regression analyses indicated that supplementation had similar effects on behavior in the two sex groups—affecting peer involvement, activity level, affect, and attention. For both sexes, the variables seeks help, involved in group activity, moderate activity level, happy, anxious, persistence, and following directions were significantly related to one or more of the supplementation measures.[6] There was evidence of two interactions. First, a significant positive association between supplementation and angry affect was obtained for boys only. CS1 was significantly associated with angry affect for boys, $F(1, 67) = 8.22$, $p < .01$, whereas there was no association for girls. Second, supplementation from birth to 2 years had significant positive correlations with a cluster of interrelated peer interaction behaviors for boys, whereas there were not significant positive associations for girls. For boys only, CS1 was associated with high rates of physical aggression, rough and tumble play, and intrudes ($rs = .24$, .23, and .21, respectively, $p < .05$), and MS predicted high rates of assertive behavior ($r = .22$, $p < .05$).

Correlations between height, weight, and behavior. In contrast to the relations between supplementation and behavior, the relations between height, weight, and behavior are inconsistent and difficult to interpret. For boys, height (last age-specific measurements were made at 48 months)[7] was not related to any of the social or emotional outcomes. It was significantly related to the following individual test scores: Persistence ($r = .29$, $p < .05$), Hidden Figures ($r = .25$, $p < .05$), Digit Span ($r = .25$, $p < .05$), Block Design ($r = .22$, $p < .10$), Concept Identification ($r = .30$, $p < .05$), and Cognitive Composite ($r = .31$, $p < .05$). Weight at age 4 correlated with negative to bid from peer ($r = -.23$, $p < .10$) and submissive ($r = -.27$, $p < .05$). It was associated also with Persistence ($r = .22$, $p < .10$). For girls, height was significantly associated with friendly interaction ($r = .34$, $p < .05$), total aggression ($r = -.34$, $p < .05$), submissive ($r = -.25$, $p < .10$), only watches ($r = -.27$, $p < .10$), no activity with environment ($r = -.23$, $p < .10$), low activity level ($r = -.29$, $p < .05$), loses control ($r = -.26$, $p < .10$), and no emotion shown ($r = -.26$, $p < .10$). For individual tests, height correlated with Persistence ($r = -.25$, $p < .10$) and Verbal Inferences ($r = .38$, $p < .01$). Weight was associated with total aggression ($r = -.30$, $p < .05$) and loses control ($r = .37$, $p < .01$) and also with Persistence ($r = -.33$, $p < .05$), Distraction ($r = .30$, $p < .05$), and Verbal Inferences ($r = .25$, $p < .10$).

---

[6]Details of these analyses are available from the first author.

[7]Height and weight measurements were also made at the time of the present data collection when all children were between the ages of 6 and 8. However, these assessments are correlated with age.

DISCUSSION

The results of the present study are by and large supportive of the hypothesis that undernutrition in early life may adversely influence the child's social functioning and emotional development. Children who received better caloric supplementation during the first years of life, including prenatal supplementation, were more socially involved, more interested in the environment, more active, and more capable of affective expression (both positive and negative) than were children who did not receive such supplementation. Further, such relationships were obtained both in a village that had received relatively high levels of caloric supplementation and in a village that had received a supplement that contained only one third the level of calories as the more enriched supplement.

The effects of caloric supplementation on cognitive functioning are less clear. Whereas quality of home living conditions and home stimulation (i.e., SES) was often predictive of performance on cognitive tasks, supplemental caloric intake tended to improve prediction of performance only for those tasks that tapped primarily attentional processes. For example, child caloric supplement intake was significantly related to the ability to persist on an impossible puzzle, to detect hidden figures, and to resist distracting stimuli. In contrast, caloric supplement intake did not predict such abilities as memory in a free-recall task (memory for objects), verbal inferences, or concept identification. Whereas there were significant relationships between supplement measures and two general measures of cognitive development (Cognitive Composite and Bender-Gestalt), as well as between supplement measures and visual representation ability (Block Design), these effects occurred only in the less well-supplemented village.

In interpreting the results of this study, we are concerned with the following issues: (a) If there are significant and consistent effects of early undernutrition on later social–emotional functioning, what are the processes that mediate these effects? (b) If social and emotional characteristics are indeed more vulnerable to nutritional stresses than are cognitive functions, why might this be so? (c) What is the significance of the timing of supplementation? (d) How can we interpret the apparent village differences in the effects of supplementation on behavior?

Processes Mediating Nutrition–Behavior Relationships

We hypothesized that chronic malnutrition would have a progressive and cumulative effect on the child's behavior and in particular on his or her interactive functioning. Research on very young infants indicates that early undernutrition results in attentional failures, apathy, and poor behavior organization and emotional control. The undernourished child is thus at risk for developing disordered interaction patterns in infancy. We suggest that the failure to learn how to interact with persons in the first years of life may inhibit the development of interpersonal skills and thus influence the course of social and emotional development in later childhood.

An elaboration of this formulation has been proposed by Lester (1979) and Rossetti-Ferreira (1978). According to these investigators, early malnutrition stresses the central nervous system of the organism and also depletes energy resources. The child is, therefore, poorly equipped to stimulate the caregiver, respond to the caregiver's social initiations, and develop a normal (i.e., synchronous and reciprocal) pattern of interaction with the caregiver. If the caregiver is also malnourished, the problem is exacerbated because he or she is not likely to have the attentional and motivational capacity to be sensitive to the child's inadequacies and to give the child the additional stimulation and support he or she needs. The result is a cycle of dysfunctional responses leading to unsatisfying caregiver–child interactions, withdrawal on the part of the child, and neglect or rejection on the part of the caregiver. Such a cycle is most likely to develop if the social–cultural milieu is also impoverished; that is, middle-class parents living in a disease-free and emotionally supportive environment would be more likely to make those efforts to be sensitive to the undernourished child that might prevent the establishment of dysfunctional interaction patterns. In contrast, under adverse social–environmental conditions, the caregiver would be less likely to provide the caregiving behaviors necessary for the baby's recovery.

The results of the present study indicate that better nutrition prenatally and during the first 2 years of life is associated with greater social responsiveness, more expression of affect, greater interest in the environment, and higher activity level at school age. These findings may be interpreted as indicating that prenatal and postnatal undernutrition lowers the capacity of the child to develop optimal social interaction patterns in early life. The result over time is a failure to develop normal patterns of social interaction with other persons, peers in particular.

Differential Effects of Chronic Nutritional Stress on Social–Emotional and Cognitive Functions

Performance on tasks that tapped higher level cognitive processes was at best only weakly predicted by the nutritional history variables. There were no relations at all (across villages) between caloric supplementation and scores on verbal inferences, memory for objects, or concept identification. Of the predictors used in our analysis, only SES was a significant predictor of any of these variables. The results raise the question of whether cognitive processes are less vulnerable to the effects of chronic malnutrition than are social–emotional competencies. The evidence from the present study is consistent with previous research. Rutter (1979), reviewing the literature on environmental deprivation and, in particular, maternal deprivation and its effects on cognitive and social–emotional development, noted that disruptions in parent–child relationships that have lasting effects on later social and emotional development in the child have tended to have insignificant effects on later cognitive functioning (cf. Tizard & Hodges, 1978; Tizard & Rees, 1974). Rutter (1979) suggested further that although the development of social competencies appears to be highly dependent on the learning of social interaction skills in the earliest stages of childhood, and thus on optimal caregiver–child interaction, intellectual development depends more on experiencing some minimal level of interaction with the environment. The implication is that this may be achieved under less than ideal interpersonal circumstances.

A second line of support comes from a review of 13 studies (Lloyd-Still, 1976) on the effects of malnutrition on cognitive development. Ten of the studies investigated the intellectual development of children over 5 years of age. Several studies showed no significant IQ deficits in the malnourished group. In all studies, IQ differences between malnourished and control children decreased over time. When malnutrition occurred as a result of neonatal illness but not in the context of poverty or environmental deprivation, there were no lasting effects of malnutrition on intellectual functioning. Lloyd-Still's review suggests that lowered cognitive performance of malnourished children relative to better nourished controls in studies that report such differences may be related to the general socioeconomic deprivation that characterizes the study populations, of which malnutrition is but one component.

It should be noted that our expectation that malnutrition would be related to attentional characteristics of the child was supported. Although the prediction of individual psychological test performance on the basis of nutritional measures was not as strong as the prediction of the social–emotional outcomes, there was generally consistent prediction of scores on those tests that measured the child's ability to attend to directions, to persist on a difficult task, and to attend to the details of a stimulus configuration. These findings are consistent with the previous research.

Timing of Supplementation

One of the questions raised by the within-village analyses is why the relative effectiveness of supplementation at different times differed for different villages. In the large protein–calorie village, the effects of supplementation tended to be greater for the periods before 2 years of age, whereas for the calorie-only village, supplementation after 2 years appeared to be more important. The question of the timing of supplementation is a major one, and one to which INCAP investigators have addressed themselves. For example, Klein, Irwin, Engle, and Yarbrough (1977) reported that in predicting cognitive functioning in preschool, prenatal supplementation was a more important predictor of cognitive development than supplementation from birth to time of measurement (36 months). The earlier findings seem inconsistent with the present results, which indicate that postnatal supplementation is a more important predictor of the child's later social–emotional development than prenatal supplementation.

There are no clear theoretical grounds for predicting the importance of one period of supplementation (or malnutrition) over another. From a neurophysiological point of view, the central nervous system is developing rapidly not only prenatally and shortly after birth (i.e., during the first year) but also well into early childhood. There are several major stages of rapid brain growth: a period of hyperplasia when new brain cells are formed: a period when the rate of increase in new cells decreases and there is a shift to hypertrophy or increase in brain cell size: and a period of pure hypertrophy (Coursin, 1972). Only the first phase, which begins prenatally at about 22 weeks gestational age, terminates before the end of the second year of life. Between the ages of 1 and 2 years when there is the shift to hypertrophy, there is a marked increase in brain weight due to elaboration of dendritic processes, myelinization, and increased input of energy and nutrients to the brain (Epstein, 1978). This period of brain growth continues for several years. What is most important is that it is assumed that the increase in brain weight reflects an increase in neural complexity and in efficiency of neural circuiting. Thus, whereas one might assume that prenatal malnutrition (and/or supplementation) would be of decisive importance for the developing organism because there is an increase in brain cell number during this period, one might also postulate a postnatal critical phase corresponding to the period of increased functional complexity and competence of neural networks. Moreover, there is some evidence that the 2nd through 4th years in particular should be tagged as crucial for later behavioral and cognitive development, since there is evidence that it is during these years that cortical specialization of the brain for language production is established (Lenneberg, 1969). Thus, one might expect that stresses on the brain (e.g., undernutrition) would have an impact on social development if they occurred during these particular years.

One other consideration relevant to the question of the timing of supplementation is a psychometric one. In the present study, during the period from birth to 2 years, the mean level of daily supplemental caloric intake in Santo Domingo, the calorie-only village was less than $\frac{1}{10}$ the magnitude of the mean intake in either of the other villages. Further, the standard deviation, in calories per day, was approximately $\frac{1}{10}$ the standard deviation of the protein–calorie villages. However, by age 2 to 4, the mean level of supplemental caloric intake in Santo Domingo had increased 10-fold, and the standard deviation was also approximately 10 times greater. Means and standard deviations increased at less than half these rates in the other villages. It may have been the case that the relative importance of CS2 (representing supplementation from age 2 to 4) as a predictor of later developmental outcomes in Santo Domingo was due largely to the fact that CS1 had insufficient variance to strongly predict the criteria.

Village Differences in Supplementation Effects

Whereas certain general effects of malnutrition on behavior have been identified (i.e., reduced social responsiveness, interest in the environment, affect, and activity level), the specific manner in which malnutrition affects the child's interpersonal functioning may depend on other factors, specifically, certain aspects of the environmental milieu. As indicated earlier, the village environments were very different. Conocaste was the least well-cared for, had the harshest climate, and had a severe shortage of water. San Juan and Santo Domingo were greener, cooler, and had no water shortage. Differences in the effects of supplementation were noted: In Santo Domingo better supplementation was associated with more prosocial behavior, whereas in Conocaste, supplementation was associated with hostile and intrusive behavior. These findings suggest a distinction between the general effects of improved energy intake on the child's ability to engage with the social and nonsocial environment, and the specific forms of child behavior that develop. The role of social learning, not otherwise discernible, becomes evident. The particular patterns of behavior are shaped by what is available and fostered in a given physical, social, and cultural environment.

A related issue is why supplementation was associated with performance on several of the cognitive measures in the village given the calorie-only supplement but not in the village given the protein–calorie supplement. One hypothesis is that only at the lowest levels of energy intake will differences in calorie supplementation be sufficient to produce differences in cognitive development. This interpretation is consistent with Lloyd-Still's (1976) position that malnutrition may have its strongest effects on mental development when environmental stimulation is also limited.

In conclusion, it appears that the child attempts to adapt to the physiological stress of nutritional deficit by developing behaviors that remove and insulate him or her from the social and nonsocial environment. These behaviors inhibit the later development of appropriate patterns of social interaction. The finding of a special vulnerability of social–emotional functions (as opposed to cognitive functions) to nutritional insult is consistent with research showing long-term effects of interpersonal deprivation on children's social behavior and affect, with less influence on cognitive development.

REFERENCE NOTES

1. World Health Organization. *Energy and protein requirements. Report of a joint FAO/WHO ad hoc expert committee* (Tech. Rep. Series No. 522). Geneva, Switzerland: Author, 1973.
2. Barrett, D. E., Yarrow, M. R., Ziegler, M., & Livingston, R. B. *Effects of early malnutrition on children's social emotional functioning at school-age.* Paper presented at the meeting of the Association for the Care of Children's Health, Toronto, May 1981.

REFERENCES

Barnes, R. H. Dual role of environmental deprivation and malnutrition in retarding intellectual development. *American Journal of Clinical Nutrition, 1976, 29:* 912-917.

Barnes, R. H., Moore, A. U., & Pond, W. G. Behavioral abnormalities in young pigs caused by malnutrition in early life. *Journal of Nutrition,* 1970, *100,* 149-155.

Bartko, J. J. The intraclass correlation coefficient as a measure of reliability. *Psychological Reports,* 1966, *19,* 3-11.

Brazelton, T. B. Tronick, E., Lechtig, A., Lasky, R. E., & Klein, R. E. The behavior of nutritionally deprived Guatemalan infants. *Developmental Medicine and Child Neurology,* 1977, *19,* 364-372.

Brozek, J. Malnutrition and human behavior. In J. Brozek (Ed.), *Behavioral effects of energy and protein deficits.* Bethesda, Md.: Department of Health, Education, and Welfare (National Institutes of Health), 1979.

Chavez, A., & Martinez, C. Consequences of insufficient nutrition on child character and behavior. In D. A. Levitsky (Ed.), *Malnutrition environment and behavior,* Ithaca, N.Y.: Cornell University Press, 1979.

Coursin, D. B. Nutrition and brain development in infants. *Merrill-Palmer Quarterly*, 1972, *18*, 177-202.

Dobbing, J. The influence of early malnutrition on the development of myelination of the brain. *Proceedings of the Royal Society of London*, Series B,, 1964, *159*, 503-509.

Dyson,, S. E., & Jones,, D. G. Undernutrition and the developing nervous system. *Progress in Neurobiology,*, 1976, *7*, 171-196.

Engle,, P. L., Irwin, M., Klein, R. E., Yarbrough, C., & Townsend, J. W. Nutrition and mental development in children. In M. Winick (Ed.), *Nutrition, pre- and postnatal development*. New York: Plenum Press, 1979.

Epstein, H. T. Growth spurts during brain development: Implications for educational policy and practice. In J. S. Chall & A. F. Mirsky (Eds.), *National Society for the Study of Education yearbook*. Chicago: University of Chicago Press, 1978.

Frankova, S. Effect of protein-calories malnutrition on the development of social behavior in the rat. *Developmental Psychobiology*, 1973, *6*, 33-43.

Frankova, S., & Barnes, R. H. Effect of malnutrition in early life on avoidance conditioning and behavior of adult rats. *Journal of Nutrition*, 1968, *96*, 485-493.

Gomez, F., et al. Mortality in second and third degree malnutrition. *Journal of Tropical Pediatrics*, 1956, *2*, 77-83.

Klein, R. E. Malnutrition and human behavior: A backward glance at an ongoing longitudinal study. In D. A. Levitsky (Ed.), *Malnutrition,, environment and behavior*. Ithaca, N.Y.: Cornell University Press, 1979.

Klein, R. E., Irwin, M., Engle, P. L., & Yarbrough, C. Malnutrition and mental development in rural Guatemala. In N. Warren (Ed.), *Studies in cross-cultural psychology*. New York: Academic Press, 1977.

Lechtig, A., Yarbrough,, C., Delgado, H., Habicht, J. P., Martorell, R., & Klein, R. E. Influence of maternal malnutrition on birth weight. *American Journal of Clinical Nutrition*, 1975, *28*, 1223-1233.

Lechtig, A., Yarbrough, C., Delgado, H., Klein, R. E., & Behar, M. Effects of moderate maternal malnutrition on the placenta. *American Journal of Obstetrics and Gynecology*, 1975, *123*, 191-201.

Lenneberg, E. H. On explaining language. *Science*, 1969, *164*, 635-643.

Lester, B. M. Cardiac habituation of the orienting response in infants of varying nutritional status. *Developmental Psychology*, 1975, *11*, 432-442.

Lester, B. M. A synergistic process approach to the study of prenatal malnutrition, *International Journal of Behavioral Development*, 1979, *2*, 377-394.

Livingston, R. B. Calloway, D. H., MacGregor, J. S., Fischer, G. J., & Hastings, A. B. U.S. poverty impact on brain development. In M. A. B. Brazier (Ed.), *Growth and development of the brain*. New York: Raven Press, 1975.

Lloyd-Still,, J. D. Clinical studies on the effects of malnutrition during infancy on subsequent physical and intellectual development. In J. D. Lloyd-Still (Ed.), *Malnutrition and intellectual development*. Littleton, Mass.: Publishing Sciences Group, 1976.

MacLaren, D. S., Yaktin,, U. S., Kanawati, A., Sabbagh, S., & Kadi, Z. The subsequent mental and physical development of rehabilitated marasmic infants. *Journal of Mental Deficiency Research*, 1973, *17*, 273-281.

Martorell, R., Lechtig, A., Yarbrough, C., Delgado, H., & Klein, R. E. Protein-calorie supplementation and postnatal physical growth: A review of findings from developing countries. *Achivos Latinoamericanos de Nutrición,*, 1976, *26*, 116-128.

Monckeberg, F. Effect of early marasmic malnutrition on subsequent physical and psychological development. In N. S. Scrimshaw & J. E. Gordon (Eds.), *Malnutrition, learning and behavior*. Cambridge, Mass.: MIT Press 1968.

Mora, J. O., et al. Nutritional supplementation, early stimulation, and child development. In J. Brozek (Ed.), *Behavioral effects of energy and protein deficits.* Bethesda, Md.: Department of Health, Education, and Welfare (National Institutes of Health), 1979.

Nie, N. H., Hull, C. H., Jenkins, J. G., Steinbrenner, K., & Bent, D. H. *Statistical package for the social sciences* (2nd ed.). New York: McGraw-Hlll, 1975.

Neumann, C. G., Jelliffe, D. B., & Jelliffe, J. Interaction of nutrition and infection. *Clinical Pediatrics,* 1978, *11,* 807-811.

Platt, B. S., & Stewart, R. J. C. Effects of protein calorie deficiency on dogs. Vol. 1. Reproduction, growth and behavior. *Developmental Medicine and Child Neurology,* 1968, *10,* 3-24.

Pollitt, E., & Thomson, C. Protein-calorie malnutrition and behavior: A view from psychology. In R. J. Wurtman & J. J. Wurtman (Eds.), *Nutrition and the brain* (Vol. 2). New York: Basic Books, 1977.

Rossetti-Ferreira, M. C. Malnutrition and mother-infant asynchrony: Slow mental development. *International Journal of Behavioral Development,* 1978, *1,* 207-219.

Rutter, M. Maternal deprivation, 1972-1978: New findings, new concepts, new approaches. *Child Development,* 1979, *50,* 283-305.

Strobel, D. A., & Zimmerman, R. R. Manipulatory responsiveness in protein-malnourished monkeys. *Psychonomic Science,* 1971, *24,* 19-20.

Strobel, D. A., & Zimmerman, R. R. Responsiveness of protein deficient monkeys to manipulative stimuli, *Developmental Psychobiology,* 1972, *5,* 291-296.

Tizard, B., & Hodges, J. The effect of early institutional rearing on the development of eight-year-old children. *Journal of Child Psychology and Psychiatry,* 1978, *19,* 99-118.

Tizard, B., & Rees, J. A comparison of the effects of adoption, restoration to the natural mother, and continued institutionalization on the cognitive development of four-year-old children. *Child Development,* 1974, *45,* 92-99.

Underwood, B. A., et al. Height, weight and skin-fold thickness data collected during a survey of rural and urban populations of West Pakistan. *American Journal of Clinical Nutrition,* 1967, *20,* 694-701.

Yarrow, M. R., Scott, P. M., & Waxler, C. Z. Learning concern for others. *Developmental Psychology,* 1973, *8,* 240-260.

27

Issues in the Psychological Care of Pediatric Oncology Patients

Donald Brunnquell and Marian D. Hall
Children's Health Center, Minneapolis

Rapid advances in medical technology have raised a new set of psychological problems for children who are surviving their struggle with cancer. This paper examines some of the issues arising for pediatric oncology patients and their families, and illustrates through case vignettes the highly complex nature of psychological care of these children.

In a recent report of the American Cancer Society,[1] cancer was cited as the disease causing the greatest number of deaths among children between three and 14 in the United States. Over 6000 new cases were expected during 1980. Of these, some would die quickly, others show periods of remission of varying length, and some live on. The five-year survival rate for all cancers in children under the age of 15, age-adjusted to normal life expectancy, is 39%. For one specific disease that has been widely researched, acute lymphoblastic leukemia, the American Cancer Society expects five-year survival in 50%–75% of the cases obtaining optimum treatment. This is a vast change from the situation in 1960, when five-year survival was extremely rare.

As a result of the enormous changes in mode and efficacy of treatment, a new population with distinct psychological needs is rapidly developing: the pediatric cancer survivor. The rigors of the medical treatment, pat-

Reprinted with permission from the *American Journal of Orthopsychiatry*, 1982, Vol. 52, No. 1, 32–44. Copyright 1982 by the American Orthopsychiatric Association, Inc.

tern of hospitalizations, remissions, and relapses, and the ever-present fear of death all require enormous psychological adjustment on the part of patients and their families. While each case presents a unique picture of strengths and difficulties, certain similarities in problems exhibited by these children are beginning to be seen.

Geist[3] referred to a "developmental lag" between provision of medical and psychological services, with medical technology advancing so rapidly that the adjustments required of the human systems are very difficult. His review of the area of psychological care of chronically ill patients provides an important basis for understanding both the patients' and caregivers' reactions. But due precisely to the stress on *all* involved, provision of optimal care is difficult. The aggression, regression, and depression of patients, as well as the feelings of guilt, helplessness, anger, and depression of the family and the staff must all be taken into account in dealing with pediatric oncology patients.

BROAD ISSUES

While the idiosyncratic nature of the difficulties in each case must be stressed, it seems that almost every aspect of cancer and ensuing treatment has implications in two broad areas: separation/loss and control/competence. While these are interrelated and mutually influencing areas, some conceptual distinctions can be made.

Separation and Loss

Most clear is the area of separation and loss. The life-threatening nature of cancer requires extensive psychological adjustment in every case. Spinetta, Rigler and Karon[10] have shown that children from six to ten years of age, supposedly unaware of the fatal nature of their leukemia, show clear evidence of awareness of the seriousness of their illness compared to chronically but not fatally ill children. The fatally ill children showed greater anxiety, told stories more preoccupied with threats to body integrity, and made more metaphorical references to death.

But what is the implication of death for children? It is, of course, different at different ages; that is, dependent on the developmental status of the child. But whether or not the child conceives of death as an adult might, it clearly implies separation from and loss of loved ones, something unknown and unknowable. When one thinks how traumatic a move of a few blocks can be for a child, the vast impact of something as enormous as death can be seen. One wonders how the child can ever adjust. It is clear why regression to a symbiotic or dependent relationship with a parent is a common problem,[7] and that issues of separation and loss must be dealt with in each case. Thus, separation from pets or objects can be immensely overdetermined events, and the seemingly minor issue of loss or change becomes a major crisis.

Control and Competence

Issues of control and competence are also present in almost every aspect of the illness and treatment. These are especially highlighted in children, since from infancy onward the child's major developmental changes are in the direction of greater control of self, of relationships, and of the surrounding environment. The psychological individuation from parents in the toddler and preschool years, the ever greater mastery of the world and (more importantly) one's own body in the elementary school years, and the formation of one's own sense of identity in adolescence are all issues of self-control that are seriously threatened by cancer. The threat emerges both from the illness and from the treatments. When we ask a seven-year-old to be confined to a single room for weeks, we disrupt his developing sense of control over his environment, which is now perceived as threatening or germ-filled, something to be avoided. Similarly, requiring that a three-year-old not eat but receive nourishment through a tube removes control of a not long established area of self-control. Furthermore, if the child cannot control such minor aspects of his life, how can he "control" the disease that is destroying him. Again, the overdetermined nature of the particular issue should be noted. Through such overdetermination even seemingly minor issues have repercussions for a child's overall psychological functioning. The major loss of control implied by the disease, and the loss of control over the particulars of one's life are extremely important.

Both the disease process and the treatments throw the child's developing sense of competence and self-worth into a state of havoc. In young children, the fantasy of disease as punishment is at times clearly present; in older children, the fantasy is more subtle and complex, but still the question, "Why me, what did I do to deserve this?", is present. Along with such basic doubts, issues such as bodily weakness, need for protection from others by isolation, and falling behind in school work throw the child's sense of competence and self-worth into question. Such massive problems may develop that the child regresses, completely abandoning competence recently achieved at one level for an earlier form of relating to the world, clearly making issues of separation and loss and control even more difficult to deal with. Here again, the "small things" can have great weight, and maintaining competence in even one area, through doing at least one small bit of homework every day, for example, can prevent such massive regression.

SPECIFIC CONCERNS

Mobility, Activity, and Isolation

A frequent problem in many hospital situations is impairment of mobility and activity. This is often so with oncology patients because of testing procedures and intravenous administration of medication, blood, fluids, or nutrients. This is, of course, in addition to any pre- or post-surgical restrictions, bodily weakness, pain, or nausea which can cause disturbance of mobility and activity. Additionally, one must consider self-imposed "psychological" restrictions.

Motor activity is an important form of self-expression for all children, and helps them develop competent relations with the world. Murphy[9] noted that "the time-space dimensionsof freedom" contribute not only to the child's bodily development but "to his inner image of the world" and his place in that world. The effects of hospitalization and interventions in this realm must therefore be carefully weighed. To older children, being in bed constantly, especially in a bed with side-rails, which is associated with babies, has clear regressive implications. In such cases, some means should be provided to help motivate greater, and more age-appropriate, activity. Simply allowing the child to wear his own clothes or to decorate the hospital room, for example, can serve this purpose:

> Jim, a very ill 11-year-old hospitalized briefly for a transfusion and medication, was not only physically weak but could, for the day, use only one arm. He was very irritable and angry through the day, finally insisting that he be brought something to do. He worked intensely on simple snap-together models of cars. While these were below his usual competence level, he accepted them and proved to himself, his parents, and nurses that he was still able to do things that boys of his age "should be able to do." After completing the models, he was able to relax considerably and cooperate more fully with the treatment.

At times, restriction of activity combines with realistic pain, the child's fears, and the parents' reactions to the child's condition to hinder recovery:

> Karl, a six-year-old with Hodgkins Disease, was very resistant to any activity following surgery. He simply lay in bed in a darkened room, with his mother constantly present and meeting all his needs. Before any progress with Karl could be made, his mother's fears of leaving him alone had to be dealt with; finally, when she was out of the room with the psychologist, the nurses were able to engage Karl to sit up, and eventually stand up to go to the bathroom. He did at first experience pain from his incision and was fearful of separation from his mother, but within two days was acting as an independent, curious, though somewhat stiff, six-year-old.

The restriction of contact and activity entered into by this boy and his mother gave clear messages of a more severe situation than existed. If not interrupted by a return to more normal activity, a much more disturbed, symbiotic situation could easily have developed.

Periods of isolation constitute a special problem for many oncology patients. This is due not only to the enforced separation from one's family and peers, but to the restriction of mobility over a long period of time. A small, private hospital room is not a stimulating environment for a child, and in time can contribute significantly to depression and fears. The restlessness that grows as children stay in such a room contributes greatly to irritability and noncooperation. Even brief excursions, if they can be safely arranged, can help alleviate "cabin fever." Since peer relations are so important to latency-age children, isolation has serious effects on their self-esteem as well. This increases the fear of never again having friends relating competently to other aspects of the environment:

> Bill, an 11-year-old boy with leukemia, was in isolation for about a week, with steady decrease in his mood and ease of relationship with staff and parents. When he was finally free to leave his room and to go outside, he said he didn't want to. This refusal continued for a time, and he was finally able to confide his fears that the air pollution would make him sick again. He held to this fear in spite of reassurance that it was unfounded, clearly indicating the broader effect on his own sense of control and competence and fears stirred up by his isolation.

Accommodations to such psychological repercussions of isolation can come in various forms, such as living-in parents or visiting sibs and friends. Two private rooms in our facility, built for isolation and often used for oncology patients, were recently slightly changed by installing a window and intercom phone. In the past, patients in these rooms have often spoken on the phone or exchanged notes and pictures. The change is intended to allow more direct contact and interaction, thereby relieving the effects of isolation to some extent.

Sequelae of Treatment and Issues of Self-Control

Because of the aggressive therapy regimens now in widespread use, side-effects of therapy present adjustment problems as great as the illness itself, and consultation is often sought to deal with the adjustment problems. Perhaps most prominent is difficulty with nausea. This is a frequent side-effect of cancer therapies, but its severity varies greatly from child to child, in part because of psychological factors. A very great difficulty in dealing with nausea is separating out the physiological and psychological aspects. Children very quickly learn that vomiting elicits immediate concern, sympathy, and attention from parents and staff. Such responses are appropriate, but quite often come to be manipulated by patients. As a psychological symptom, nausea is very closely tied to issues of self-control, regulation of relations with others, and one's sense of competence:

> Michael, a 15-year-old with an abdominal tumor, had developed a habit pattern that involved vomiting as a major vehicle for relating to other people. He would lay in his bed curled around an emesis basin. When a nurse or visitor said they were going to leave, he would begin to wretch violently. Similarly, when emotionally difficult topics were raised, he would immediately complain of nausea and begin to throw up, requiring that nurses clean him up. He had a great need for affective physical contact, and used his nausea as a means of achieving that contact. He once told a nurse to come back to talk to him in 20 minutes, because he knew he would throw up then if she didn't come back.

This boy, having lost the more positive, age-appropriate means of relating to other people, used his nausea, in part a real physical side-effect, to manipulate others. This tied in to other regressive aspects of his case (lack of activity, no ongoing peer relations, and no eating), and presented a major problem to the staff. It was handled, after determining no medical cause for frequent vomiting, by removing "rewards" of attention and physical contact, and restoring self-control by requiring the boy to clean himself. The emesis basin was removed (he was allowed to have towels, but had to dispose of them himself, leading to more activity) and staff and family did not stay with him during his vomiting, but returned afterward to engage him in positive interaction.

Eating is frequently an issue, as a result of nausea or of surgical requirements or protocol. It should be noted that eating is the quintessential instance or example of nurturance and self-control, and any change of eating patterns can be expected to raise psychological issues. For children up to age seven or eight, feeding one's self is an issue of considerable importance simply because it is a relatively new learned skill; as children grow up, the complexity of their feeding themselves increases, and they are frequently told to "eat like a big boy (or girl)." When they are suddenly told not to eat and are fed passively through a tube, a great blow to their self-esteem has been struck. When they can again eat, children sometimes are eager and cooperative; at other times, because of specific fears or a more general regression, eating becomes an activity laden with many affective and control issues (they can make me take the medicine, but they can't make me eat!):

> Peter, an eight-year-old who had been transferred from two previous hospitals, was now many miles from his home. He had become increasingly withdrawn and irritable after many procedures and considerable difficulty with IV sites. The last straw came when he was placed on a no-food regimen. After this he became extremely uncooperative and almost totally uncommunicative. He eventually was set to be transferred to yet another, more specialized hospital. He said he did not want to go, but raised little fuss until the morning of his transfer, when he wrapped his legs around the bed and refused to let go until he had something to eat. He said even one bite would be enough. His doctor talked with him and agreed to let him have one pancake; he ate only half and was afterward very cooperative.

This illustrates the importance both of eating and of small accommodations when they are medically feasible. Unusual requests often are made around food, and can have a positive as well as negative meaning:

Bill, mentioned above, had had no food for almost a week. When asked what he would like to eat, he refused the standard fare for a few days. Eventually, on his own time, he said he was ready to eat something, and chose a very salty fish dish that was traditional holiday fare for his family. He surprised his family and staff by not only eating and keeping it down, but by asking for seconds. While some difficulties continued, this signaled his desire to move back to more normal patterns of eating, self-control, and relating to his family.

It should be mentioned here that intake of fluids is also a frequent problem, and has much of the same significance as intake of solid foods. Often issues of food or beverage intake become confrontations with staff or parents, in which the child takes a stand based on not eating as an assertion of self-control. Helping the child formulate his concern around eating, so that the activity implying greater self-control is the act of eating, is a useful strategy in dealing with this problem.

The issue of "cares and procedures" also relates clearly to the treatment and to the child's sense of competence and control. Oncology patients are constantly bombarded by cares and procedures that invade their body—IVs, dressing changes, bone marrows, spinal taps, biopsies, NG tubes, and -oscopies, -ostomies and -ectopies of various sorts. It is little wonder that the issue of bodily control is a major one. Certainly fears play a major role in the child's reaction, ranging from fear of disfigurement to fear of all their blood running out, to fear of bursting like an overfilled balloon. These must be dealt with, but are in general much more obvious than the insidious loss of control and of self-esteem occasioned by constantly "having things done" to them. This can be among the strongest forces pushing children towards aggression, dependence, and depression. In every case it is important to enlist the child's involvement as much as possible. This is especially important in light of the feeling of loss of control over the body occasioned by any disease, but especially by cancer. Even small acts of cooperation can help the child maintain such feelings of control and thus a cooperative and helpful attitude toward the treatments:

Peter, mentioned above, had been on the receiving end of so many procedures and changes, at three different hospitals, that he had no sense of having any role at all in his care, and would complain about and make more difficult the regular nursing tasks. Before long, the nurses here discovered that by explaining what had to be done and letting him do as much as possible, the cares could be accomplished with little struggle. While the cares took longer overall for the nurses to perform, enlisting his help made the cares easier and began to engage Peter in an active way in fighting his disease. He thus helped with changing tape, dressings, and even, under close supervision, IV changes. When his help was engaged, the cares went smoothly; when done "to him," he made them extremely difficult.

Related to the issue of control in the face of numerous procedures are issues of control in the face of sedative or antinausea drugs, with side-effects of drowsiness, loss of awareness, or dyscoordination. These can be very frightening to a child, and are highly overdetermined fears since they reflect in great detail fears of separation, loss, and death. Children's fantasies about the loss of control involved in death often include effects similar to the loss of awareness or control that are side-effects of tranquilizers:

Cindy, an eight-year-old receiving extremely high chemotherapeutic doses, was very fearful of, and resistant to, receiving doses of Thorazine to help reduce nausea and promote relaxation. At other times she had described her feelings while receiving these as "talking to angels" and "thinking she'd gone up to Heaven." She did not want to "have to" go to sleep unless she wanted to, and was extremely resistant to receiving the medication. Rational explanations, while important to give, were not sufficient to allay her fears, which clearly reflected her larger fear of death.

While this girl was able to receive the medication with some working through, the panic that the spectre of loss of control raised is important to note. In her case, where other issues of control were not major problems, she was able, with support, to handle her fears.

Interpersonal Issues

As in all areas of functioning, a child's social relations are often greatly altered by disease, hospitalization, and treatment. Issues of a balance of dependence and independence are extremely difficult, not only for the children but for family and staff. Yet a balance of those forces appropriate to the child's developmental level must be reached if the child is to maintain self-control and feel competent in the world:

> Michael, mentioned above, who had developed a manipula-
> tory pattern with vomiting, had been very adept at using the
> sympathy of staff to maintain such patterns. At another hos-
> pital, the staff and family, feeling great sympathy for a young
> man with a terminal illness, had begun to take care of his
> every need. In an attempt to remove "burdensome cares"
> from him, they removed his active role in caring for himself,
> giving him an indication of their own hopelessness. He re-
> sponded by insisting on more and more cares carried out by
> staff, until he was very regressed. His need for physical af-
> fective contact recalled that of a toddler. By yielding to and
> encouraging natural regressive tendencies (in a situation in
> which he must in part be dependent) rather than encouraging
> his independence or maintenance of the developmental mile-
> stones he had achieved, his regression was massive and re-
> quired great effort to overcome. As he became more regressed,
> he became more fearful of his state and more depressed,
> leading to still further regression.

That cycle of dependence, regression, being frightened by the regression, and becoming more regressed and dependent is present in some
way in almost every case, and must continually be prevented by careful
staff monitoring of their own and family behavior.

One frequent issue in a complex case is the sheer number of professionals involved. Effective team relations is an important issue,[5,8] complicated by growing numbers of disciplines concerned in total care
management. A young child's natural fears of separation from parents
can easily be compounded by many professionals trooping in and out,
no matter how caring those people are. They can heighten fears of being
left at the hospital or taken away from parents. Frequent disturbance
can also prevent a child from forming the close relationship he needs
with a select few staff members in whom he might confide. Every person
who interacts with the child places further emotional demands on him;
demands as simple as polite conversation can prevent a child from working through the more significant issues at his own time or speed. Simple
numbers also increase general confusion and stress level for patients and
their families.

Of special importance is consistency in nursing care. The trust that
develops between a long-term patient and a nurse can be a major source

of strength for the child in times of particular stress. The assignment of the same nurse to a child regularly in the course of a hospital stay and on return visits is extremely valuable. It is, of course, also more taxing on the nurse, since it leads to a closer relationship to the child and family. This can at times be a treatment issue, and therefore must be watched closely by the nurse and her peers; provision of support for nurses dealing frequently with chronically or terminally ill patients must be made.

Another frequent issue in this area is open discussion of the patient's condition. Discussions among staff or between staff and parents often take place in a child's room. While it is important for the child to see doctors and parents communicating and to have a chance to be informed, a number of complications can arise. Children frequently misinterpret technical or jargon terms and invent very frightening explanations for routine events. Due to their not fully developed sense of time, misunderstandings can occur. Events that are in fact difficult, but which with proper verbal preparation can be adequately handled, are raised before the preparation can occur. Parents' reactions to new information can be anxiety-provoking to the children in an unnecessary way. Finally, the child's sense of exclusion from control can be emphasized by a discussion in which the child feels more like an object than a person. All of these issues frequently arise:

> Claude, present during discussion of a minor surgical procedure on his leg between surgeon and mother, interpreted the talk to mean that his leg would be cut off. While not reporting this fear to parents or nurses, he raised considerable fuss whenever any procedure was done, even long after the event that was originally misinterpreted, continuing to fear that his leg would be removed. Eventually he did, in panic, express his fear, and the misunderstanding was dealt with.

This incident points out not only the danger of discussion in front of children, but the need for careful and frequent work with them to help understand what will be done. Fantasy can always be, and often is, worse than the fact. It is therefore of great importance to help children deal with the facts without providing further grist for fantasy. A routine of the doctor talking alone to the patient and alone to the parent, and sharing information appropriately with each can be useful.

It is furthermore important to mention that discussions in the presence of "sleeping" children are a real problem, precisely because both staff and parents feel more free when the child "can't hear." Leaving aside the issue of incorporation of environmental events into sleep and dreams, children waking up or feigning sleep is a frequent occurrence when such discussions are taking place. Parents have reported numerous times that the child "could not have known, since he was asleep when it was discussed." Once again, care and consideration are constantly important in this regard. We do not advocate hiding information from children. One must, however, be aware that giving even "correct" information in confusing ways, or at times when it will be misinterpreted or not open to discussion, is tantamount to giving incorrect information. There is, of course, a need to answer questions that arise, based on the child's cues of his or her readiness for the information. This must be done honestly, to maintain trust and open communication, but in such a way that hope is maintained and adaptation facilitated. Flexibility and attentiveness to the child's need to know are the basic principles.

Interaction with other oncology patients is a frequent issue. While such contact can be extremely valuable, it must be approached and handled with extreme sensitivity. The affected children can offer each other a type of support that no one else can offer, and, as friendships develop, patterns of dealing with the disease and treatments are exchanged, including coping strategies, fears, anxieties, and possible misconceptions. It is not a priori bad for children to discuss their fears with one another, and in fact is often helpful. But all of the factors affecting relationships of children in more usual circumstances are at play here, including rivalry, comparison of condition, and selfish motivation as well as sharing, exploring, and growing. Of course, the physical condition of a child influences his feelings, and a child who is very weak, withdrawn, and depressed may not want to be with other children, or may frighten other children. Difficulty also arises in informing children of the relapse or death of a friend. It is unfair to expect any child to relate always in a positive, uplifting manner; adults must be careful not to expect one child simply to minister to or support another. Their relationship will, of necessity, be more complex. None of these difficulties is reason for discouraging friendship among oncology patients; in fact, the difficulties can become growth experiences. Parents and staff should, however, remember that such difficulties may arise and be prepared to deal with them.

Fear of Disfigurement

This very real fear for all hospitalized children is especially intense among oncology patients because of hair loss, weight loss, and tubes or apparatus necessary on a long-term basis. The fear of hair loss is often the most intense of these, and for many children is the single most difficult adjustment issue. While some children adjust easily, for others "being bald" is frequently used as a tease among children, and actual hair loss can mark a child for extreme teasing. While some children seem to adapt well by taking an almost aggressive approach, as the girl who would pull off her wig and chase people at the slightest indication of their discomfort, others find it extremely painful. It should be noted that hair loss is a subject parents find extremely painful as well, and they must be helped to deal with their own feelings on the subject:

> Gail, an 11-year-old, had been well informed about her leukemia, its prognosis, the necessary therapies, and their effects, with the exception of hair loss. Her parents explained they did not want to burden her with that before it was necessary, and when the time came decided to allow her to read about it rather than tell her directly. On reading of it, she called her mother into the room and angrily demanded an explanation, not of the hair loss, but of why her parents had not told her about it. Afterward, Gail confided that she hated losing her hair, but what made her feel worse was that she had not been told by her parents.

There is no standard or easy way to deal with this subject but professionals must be aware that, for many children and parents, the hair loss can come to be a constant reminder of the patient's condition and separation from other people, and can have much more significance than simply loss of a "nonessential" body part. It comes to represent social acceptability and normal functioning in a way that is difficult for adults, who tend to give up learning about the world through their bodies, to understand.

Fear of disfigurement through weight loss and various medical devices is also frequent. With the advent of the "bionic" man and woman, such devices tap into deep fantasies about power and survival. While all children fantasize about such matters, it is the rare child who wants to be different from others by having those fantasies realized in any way, including IVs, deep-line tubes, nasogastral tubes, colostomies, etc. Fear of being seen by other children while experiencing such procedures frequently causes great anxiety and effects such as school phobia or social withdrawal. This implies that staff and parents should be ready to deal with such reactions and encourage children to express their fears, fantasies, and wishes in play and in words.

Time, Change, and Adjustment

Because of the severity of the disease and the necessity of immediate intensive treatment, many of these children are exposed, especially in a first hospitalization, to many major changes with great rapidity. Some of these have been noted above—isolation, mobility restriction, medical procedures, complications with eating, chemotherapy, disfigurement, large numbers of strangers, a new environment, and the life-threatening nature of the disease itself. Adjustment to each of these factors takes time. For some children almost all of these occur simultaneously, with many additional difficulties such as surgery and anesthesia complicating the picture. The greater the number of changes instituted at a given time, the more difficult the adjustment period generally is. Modulating the pace of such adjustment, when possible, can be extremely important to the child. For example, a child confused and bewildered because of isolation, bone marrow and other procedures, and an exploratory surgery has many adjustments to make; beginning chemotherapy immediately can affect the entire course of treatment in major ways. If adjustment problems are evident, consideration should be given to a brief delay in adding the new procedure, during which time the child receives help in adjusting to what has happened. This may permit a more mature reaction to the therapy, which can significantly affect long-term adjustment:

Amos, a three-year-old with a lymphoma, underwent exploratory surgery shortly after initial hospitalization. Two days after that, a second surgery was performed to make a vein available for IV work. His return to normal mood and activity after the second surgery took much longer, and was in fact not complete before a third surgery, for the same reason as the second, was undertaken. After this third surgery, the boy was extremely depressed, showing almost no activity, withdrawal, general dysphoria, refusal of food, and very little verbalization outside of whining. Long after the physiological effects of the third surgery had disappeared, his depression remained as the only adjustment he could make to the rapid and continued major changes to which he was subject. Such massive disruption so overwhelmed this usually talkative, expressive boy that no adaptive adjustment was possible; instead he withdrew from any interaction with external events or persons.

In every case, one must keep the pace of change and adjustment in mind; the more changes, the greater the adjustments that are necessary, the longer they will generally take. This cumulative impact must be taken into account in the total care picture of the patient. The child's sense of control and competence is affected by the quantity of change as well as the specifics of each individual adjustment.

Family Issues

While this paper has in general been focused on the direct care of children, it is clear that total care involves provision for helping families meet stress. Only then can optimal care be provided to the child. Parental difficulties have been more clearly dealt with than those of the child,[2,4,6] so will be only briefly mentioned here.

First, the necessity of adjustment time for parents should be noted. Hearing a diagnosis of cancer, no matter how gravely ill the child has been, is always a shock, and staff must be careful to allow time for the diagnosis to "sink in." One should not expect parents to hear and to fully comprehend complicated statements or considerations, for the largest part of their energy will be involved in dealing with their own emotional reaction. Parents have reported recalling not a word from long meetings, aside from diagnosis, even though points were frequently repeated. It is therefore important that some person with whom parents can talk after the doctor leaves, a nurse or other frequently available staff person, be present to hear what is said and help parents reconstruct and understand it. It is not uncommon that days will elapse before parents fully grasp the situation and can return to being competent, involved decision-makers and caretakers. Provision of time between learning of the diagnosis and being with the child is also often helpful to permit parents to compose themselves and share their reactions with other adults.

Given the frequency of cancer in our society, previous experiences with cancer can greatly color a parent's reaction to the child's disease. Friends or parents who have died from cancer, whether it be the same form as the child's or not, have set expectations of both the prognosis and quality of life for "cancer patients." These images and expectations can come flooding back to parents in unexpected moments and with great strength, and can considerably complicate the parent's relation to the child:

> The father of a 12-year-old girl recalled that one day, in
> talking to his daughter, he was reminded of his own mother

who had died of cancer six months previously. Some expression that the daughter had used brought back the image of his mother in her final days in the hospital bed. The father reported that, after that flashback, it was very difficult for him not to think that his daughter would die soon, just as his mother had; he could not shake the thought for days, even though rationally he knew the daughter's prognosis was good.

When taking histories from parents, staff should help those who have had experiences with cancer understand that such memories are natural and that it is important to focus on how their child's case is different.

The difficulties and stresses of parental separation, either because of distance or frequent trips between a local hospital and home, should also be dealt with. Many cancer treatment centers draw from a geographically large area, and one parent at home working or taking care of other children creates a separation of the strongest base of support for a parent—the other parent. In such cases, it may be necessary for the staff to help provide extra support, or to encourage and help parents to take time alone together, away from the hospital. This is difficult for many parents, who don't want to "abandon" their sick child. Helping them to understand the necessity of their caring for themselves as well, at least to some degree, is in the best interest of the child.

Closely related to this issue is care of the siblings of cancer patients. Because of the time involvement with the patient, disruption of the normal patterns of relating to sibs often occurs. Over a short time, families can often make such an adjustment with relative ease, but given the chronic nature of the disease, major changes are often present. Anger on the part of siblings and guilt on the part of parents are frequently seen, and should be dealt with by the staff. The tension that can come to exist in the home can be a major complication to successful treatment of cancer. Patients can develop guilt feelings in relation to siblings as well, and signs in the patient or the family of such disturbance are worthy of attention.

CONCLUSION

Each of the specific issues raised above comes up frequently in dealing with a pediatric oncology population. The case examples were chosen to illustrate the specific problem under discussion. But, as is implied in the fact that some cases were used more than once, these problems generally do not occur singly. Rather, a given child is likely to have greater or lesser difficulty in many of the specific problem areas. Further, each of the specific problems has some implication for the two major areas of impact cited early in the paper, the threat of separation and loss, and the diminished sense of control and competence. Each problem and each child weights the impact in these areas differently, but almost any individual incident or situation will involve both to some extent. In other words, the complexity of each case is enormous, and no focus on a single issue is possible. One cannot expect a child or parent to comprehend the larger situation and integrate the impact of the various individual events. That difficult task is left to the staff, mental health consultants especially but other staff as well. Only by realizing the cumulative significance of the seemingly inconsequential specifics can we deal with the broader issues of the total care of the child. This occurs over time and through frequent contact with the patient, the family, and other involved staff members.

Similarly, no quick or easy solutions exist. Regression, depression, loss of self-esteem, and fear of death cannot be magically done away with. They may be resolved by careful work in very specific ways which meet the individual patient's needs: finding a toy model to build, working through fears of sedation, allowing a child to change his own tape, and so on. The complexity of the solution mirrors the complexity of the problem. Only by engaging the entire staff, the entire family, and the patient in his own care can one deal with the issues of control and competence, and of separation and loss. These issues cannot be permanently resolved, for they will certainly arise in new ways with each new situation in which the patient is placed. If a high quality of life is to be maintained for the growing number of long-term cancer patients, such issues must be faced by all involved—patient, family, and staff.

REFERENCES

1. American Cancer Society. (1979). *Cancer Facts and Figures 1980.* American Cancer Society, New York.
2. Bruhn, J. (1977). Effects of chronic illness on the family. *Journal of Family Practice,* 4:1057–1060.
3. Geist, R. (1979). Onset of chronic illness in children and adolescents: Psychotherapeutic and consultative intervention. *American Journal of Orthopsychiatry,* 49:4–23.
4. Gogan, J. et al. (1977). Impact of childhood cancer on siblings. *Health and Societal Work,* 2:42–57.
5. Koocher, G., Sourkes, B. and Keane, W. (1979). Pediatric oncology consultations: A generalizable model for medical settings. *Professional Psychology,* 10:467–474.
6. Lansky, S. et al. (1978). Childhood cancer: Parental discord and divorce. *Pediatrics,* 62:184–188.

7. Lansky, S. and Gendel, M. (1978). Symbiotic regressive patterns in children with malignancies. *Clinical Pediatrics*, 17:133–138.
8. Lansky, S. et al. (1976). A team approach to coping with cancer. In *Cancer: The Behavioral Dimensions*, J. Cullen, B. Fox and R. Isom, eds. New York: Raven Press.
9. Murphy, L. (1956). *Personality in Young Children*, Vol. 1. New York: Basic Books.
10. Spinetta, J., Rigler, D. and Karon, M. (1973). Anxiety in the dying child. *Pediatrics*, 52:841–845.

28

Psychiatric Consultation to the Child With Acute Physical Trauma

Kent Ravenscroft

Children's Hospital National Medical Center, Washington, D.C.

A child or adolescent suffering physical trauma is simultaneously plunged into acute emotional and social crisis. Patient and family go through several predictable phases—shock, denial and panic, protest and regression, oppositionalism, mourning, and readjustment. This paper outlines principles for the effective medical, surgical, and ward team management of the traumatized pediatric patient and family, and offers clinical illustrations of their application.

The psychological management of the acute trauma patient closely follows the basic principles discovered by military psychiatry,[12–15,18,26] which emphasize primary prevention through maintenance of high group morale and cohesiveness; early intervention at the scene of trauma, during transport and emergency hospitalization; and, finally, intensive psychological management close to the front with early return to one's company for support and reinforcement of recovery. When the victims of trauma are children and adolescents, certain age-appropriate modifications of this general approach provide the basis for effective surgical management of children in their family group. The aim is the same: successful hospitalization, rehabilitation, and return to home, friends, and community.[11,23,29]

In addition, developmental and maturational factors must be taken into account for child and adolescent trauma victims, both in terms of

---

Reprinted with permission from the *American Journal of Orthopsychiatry*, 1982, Vol. 52, No. 2, 298–307. Copyright 1982 by the American Orthopsychiatric Association, Inc.

how they react to the physical and emotional stresses, and how these reactions are managed by staff and family. Somatopsychic aspects of the injury interact with psychosomatic aspects of the stress reaction. And both interact with the emergent psychosocial processes unfolding between child and family, and within the medical milieu.

Consultation to the traumatized child or adolescent, the family, and the milieu is based on understanding of all these factors, as well as their predictable sequence of appearance. This paper will focus on the interplay of these factors as well as the expectable milieu processes unfolding on the ward. Anticipatory preparation utilizing the principles of signal or anticipatory anxiety is stressed throughout the paper. In addition, since an effective consultant is also performing liaison support and teaching functions, the educational priorities for maximizing surgical implementation of mental health principles on the front line are emphasized. The consultant cannot be present for all emergency cases and often is called in late in such cases around behavioral complications. Since training in surgical consultation liaison work is important for residents and child fellows, as well as other disciplines, this paper also provides a conceptual basis for training in surgical consultation liaison work around emergency hospitalizations.

REACTIONS TO INJURY AND THE EMERGENCY ROOM

The initial reaction of an injured child or adolescent is a function of several factors: direct or indirect CNS involvement (degree of encephalopathy and consciousness), the severity and nature of the trauma (the degree to which this is perceived and experienced, including pain), the child's age and personality (degree of maturity), and the reaction and involvement of parents or surrogates (degree of aid and support versus parental injury and panic). Initial management techniques employed by paramedical and medical personnel, at the scene of the accident, during transport, and in the emergency room are highly important.

While lifesaving procedures take priority, it is crucial for staff to support parents, siblings, or other persons accompanying the conscious child throughout all procedures to reduce psychological trauma and to insure maximum patient cooperation. For the young child experiencing multiple trauma, separation from a loved one can be more traumatic than the pain and injuries themselves. Agitation of a frightened child may result in musculoskeletal, respiratory, and blood pressure problems. A member of the care team should talk frequently with the parents to reduce their panic, orient them, and assist them in calming and diverting the child. If parents are too upset initially to attend certain emergency procedures, a nurse or paramedic should be substituted specifically for this function while the parents are kept appropriately informed. The principle of using a family member to support the child is also effective with older children and adolescents, in conjunction with appealing to their greater maturity to maintain cooperation and self-control.

Every significant injury affects brain functioning to some degree, ranging from direct head trauma to systemic pathophysiologic effects.[1,8] This can lead to gross loss of consciousness, or more subtle alterations of behavior, memory, perception, judgment and orientation.[30] Such traumatic, toxic, and metabolic effects interact with predictable psychophysiologic effects of the acute psychological stress reaction and must be considered in any differential diagnosis and management plan.[4] To illustrate:

> Rodney, seven years old, sustained a 50% deep second and third-degree burn to his anterior neck, chest, abdomen and thighs secondary to flammable pajamas. On the third night of his hospitalization, he was noted to be only slightly febrile but obviously delirious, claiming to see rats coming down the curtain and cockroaches on his bed. He was felt to have the beginning of a burn encephalopathy.

> Michael, age nine, with a 20% deep second-degree facial and anterior neck and upper trunk burn, became convinced on the seventh day that the physical therapist who was fitting a cervical traction collar was trying to hang him, and that the nurse bathing him was attempting to drown him. Prior to admission he had a history of being fearful and slightly suspicious, and felt very guilty about the burn.

PHASES OF ACUTE STRESS REACTION

Characteristically, there are several phases to an acute psychological stress reaction. Usually at the scene of the accident and in the emergency room the patient is initially stunned or in a state of emotional *shock*. This rapidly gives way to a reaction of *denial*, characterized by avoidance of physical manifestations of the injury and general withdrawal. Breakthroughs of fearfulness, tearfulness, and *panic* occur episodically, usually precipitated by pain, unexplained medical procedures, or separation from parents or other supportive figures.

Younger children can deny gross injury and even pain, avoiding looking at obvious mutilated or missing parts of themselves, remaining oblivious or seemingly "hypnotized" by their parents. Older children or adolescents can react to a partial awareness of their injuries by denying underlying fear. Instead, they can become agitated, defiant, and "fearless." For example,

> Chucky, a 16-year-old boy with a severe 10,000-volt electrical burn to arm and trunk and a badly fractured pelvis, sustained in his fall from the top of a utility pole, threatened to "get up and walk out of the emergency room because nothing is wrong, and I can take care of it better at home."

While psychological defenses of denial and avoidance must be respected, especially at first, the patient's impulse to take "fearless" unrealistic action must obviously be resisted with firm verbal limits and even physical restraint—while constantly leaving open the option to maintain self-control. Rather than stirring up the adolescents' underlying fears about their injuries, one should compliment their "strength to survive and endure" and persuade them that they can show "greater strength" by controlling themselves and assisting in treatment. To this end, constant supportive talk may be required for an action-oriented adolescent. Additionally, immediate back-up psychiatric consultation should be available in the earliest phases of severe pediatric trauma care. Psychotropic drugs are useful in specific clinical circumstances if compatible with the patient's medical-surgical status.

It is important to inform all children over one year of age about any impending procedure or transport to another part of the hospital, so they can anticipate the event and prepare themselves. The sudden loss of control over their own bodies through traumatic injury and submission to medical-surgical procedures is frightening, as is the radical alteration of their social situation through forced dependency on their parents and strange new hospital personnel. Beyond this, the psychophysiologic stress of this trauma has threatened the child's psychological control; sound surgical management, therefore, avoids adding the further psychological trauma of sudden unexpected introduction of any but the most critical procedures. If the child is conscious and there is time, every effort must be made to talk with the child, asking what happened, telling what you plan to do and why, and showing the child what you are going to do it with and where. Since injured children and adolescents are confused, upset, and misperceive their surroundings, care should be taken about what surgical and nursing staff say within earshot of the patient, as well as the family. Since parents are the main psychological buffers, mediators, and interpreters for their child, they, too, need time to prepare themselves before preparing their child. Only if time does not permit or the child will not settle down should the surgeon resort to significant restraint and sedation, since a psychological price will be paid for this during recovery and return home. Explain the need for restraint and sedation to the child and parents in advance.

MANAGING THE FAMILY

Implicit in the care of the injured child is a strategy for management of the whole family, since the trauma to the child is traumatic to the entire family.[20] If a car accident or fire has been the cause, often more than one member of the family is involved, and the family may already be dealing with death or injury to other members. It is essential, then, in the immediate situation to establish rapport with the family and provide them with support and information—setting the stage for hospitalization and rehabilitation. How the family reacts to the trauma, the emergency room, and the initial staff encounter will have a major effect on how the patient reacts to the injury and subsequent hospitalization.

For parents and other siblings, as well as for the injured child, the emergency room is a confusing, frightening place that induces feelings of helplessness and ineffectiveness at the very time their child needs them the most. Some parents withdraw; others become disorganized; most need support to come into the treatment arena. The presence of a parent is a major strength unless the parent is visibly and uncontrollably anxious and agitated. Some parents become angry, intrusive, and demanding. They may insist on unnecessarily fast care, demand details, criticize the staff, and inadvertently interfere with staff morale and function. These defensive maneuvers spring from similar anxiety and guilt, and require special staff intervention to help parents mobilize their own resources on behalf of the child and staff.

REACTION TO THE HOSPITAL SETTING

After completion of the first phase of emergency care the injured child may be moved into the intensive care unit (ICU), the burn unit, or a surgical ward. Procedures ranging from X-ray and minor surgery to a major emergency operation may have intervened. In addition to the toxic metabolic effects of the burn or injury are added the effects of anesthesia, surgery, drugs, and the stress of the entire experience.[7,10,18,22] Bodily and social routines and setting are radically altered. A major antidote to this chaotic new world, where a young child's parents are no longer in charge and protecting the child from pain and fright, is an arrangement that allows parental sleeping-in, coupled with a generous and flexible visiting policy for family, older siblings, and friends to reduce disorientation, separation anxiety, and loneliness.[6,27]

For the child and parents, the culture shock of entering an intensive care unit is exceeded only by the emergency room. Therefore, in addition to the preparation for transfer which is effected by the physician in the emergency room, it is important that the ICU (or ward) nursing staff orient the injured child and the parent appropriately. Early designation of a primary nurse for the child is particularly effective in reducing the impersonality of care in the ICU setting through nursing continuity.

Because the ICU or burn unit operates three shifts 24 hours per day, with lights on, monitors and machines going, and patient crises occurring, the environment is not only frightening and confusing, but physiologically and psychologically disorganizing. Although the initial phases of shock and denial may wear off, there is often a transient return of these states with each major transfer, especially into the ICU or burn unit. The cumulative impact after several days may be an "ICU or burn unit psychosis," similar to postsurgical psychosis,[3,28] manifested by disorientation and hallucinations with an organic flavor. Unreasonableness, rambling speech, and agitation may occur. Often representing toxic, metabolic, febrile, and drug effects as well as psychological stress, this may also have contributions from "sleep and sensory deprivation."[21,31] Transfer, if possible, to a location permitting sleep and a more routine day-night environment is indicated. During the necessary time in the ICU or burn unit, the psychosis can be managed by the use of frequent, regular brief parental and nursing visits, the use of screens to provide privacy from other patients, and normal music and voice via radio or television played quietly. Permitting the child to have personal toys and familiar clothing often helps. Sleep medication such as paraldehyde, chloral hydrate, or flurazepam hydrochloride can help regularize the sleep cycle if compatible with medical-surgical regimen and management. Regular contact, through continuity of nursing and parental care, are the most important elements. Children are so prone to personalize overheard comments, distort and fantasize about experiences, and enter into guilty magical thinking that frequent verbal ventilation and realistic reassurance are essential. Since respirators, monitors, and "tubes" can pose a frightening and isolating barrier to parent-child contact, the staff must reassure the family and help them reach the child through this forbidding maze of machinery.

Episodic nightmares and panic attacks may occur in the ICU or other special care units during the first few days. Similar to a "traumatic war neurosis,"[2,9] these periodic breakthroughs of panic represent emergence into dreams or consciousness of the "psychologically undigested" suppressed memories of the traumatic accident and emergency procedures experienced by the semiconscious child or adolescent:

> Debbie, age eight, who sustained a closed cerebral concussion with loss of consciousness for two weeks, awakened with obvious posttraumatic encephalopathy, aphasias, and immaturity which cleared slowly over several weeks. However, in listening to her, when psychiatric consultation was requested because of continuing "bizarre behavior," it became evident that a certain proportion of her "incoherent" mumblings, strange phrases, and repeated pantomimes of "you dead, it's coming closer, blood, test you, face mush, voices" represented frightening memories of dimly perceived actual experiences while she was semicomatose, and people talked around her and performed procedures thinking she was unconscious.

> Peter, age 18, broke both thighs in a car accident in which his girlfriend was killed. He remained awake but stuporous and unresponsive, except for repeated fleeting moments of painful moaning which always culminated in a shriek and burying his face. He was given Demerol for this pain, and the staff soothed him, and helped him to sleep. He was thought to have "fat emboli" and encephalopathy. When this behavior didn't stop, and he remained "withdrawn" despite a normal neurological on the eighth day, a psychiatric consultation revealed he was avoiding the images of his girlfriend dying 15 feet away while he was lying there unable to help her. The images would recur in his mind's eye, causing so much pain he would moan and shriek, banishing it from his consciousness. Simple support and encouragement allowed him to tolerate it enough during one session that he began to cry and mourn. His recovery was uneventful thereafter with supportive parental and nursing work.

Traumatic reactions in youngsters are managed by first orienting the children and getting their attention, letting them talk out their feelings while reality-testing the memories, and reassuring them—all the time providing firm verbal and behavioral limits so that they know who *you* are and recognize that you will help them regain *their* control. At times, sparing use of tranquilizers may be helpful to minimize anxiety without suppressing a child emotionally, since it is essential the child "work through" the frightening experiences, and not avoid them.[16]

SUBSEQUENT PHASES OF REACTION

As the shock, denial, and novelty wear off during the first few days of hospitalization, patients usually enter the phase of *protest*, as they start to regain some defenses and composure. At the same time, their injuries, mutilation, missing parts, altered appearance, and lack of physical capacity begin to penetrate their denial and avoidance.[5,17,25] Because this awareness is so painful psychologically, and the feelings of anxiety, guilt, fear, and rage so powerful, there is a marked increase in the tendency to blame and accuse parents and staff, paint them with distorted or imagined motives, and distort what they say or do. This use of the defense mechanisms of projection and displacement, called scapegoating, can result in mounting staff frustration and impatience, if not outright anger, since they seem to receive nothing but harrassment for all their efforts. With difficult patients posing challenging management problems, including physical and sexual threats, staff can become demoralized and disorganized in their treatment efforts. Nobody wants to be assigned such a patient. At times, patient transfer to another ward or hospital may be contemplated by staff for emotional reasons, though covered by surgical or nursing language. Although sufficiently serious psychosocial management problems are valid reasons for transfer, if beyond the management capacity of staff, it is important that this be a conscious and rational decision, rather than an overreaction to what may be a transient adjustment problem of the staff.

Since the child or adolescent has been stripped of all independence, autonomy, and control, and is forced to comply with all routines and submit to painful procedures, this phase of protest, testing, and scapegoating also ushers in a wave of *negativism* and *stubbornness*. The young patients will attempt to bargain about the true extent of their injuries, and will attempt to manipulate and rebel against necessary restraints, procedures, and routines:

Jimmie, a 16-year-old who grabbed the high-tension line on top of an electrified train, sustained exit burns of both feet, requiring below-the-knee amputations bilaterally. Depressed, sullen, and oppositional, he was awaiting a delayed stump revision one afternoon, thus having been restricted from consuming any solid food since the previous midnight. An unsuspecting student nurse happened by, and hearing him moaning thought he was back from his 11 a.m. procedure. When she entered the room, he slyly got her to give him a chocolate bar, aborting his surgery for that day. During this same period, he was refusing physical therapy, never wearing his splints, and not eating, claiming the hospital food was "crap." Five weeks earlier the food had been "fantastic."

This is, in part, a normal and healthy phase of recovery. It represents the first awkward return of self-assertion and independence, but may be frustrating and irritating for staff. Treatment procedures must be carried out, of course, but within these firm realities and limits the staff must respect this new, if misguided, energy of the patient and help to channel it into constructive action while allowing the patient to ventilate opposition and frustration verbally. Respectful firmness, careful listening, and reality-testing can help.

Beyond this, though, it is essential that every possible way be found to give the patient realistic control and choices within the necessary routines and procedures. This requires ingenuity on the part of all members of the care team. Other creative outlets for self-assertion, self-control, and activity may be found through Child Life or Activities Programs, which can drain off some of the excess frustration and energy in this phase of recovery.

Often this phase blends into the final stage of a child's acute reaction to trauma and hospitalization. Anger and rebellion are a protest against the injustice of the injury and cover the grief and sadness of the slowly dawning recognition of how seriously hurt, mutilated, and limited the patient has become. The anger and protest are defenses against *mourning* what has been lost physically and functionally.[19] Patients may break down, lose their nerve and resolve, and become moody or withdrawn at times. The work of mourning takes energy, is painful, and is done in brief repeated stages,[24] as illustrated by the case of Peter, mentioned earlier. While treatment and rehabilitation must go on, a sensitive mixture of support and firmness, along with respect for the patient's limitations and need for separateness, is required to facilitate mourning.

PARENT AND STAFF REACTIONS

Parents and staff go through a mutual grieving process with the patient, but there is a hazard of getting out of phase. They can either lag behind or try to push the patient ahead too fast. They can collude with a patient stuck in one of these phases. When an injury is severe, such as a burn in which an extremity is lost or there is grotesque loss of facial and body skin, parents and even staff hesitate to look or tend to intellectualize their reactions. Often, they overlook the patient's own hesitation; psychologically, no one wants to look *with* the patient. At other times, parents and staff may confront the patient prematurely and impatiently, expecting the patient to face things too rapidly. Timing, sensitivity, and mutuality are crucial in an approach that minimizes psychological scarring, and sets the stage for the subacute and chronic phases of hospitalization. Judgments must be made about when to respect the patient's defenses and pace, and when to initiate psychological work with a patient who will not make use of strengths.

In each setting—ICU, burn unit, or ward—the patient and family settle in, adjust, and form trusting relationships with staff, some of them very deep and intense because of the seriousness and duration of the situation. Therefore, any transfer to another setting involves a major loss, crisis of confidence, and anxiety about the future. The parents and child must be given ample warning and rationale, and even participate in a planning conference, to minimize the inevitable behavioral regression, and to set in motion the process of separation while preparing for the challenges of a new setting. Staff members also go through a mutual process because of their deep attachments, and need time to work it through with parents and child while orienting the new staff receiving the child to assure continuity of care. Similarly, any major procedures, such as reconstructive surgery or skin grafting, represent intercurrent crises requiring anticipatory preparation and post-procedure care.

LONG-TERM IMPLICATIONS

During the long days of rehabilitation, punctuated periodically by major procedures, patient, staff, and family work along, settling into a routine. Depending on the psychological maturity and strength of the patient and the resources and resilience of the family, routine surgical nursing may be sufficient. But this should be supplemented where possible by medical social work for the parents, and primary nursing or counseling for the seriously damaged long-term patient. Psychiatric consultation and even supportive therapy for the patient, with careful regular collaboration with the whole team, would be the ideal. This kind of integrated communication and monitoring minimizes the risk of patient, family, or staff getting seriously out of phase, permits anticipatory planning, and facilitates continuous total care planning as the patient moves from phase to phase, procedure to procedure, ward to ward.

From a developmental point of view, each patient age-group should have a special approach. For preschoolers, parent involvement and play activities are important; for school-age patients, peer involvement and school activities must be added, as well as provisions for siblings and friends to visit; for adolescents, with their emerging sexuality, independence, rebelliousness, and propensity for acting out, special adolescent ward groups and activities, with appropriate supervision, are essential additional ingredients.

Because of the prolonged, intense, and special care all patients get in the hospital, with sensitive acceptance of their appearance and problems, a deep institutional dependency develops within this special protected community. As a result, visits home, trips outside the hospital, and discharge to outpatient status represent major turning points. Anticipatory planning becomes crucial; even so, major breakdowns in follow-up care can occur. The patient and family must be prepared for and supported through this critical movement back into home and community, lest the painful progress of physical and psychological rehabilitation be set back or lost. Despite the initial positive anticipation of going home, seeing other family members, being in familiar surroundings, and venturing out into the community, the patient and family find themselves confronted suddenly with having to take on many of the tasks carried out by staff, while experiencing the loss of staff support on an hour-by-hour basis. Moreover, the patient is powerfully reminded, through memories and hard realities, of what has been lost; the reactions of friends and strangers reinforce this new self-understanding: physically and socially, the patient has become a different person, a person with handicaps.

> Jimmie, the previously mentioned 16-year-old double-amputee, steadfastly denied for weeks any worries, fears, or sadness about his missing feet, saying he'd "walk out of here, just watch." After much work by nursing staff, with psychiatric assistance and social work support for mother, he was beginning preparations for the first pass home. He was also clearly nowhere near walking. He had not even been fitted for his prostheses yet. Finally, he broke down and cried, wanting his

legs back, wondering "where are they now, oh, God will give me new ones. I feel so worthless, so helpless, they'll all make fun of me." Shortly afterward, he reiterated his deep desire to go home, but stopped eating again, ceased his resumed OT and PT so essential to his rehabilitation, and began to talk of "lighting his curtains on fire, what will you nurses and the kids do." This behavior revealed his fear of going home, his desperate, provocative (and secretly suicidal) state. His pass was delayed temporarily to work these issues through, permitting further mourning and better self-control. His mother became convinced of his ambivalence at this point, and began to relate to his hard, sad task much more realistically, which helped him immensely.

The impact of these realities compound the continuing, slow, painful outpatient rehabilitation, and usually lead to depression, withdrawal, or acting out. The parents and family experience a similar reaction and yet must also support the patient through this period. Therefore, the most painstaking attention must be paid to arranging outpatient follow-up appointments, training for home rehabilitation, tutoring and special school placement, home equipment, visiting nursing, financial and social support, with a continuing team approach to total patient and family care. The most risky period for continuity of care is at the time of discharge, although there will be episodic crises throughout the long road to complete outpatient rehabilitation.

CONCLUSION

Children or adolescents suffering physical trauma are plunged simultaneously into acute emotional and social crisis as they and their families react to the emergency. From the scene of the accident, through the emergency room and acute hospitalization, to discharge, this type of crisis has several predictable phases (shock, denial and panic, protest and regression, oppositionalism, mourning, and readjustment). Somatopsychic aspects of the injury interact with the psychosomatic aspects of the acute stress reaction. Both interact with the emergent psychosocial processes unfolding in child and family, and within the medical milieu. As a result, each phase of acute pediatric hospitalization has expectable neuropsychiatric aspects leading to important surgical management approaches. Effective medical, surgical, and ward team management of the traumatized pediatric patient and family is based on consistent application of these principles by the entire pediatric surgical team. Psychiatric consultation liaison work in surgery, where a majority of cases are traumatic or emergent, is dependent on application of these principles in work with staff, patients, and family.

REFERENCES

1. Auerbach, A. et al. (1960). The psychophysiologic sequelae of head injuries. *American Journal of Psychiatry*, 117:499.
2. Baker, S. (1975). Traumatic war neurosis. In *Comprehensive Textbook of Psychiatry*, A. Freedman, H. Kaplan and B. Sadock, eds. Baltimore: Williams and Wilkins.
3. Blacher, R. (1972). The hidden psychosis of open heart surgery. *Journal of the American Medical Association*, 22:305.
4. Brosin, H. (1959). Psychiatric conditions following head inury. In *The American Handbook of Psychiatry*, S. Arieti, ed. New York: Basic Books.
5. Cath, S., Glud, E. and Blane, H. (1957). The role of the body-image in psychotherapy with the physically handicapped. *Psychoanalytic Review*, 14:34.
6. *Clinical Proceedings*. (1976). The hospital experience. 32:11.
7. Eliel, L., Pearson, O. and Rawson, R. (1950). Postoperative potassium deficit and metabolic alkalosis. *New England Journal of Medicine*, 243:471–518.
8. Engel, G. and Romano, J. (1959). A syndrome of cerebral insufficiency. *Journal of Chronic Diseases*, 9:260.
9. Fetterman, J. (1935). The neuroses associated with trauma. *Industrial Medicine*, 4:4.
10. Fox, H., Rizzo, N. and Gifferd, S. (1954). Psychological observations of patients undergoing mitral surgery. *Psychosomatic Medicine*, 16:186.
11. Galdston, R. (1972). Burning and healing of children. *Psychiatry*, 35:57–66.
12. Glass, A. (1952). Psychological considerations in the rehabilitation of battle casualties. Symposium on Treatment of Trauma in the Armed Forces. Washington, D.C.: Walter Reed Army Medical Center.
13. Glass, A. (1953). Preventive psychiatry in the combat zone. *United States Air Force Medical Journal*, 4:683.
14. Glass, A. (1955). Principles of combat psychiatry. *Military Medicine*, 117:27.
15. Golden, J. (1966). Psychiatric management of acute trauma. In *The Early Management of Acute Trauma*, A. Nahum, ed. St. Louis: C. V. Mosby.
16. Hackett, T. and Weisman, A. (1960). Psychiatric management of operative syndromes. II: Psychodynamics factors in formulation and management. *Psychosomatic Medicine*, 22:356.
17. Hamburg, D. et al. (1953). Clinical importance of emotional problems in the care of patients with burns. *New England Journal of Medicine*, 248:355.
18. Janis, I. (1958). *Psychological Stress*. New York: John Wiley.
19. Kubler-Ross, E. (1969). *On Death and Dying*. New York: Macmillan.
20. Langsley, D. and Kaplan, A. (1968). *The Treatment of Families in Crisis*. New York: Grune and Stratton.
21. Leiderman, H. et al. (1959). Sensory deprivation: Clinical aspects. *Archives of Internal Medicine*, 101:389.
22. Le Femine, A. et al. (1957). The adrenocortical response in surgical patients. *Annals of Surgery*, 146:26.

23. Lewis, M. and Lewis, D. (1973). Pediatric management of psychologic crises. *Current Problems of Pediatrics*, 3(12):3–47.

24. Lindemann, E. (1945–45). Symptomatology and management of acute grief. *American Journal of Psychiatry*, 101:141–148.

25. Long, R. and Cope, O. (1961). Emotional problems of burned children. *New England Journal of Medicine*, 264:1131.

26. McLaughlin, H. (1959). Emotional response to injury. In *Trauma*, H. McLaughlin, ed. Philadelphia: W. B. Saunders.

27. Mason, E. (1965). The hospitalized child: His emotional needs. *New England Journal of Medicine*, 272:406–414.

28. Miller, H. (1939). Acute psychoses following surgical procedures. *British Medical Journal*, 1:558.

29. Morrison, G. (ed.) (1975). Emergencies in child psychiatry: Emotional crises of children. *Youth and Their Families*, Springfield, IL: Charles C Thomas.

30. Ruesch, J. and Bowman, K. (1945). Prolonged post-traumatic syndrome following head injury. *American Journal of Psychiatry*, 102:145.

31. Wexler, D. et al. (1958). Sensory deprivation: A technique for studying psychiatric aspects of stress. *Archives of Neurology and Psychiatry*, 79:225.

PART VI: CLINICAL ISSUES

29

Somnambulism in Childhood—Prevalence, Course and Behavioral Correlations

Gunnar Klackenberg

Clinic for the Study of Development and Health in Children, Karolinska Hospital, Stockholm, Sweden

The occurrence and course of somnambulism and its correlations with behavioral variables have been investigated annually from 6 to 16 years of age in a sample recruited by random means. The prevalence was highest at 11–12 years. No sex difference was found. Apart from sporadic occurrences, the longitudinal data reveal a group of children for whom somnambulism is rather persistent. But even in this group the somnambulism is usually unrelated to other sleep disturbances (apart from "bad" dreams), deviant behavior or known environmental factors. These children have more inhibited aggression and a more developed mental defense against anxiety as determined by Rorschach tests. At school they appear to be more popular than other children.

Research in recent decades from sleep laboratories has assigned somnambulism to the group of sleep disturbances known as "disorders of arousal" (1). The group also includes genuine night terror (pavor nocturnus) and nocturnal enuresis.

Somnambulism's typical charcateristics are considered to be an abrupt onset early in the night, veiled consciousness, coordinated movements,

Reprinted with permission from *Acta Paediatrica Scandinavica*, 1982, Vol. 71, 495–499.

The author wishes to express his gratitude to the Rädda Barnen Research Foundation for economic support of this study.

fairly brief duration, spontaneous cessation and poor recall of the night's events on waking up next morning (1, 2, 3). Episodes are elicited in conjunction with special activity in stages 3–4 of NREM sleep (1, 2, 3, 4). The view that sleepwalking and night terror represent an acting-out of dreams has not found support in laboratory studies but the results are not clear-cut concerning the initiation of attacks (1, 5). Periods of REM sleep in somnambulists do not differ from those in other children from the same age group (2, 4, 6).

Somnambulism has been studied as a rule in selected groups and the disorder's prevalence has accordingly been reported very differently, ranging from 1 to 15% (2, 6). There are certain indications that children are afflicted more commonly than adults and boys perhaps more than girls (2, 3). The few studies which deal with somnambulism's relationship with psychological factors have yielded widely differing results, depending on whether the subjects were adults or children. Among adults sleepwalking is associated with psychopathology to a substantial extent (7), whereas the children do not belong to any particular personality type or other behavioral class (8). The commotion that child somnambulism is liable to generate mostly comes from the child's surroundings, e.g., questioning parents. The child feels perfectly healthy. Somnambulism has been known to give rise to accidents but this seems to be very rare.

This study is concerned with the prevalence of somnambulism in a sample recruited by random from a child population, the course over a period of years (from 6 to 16) and any correlations with behavioral variables. No such prospective longitudinal study could be found in the literature.

MATERIAL AND METHODS

The data come from the prospective longitudinal Solna study, which has been presented earlier (9).

The numerous questions concerning behavior which the parents, usually the mother, had to answer at each annual study between the ages of 6 and 16 included one on somnambulism: Has he/she ever sleep-walked? The alternative replies were graded: never, seldom (1–2 times/year), sometimes (3–6 times/year), often (7–12 times/year) and frequently (more than 12 times/year). The occurrence of "bad" dreams was also recorded. The behavioral variables, usually on 5-point scales, that have been used to compare the somnambulists and other children are described in earlier publications (10).

The structured assessments obtained from teachers in grade 5 (at 12 years) comprised all the pupils in the relevant child's class without the teacher knowing which child/children belonged to the growth study. The sociometric studies in grades 3, 4 and 5 likewise cover a great many classes where the children ranked each other without knowing who were the actual subjects.

The Rorschach interpretations have been made by a specialist in this test, without access to any data except age and sex. The tests were made at the age of 10.

RESULTS

Prevalence

Between 6 and 16 years of age the symptom was reported for 31 girls and 44 boys. The annual frequency varies from once in a particular year to at least once a month. The prevalence of somnambulism of varying frequency is highest at 11–12 years (16.7% at 12 years, see Fig. 1). At this age, however, only 2.5% had a frequency of at least once a month. There are no significant differences between boys and girls.

Of the 75 children for whom somnambulism was noted at least once between 6 and 16 years of age, 40 had the symptom only very occasionally—either once only (26 children) or two or three times at intervals of several years (14 children). When testing persistence and covariation with behavior, these children were excluded lest they conceal a profile for the remaining 35 children. The sleepwalking group thus consists of children graded for this symptom as "sometimes" or "often."

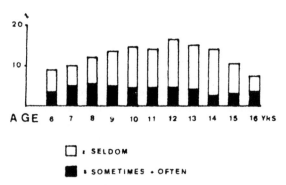

Fig. 1. Prevalence of somnambulism.

Persistence

Somnambulism commonly occurs year after year in the same child, though at different intensities. There were 6 children who had walked in their sleep over a period of about 10 years and 23 had done so for more than 5 years. Such occurrences over a series of years were independent of the annual frequency. The ø-coefficients for the correlations between years are given in Table 1 (ø = phi coefficient).

Correlations with behavioral and environmental factors are presented in Table 2. Somnambulism does not covary significantly with such nocturnal disturbances as frequent wakening, resistance at bedtime and the habit of moving into the parents' bed. Neither is there any link with fear of the dark, shyness, defiance or fits of anger. Nor does the occurrence of somnambulism seem to be connected with the mother going out to work or a new situation for the child on separating from one of his parents. A separate bedroom did not give a greater propensity for somnambulism.

The teachers' assessments of school performance, of the child's ability to get on with peers, his propensity to start trouble and to act as leader did not distinguish the somnambulists from the other children. It seems, on the other hand, that the somnambulists were appreciated more by the teachers (in grade 5, $p = 0.10$) as well as by their peers in the sociometric test (in grade 3, $p = 0.05$).

According to the Rorschach test, done blind at 10 years of age, the somnambulist group had significantly more inhibited aggression ($p = 0.05$) as well as more pronounced anxiety-suppressing mechanisms ($p = 0.005$) than the other children. Their anxiety is mostly contained by various psychological defenses. However, the strength of aggression and anxiety loadings did not differ significantly.

Table 1

Persistence of somnambulism—ø correlation coefficients for different intervals in years

1 year's interval (years 11 and 12)	0.8
2 years' intervals (years 6 and 8)	0.7
8 and 10	0.7
10 and 12	0.6
12 and 14	0.6
3 years' interval (years 6 and 9)	0.6
4 years' interval (years 8 and 12)	0.4
6 years' interval (years 8 and 14)	0.4

Table 2

Somnambulism related to behavioral and environmental factors at 12 years of age (except where other ages are indicated)

Variable	Probability of co-variation
Sleep	
Night-awakening	NS ($\chi^2 = 1.3$)
Difficulties in getting to sleep	NS
"Bad dreams"	0.02 ($\chi^2 = 5.468$)
In parents' bed part of night	
(at 10, 11, 12 yrs)	NS
Fits of anger	NS
Fear of the dark	NS
Defiance	NS
Shyness with children	NS
Shyness with adults	NS
Nailbiting	NS
Delayed speech development	
(at 3 yrs)	NS
Mood	
Serious-glad (3-point scale)	NS
Lively-calm (3-point scale)	NS
Sensitive-robust (3-point scale)	NS
Teacher assessment (grade 5)	
School performance	NS
Popularity among peers	NS ($\chi^2 = 3.512$)
At ease with peers	NS
Trouble-maker	NS
Leader	NS
Sociometry	
Grade 3 (10 years)	0.05 ($\chi^2 = 4.243$)
Grade 4 (11 years)	NS
Grade 5 (12 years)	NS
Grade 6 (13 years)	NS
Mother out to work	NS
Change in family situation	NS
Separate bedroom	NS
Rorschach (at 10 years)	
Aggressive loading	NS
Inhibited aggression	0.05 ($\chi^2 = 4.917$)
Anxiety loading	NS
Defense against anxiety	0.005 ($\chi^2 = 10.472$)
Maturity	NS
	NS

NS = not significant

DISCUSSION

Although up to 16% of the families reported that the child had sleep-walked once or several times, it is much less often that the frequency of episodes at a particular age warrants the epithet habitual. There is no means of determining whether every reported occasion matches the full definition of somnambulism. The main features of the symptom are familiar to observant parents. For this study sleep disturbances have been evaluated as follows. A child who, without waking up, sits up in bed and moves his arms or talks in his sleep has not been counted, even though such signs are sometimes classified as abortive somnambulism (4). If bed behavior is marked by facial and other gestures indicating intense anxiety and the child is difficult to wake up, the disturbance is by definition pavor nocturnus which was uncommon in the present material. If the child wakes up spontaneously in connection with a dream and is able to relate or suggest a frightening experience, this is classified as a nightmare. Children who walk in their sleep usually do so calmly without any observable fear.

Not one of the children was taken to a doctor on account of the sleepwalking. This tallies with pediatric experience and studies by others (2). Somnambulism is seldom considered to be sufficiently alarming to warrant a consultation for this alone, even when the symptom persists for several years and the nocturnal events may seem bizarre. The correlations for persistence and the longitudinal picture support the existence of a small group of children with years of a propensity for this form of sleep disturbance.

Perusing the records from year to year failed to reveal distinguishing characteristics in most respects for the group of sleepwalking children. Many symptoms and environmental variables have been tested. It seems to be an arbitrary matter which children walk in their sleep and the same applies to the age at which they start. Their experiences do not differ by and large from those of other children. An exception is that the future somnambulists, at the age of 4–5 years, had a more than random covariation with restless sleep interpreted as "bad" dreams; the level of significance is 0.05 at 4 years and 0.025 at 5 years. Furthermore, reports of such dreams among the sleepwalking group during periods of somnambulism show a more than random coincidence ($p = 0.02$) compared with their dreaming in non-somnambulist periods. As neither somnambulism nor "bad" dreams are markedly frequent among the sleepwalkers, these children by no means suffer from poor sleep in general. Between the occasional incidents their sleep is reportedly good, with no clusters of nightawakening.

Somnambulism and wakening dreams are elicited in different stages of sleep with no mutual relationship. Still it is worth commenting on the statistically demonstrated simultaneity in particular individuals. The correlation is weak but support for it is to be found in laboratory evidence that NREM sleep is not necessarily cut off from demonstrable psychic experiences. A high concordance has been found, for instance, between the content of talk during a typical NREM stage of sleep and what is related immediately after awakening from this sleep (11). Similarly, another state that is initiated in the NREM stage—pavor nocturnus—has been associated on certain occasions with concurrent mental activity (5), though this is not usually the case (1). It has also been demonstrated that both pavor nocturnus and somnambulism can be elicited in predisposed persons by external stimuli, the former by loud noise (5) and the latter by passively generated leg movements, which leave no trace on the sleep curves of nonsomnambulist children (4). Another indication that somnambulism is susceptible to environmental factors is that individuals who have not displayed signs of somnambulism for a long time can do so under stress (6) or in connection with a febrile disease (12).

A sleepwalking propensity has been interpreted as a manifestation of the nervous system's immaturity. Anders & Weinstein (6) note that the EEG changes characteristic of the start of a sleepwalking phase sometimes appear both without a clinically observable attack materializing and in young children who are not somnambulists. In such cases the changes are reported to be less frequent and briefer. Their frequency decreases with age and they are said not to occur in normal children after the 9th year. These findings, coupled with the clinical observation that even the sleepwalking child apparently grows out of the habit without presenting substitute symptoms, point to a maturity factor. However, such an interpretation implies that somnambulism should be relatively more common below than above the age of 9, which this study does not confirm. There is of course the possibility, as pointed out by Jacobson et al. (4), that "subsomnambulistic" activities tend to be overlooked by parents. A contribution from a genetic disposition has been indicated by a twin study (13), where monozygotic twins were concordant for sleepwalking considerably more often than dizygotic ($p = 0.04$).

Somnambulism and nocturnal enuresis are reported (1) to occur quite often in the same child. As shown earlier (14), the relationship is not definitely established in the present sample, in which both variables have been followed continuously.

It is not clear how the Rorschach findings should be interpreted. Some of the somnambulists' parents are known to have a notably dominant relationship with their child but this is not so for the majority. Perhaps a psychodynamic explanation comes closest to the mark. Suppressed impulses that usually find a nocturnal outlet in dreams are not always allowed—on account of their threatening character—to find expression in this way. Psychoanalysts refer to this as dream censorship. In the children with a strong built-in defense against feelings of anxiety (according to the Rorschach interpretation), other sleep disturbances such as somnambulism or night terror are elicited unconsciously and without noticeable memory traces.

REFERENCES

1. Broughton, R. J. (1968). Sleep Disorders: Disorders of arousal? *Science*, 159:1070–78.
2. Jacobson, A., Kales, J. and Kales A. (1969). Clinical and electrophysiological correlates of sleep disorders in children. In *Sleep Physiology and Pathology*, A. Kales, ed. Philadelphia, Toronto: Lippincott, pp. 109–18.
3. Kales, A. and Kales J. (1974). Sleep disorders. Recent findings in the diagnosis and treatment of disturbed sleep. *New England Journal of Medicine*, 290:487–99.
4. Jacobson, A. and Kales, A. (1967). Somnambulism: All night EEG and related studies. In *Sleep and Altered States of Consciousness. Res. Publ. Assoc., Res. of Nerv. Ment. Dis.*, Vol. XLV. Baltimore: Williams and Wilkins, pp. 424–48.
5. Fisher, C., Kahn, E., Edwards, A., Davis, D. and Fine J. (1974). A psychophysiological study of nightmares and night terrors. III. Mental content and recall of stage 4. *Journal of Nervous and Mental Disease*, 158:174–88.
6. Anders, I. and Weinstein, P. (1972). Sleep and its disorders in infants and children: A review. *Pediatrics*, 50:312–24.
7. Sours, J. A., Frumkin, P. and Indermill, R. (1963). Somnambulism. *Archives of General Psychiatry*, 9:400–13.
8. Kales, A., Paulson, M. and Jacobson, A. (1966). Somnambulism: Psychophysiological correlates. *Archives of General Psychiatry*, 14:595–604.
9. Karlberg, P., Klackenberg, G., Klackenberg-Larsson, I., Lichtenstein, H., Stenson, J. and Svennberg, I. (1968). The development of children in a Swedish urban community. A prospective, longitudinal study. Introduction, design and aims of the study. *Acta Paediatrica Scandinavica*, Suppl. 187.
10. Klackenberg, G. (1971). A prospective, longitudinal study of children. Data on psychic health and development up to 8 years of age. *Acta Paediatrica Scandinavica*, Suppl. 224.
11. Arkin A. M., Antrobus, J. S., Toth, M. F., Baker, J. and Jackler, F. (1972). A comparison of the content of mentation reports elicited after NREM-associated sleep utterances and NREM "silent" sleep. *Journal of Nervous and Mental Disease*, 155:427–35.
12. Kales, J., Kales, A., Soldatos, C., Chamberlin, K. and Martin, E. (1979). Sleep walking and night-terrors related to febrile illness. *American Journal of Psychiatry*, 136:1214–15.
13. Bakwin, H. (1970). Sleep walking in twins. *Lancet*, 11:446.
14. Klackenberg, G. (1981). Nocturnal enuresis in a longitudinal perspective. *Acta Paediatrica Scandinavica*, 70:453–57.

Part VII

FETAL METHADONE AND ALCOHOL SYNDROMES

There has been increasing concern in recent years over the effect of potentially toxic substances utilized by the mother on the fetus, whether these be tobacco, drugs, or medications. The dramatic effects of thalidomide are horrible examples of how extreme the destructive effects can be.

In this section, studies of the effects of methadone and alcohol on the fetus are reported. The paper by Marcus and his co-workers details data on the motor and state functioning in a group of newborns whose mothers were on methadone maintenance therapy. The results suggested that methadone acts differentially on CNS functioning, with strong effects on neuromotor functioning.

Rosen and Johnson carry this issue further with a follow-up to 18 months of the children of methadone-maintained mothers. They report a number of findings of concern, including a higher incidence of certain physical symptoms such as small head circumference, lags in physical development, neurologic findings, and significantly lower scores on the Bayley developmental indices.

Similarly, Steinhausen and his co-workers, in a study of German children, report a broad scale of developmental hazards and psychopathologic symptoms indicating the long-range effects of alcohol abuse during pregnancy.

These studies indicate the need for a major commitment in research funding to this vitally significant issue of the effects of substance abuse and special drug intake by the mother on the fetus. Studies in this field are complicated, because such mothers are likely to be ingesting other potentially toxic substances. Also, their substance abuse may reflect significant psychopathology or sociocultural pathology, which may also conceivably affect the fetus or newborn. These possibilities may confound

471

the problem of isolating the specific influence of an individual substance, such as methadone or alcohol, but they do not alter the importance of this area of research, both for its theoretical and practical implications.

PART VII: FETAL METHADONE AND ALCOHOL SYNDROMES

30

Differential Motor and State Functioning in Newborns of Women on Methadone

Joseph Marcus, Sydney L. Hans, and Rita Jeruchimowicz Jeremy

University of Chicago

Motor and state functioning of 20 infants born to methadone-maintained women and 25 born to controls was assessed at 1 day and 1 month of age using Brazelton Neonatal Behavioral Assessment Scale with Kansas Supplements (NBAS-K). The infants were of mothers who were Black, of low SES, between the ages of 18 and 35 years, and who had good prenatal care. Motor behaviors were scored on NBAS-K items: General Tonus, Motor Maturity, and Tremulousness. State behaviors were scored on 2 items: Alertness and General Irritability. Guttman's Multidimensional Scalogram Analysis (MSA) of individual profiles revealed an orthogonal relationship between motor and state functioning, with motor functioning being a much clearer discriminator between methadone and non-methadone infants than state functioning. With age, both groups generally improved, but non-

Reprinted with permission from *Neurobehavioral Toxicology and Teratology*, 1982, Vol. 4, 459–462.

This research was supported by NIDA Grant PHS5R18DA-01884 and the Irving Harris Foundation.

The authors acknowledge the help of Victor Bernstein, Susan Lutgendorf, and Wendy Rabinowitz-Munson in the collection of data, and Patricia Huetteman and Terrence Joyce in the preparation of the manuscript. Special thanks are due to Professor Louis Guttman, The Hebrew University of Jerusalem, and Leland Wilkinson, Chairman, Methods and Measurement Division, Department of Psychology, University of Illinois, Chicago, for their invaluable consultations on methodology and data analysis.

*methadone infants maintained some of their advantage in motor func-
tioning. Both groups showed a variety of behavior patterns during
the neonatal period. The results suggest that methadone acts differentially on CNS functioning, with strong effects on neuro-motor functioning.*

Many newborn infants exposed to opiates *in utero* develop a variety
of medical conditions and behaviors that include gastrointestinal dysfunction, elevated basal temperature, respiratory dysfunction, frantic
but weak sucking, high-pitched crying, tremulousness, irritability, and
hypertonicity (cf., [4, 7, 8]). Because many of these behaviors bear a close
resemblance to withdrawal symptoms observed in adult narcotics addicts,
their presence during the neonatal period has generally been described
as generalized hypersensitivity of the central nervous system (CNS) due
to withdrawal from opiates and has been termed the neonatal abstinence
syndrome.

Neonatal abstinence syndrome is known to manifest itself in different
ways in individual infants. The time of onset of the syndrome varies
widely, as well as its severity and duration. Even though the range of
symptoms seen in the syndrome has been well described, little is known
about the meaning of these symptoms in terms of underlying biological
function and what variation in the symptoms means for the prognosis
of an individual infant or subgroup of infants. Withdrawal signs such
as tremulousness and hypertonicity are "soft" indicators of dysfunction
that do not pinpoint a precise source of biochemical or structural abnormality. They are also warning signs commonly seen in children who
have other kinds of CNS dysfunction not associated with maternal narcotics use. Thus the presence of such symptoms during the neonatal
period could be an indication of a temporary state of withdrawal from
drugs or of an underlying and more permanent CNS dysfunction. Such
dysfunction could be due to the toxicological effects of drugs *in utero*,
to complications of birth associated with drug use, or even to inherited
dysfunction. Only longitudinal study of infants exposed to drugs, with
careful consideration to the patterning of symptoms in individual infants, can reveal the meaning of such behaviors during the neonatal
period.

METHOD

Overall Description of the Study

We presently are engaged in a longitudinal study at The University of Chicago of the behavior of infants born to methadone-using women. Pregnant women are recruited to the Project through the obstetrical clinics at Chicago Lying-In Hospital. Extensive data are collected about the medical and psychiatric history of these women and the fathers of their babies. Their infants are assessed by a battery of medical, neuro-behavior, psychophysiological, and social measures made soon after birth and at regular intervals through two years of age.

Subjects

This paper will report on the first 45 infant participants of this Project: (1) those whose mothers were maintained on methadone for the treatment of heroin addiction (methadone group, N = 20) and (2) those whose mothers were of approximately the same age, social class, and education but were not abusers either of opiates or alcohol (non-methadone group, N = 25). The methadone dosages of users during pregnancy ranged from 10 to 40 mg per day, with a median of 15 mg. A small number of the methadone-group mothers were found to occasionally use other drugs in addition to methadone, most commonly alcohol, marijuana, and heroin. All the women were Black, from low-income inner-city neighborhoods, and between the ages of 18 and 35 years. All received good prenatal care.

Five minute Apgar scores of the infants ranged between 6 and 10 for the methadone infants and between 8 and 10 for the non-methadone newborns. The methadone group contained one set of monozygotic twin girls (#35 and #36) and one pair of non-twin sisters (#15 and #16); the non-methadone group, one set of dizygotic twin girls (#22 and #23). All infants were full term except four methadone infants who were born at less than 38 weeks gestational age. The median birth weight of the methadone infants (excluding the 4 preterm infants) was 2740 g; of the non-methadone infants, 3327 g. No methadone newborn in this sample except one required pharmacologic treatment for withdrawal symptoms. The single case (#36) received one dose of phenobarbital; this infant died of Sudden Infant Death Syndrome before her 1-month exam.

Procedure

The Brazelton Neonatal Behavioral Assessment Scale with Kansas Supplements (NBAS-K) [1, 5] was used to examine the infants at approximately 24 hours of age in the hospital and, again, one month later at our Project infant laboratory. The preterm infants were first examined at their calculated 40-weeks gestational age, and again, one month later.

All Brazelton examinations were conducted by two staff members—the primary examiner being always "blind" about an infant's background.

RESULTS

The Kansas version of Neonatal Behavioral Assessment Scale contains 32 behavioral items, assessing a broad spectrum of infant functioning. Based on previous work with this instrument, we know that the items measure three general categories of behavior: state, motor, and perceptual-cognitive functioning (Marcus, Hans, Jeremy, Bernstein, and Patterson, unpublished manuscript, 1981). For analysis in this report we chose to look at only state and motor functioning; perceptual-cognitive items on the Brazelton test typically have extensive missing data.

Previous analyses (Marcus, Jeremy, Hans, submitted for publication) showed that three items from the Brazelton examination best represent motor functioning; (1) #11. General Tonus—the amount of muscle tone felt by the examiner during handling throughout examination, (2) #12. Motor Maturity—the smoothness of an infant's limb movements, and (3) #21. Tremulousness—the extent to which tremors are observed during different behavioral states. Two items best represent the infant's control of biological state: (1) #10. Alertness—the degree to which an infant displays sustained periods of responsiveness to the environment, and (2) #31. General Irritability—the degree to which an infant becomes fussy and irritable to standard stimuli of gradually increasing intensity and the ease with which an infant returns to lower states of arousal.

Because the Brazelton items are only ordinally or categorically scaled, we chose to use nonmetric techniques of data analysis. In addition, we wanted to look at individual profiles of behavior on different functions simultaneously. To meet these specifications we chose to use Guttman's Multidimensional Scalogram Analysis (MSA) [6, 9] on the five items described previously. This procedure plots subjects in Cartesian space according to the similarity of their profiles. Examination of the scalogram revealed two independent dimensions. The three motor items, as we had found previously, scaled together in one direction, and the two state items scaled in an orthogonal direction.

In Fig. 1 each infant is plotted by his or her scores at one day of age. Curved lines have been drawn to indicate the meaning of the regions according to state and motor functioning. The profiles of those infants in the upper left corner (separated by a broken line) are characterized by poor state functioning—extreme irritability and poor alertness. Those in the lower left corner (separated by a solid line) are characterized by

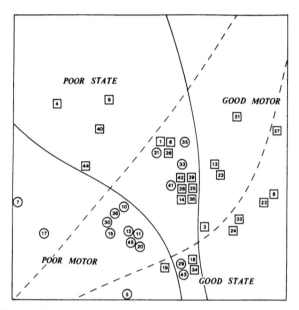

FIG. 1. MSA map of individual behavioral functioning at 1 day.
○=methadone; □=non-methadone.

poor motor functioning—hypertonicity, jerky movements, and extreme tremulousness. There is an overlapping region in the middle left of infants with both poor motor and poor state functioning. Infants on the right side (separated by a solid line) are characterized by good motor functioning—moderate muscle tonus, smooth limb movements, and almost no tremors. Those on the lower right side (separated by a broken line) are characterized by good state functioning—low irritability and good alertness. The lines on the plot allow one to identify each infant by type of both motor and state functioning. For example, Infant #5 showed poor motor functioning with good state functioning; Infant #34, good state functioning with moderate motor functioning.

On Fig. 1 the methadone infants are identified by circles, the non-methadone infants by squares. Note that in the region of both poor state and poor motor functioning there are only two infants—both exposed to methadone. In the region of both good state and good motor functioning, there are 5 infants, all non-methadone infants. Of the 12 infants showing poor motor functioning, 11 are methadone infants. Of the 9 infants showing good motor functioning, none are methadone infants.

Thus, methadone infants can be clearly discriminated from non-methadone infants on the basis of motor functioning at one day of age.

On the other hand, state functioning, including both alertness and general irritability, does not discriminate the methadone infants as clearly. Of the six infants showing poor state functioning, only 2 are methadone infants. Likewise, about one-fourth of the infants showing good state functioning are methadone infants. Thus, methadone has a different effect on state and motor functioning of the neonate.

Figure 2 presents the infants one month later, plotted according to the same regions. Again, all the infants showing poor functioning in both domains are methadone infants. However, half of the infants showing good functioning in both domains are now from the methadone group. Of infants with poor motor functioning five out of the six are from the methadone group. Again, it is motor functioning that most clearly discriminates the methadone infants.

Comparison of the one-day and one-month data reveals that with age, more infants are showing profiles of good functioning. There is movement toward better functioning for both methadone and non-methadone infants—but the advantage in motor functioning for the non-

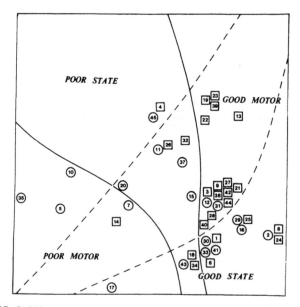

FIG. 2. MSA map of individual behavioral functioning at 1 month.
○=methadone; □=non-methadone.

methadone infants shown at one day remains at one month, although considerably reduced.

The overall impression of these data is of the great variety of behavior types typical of infants during the neonatal period, including methadone infants. Two-thirds of our methadone infants showed poor motor functioning at one day, but one third showed normal functioning. At one month the methadone infants showed an even broader range of functioning from very poor to very good.

DISCUSSION

The original work of researchers at medical centers in Chicago, Detroit, Houston, New York, Philadelphia, and New York has led to the identification of a set of clinically observable behaviors typical of neonates born to narcotics-using women. These behaviors have commonly been described as "generalized CNS hyperirritability" due to the effects of withdrawal from the narcotic drug and the body's adaptation to a new type of homeostasis.

The data reported here show that although infants born to methadone users display heterogeneous patterns of behavior during the neonatal period, motor behaviors are strongly affected in these infants. At both the one-day and one-month assessments, we found many cases of methadone infants who were hypertonic, tremulous, and had jerky movements. Almost no non-methadone infants showed this pattern of extremely poor motor behavior. However, general hyperirritability and poor alertness, as measured here by selected items from the Brazelton examination, were independent of poor motor functioning, with as many non-methadone infants as methadone infants showing this type of poor state functioning. Many of the methadone infants showing extremely poor motor functioning (including hypertonicity and tremulousness) actually displayed quite normal degrees of general irritability and alertness. These data indicate that while methadone infants may show hyperirritable motor responses, this hyperirritability is not necessarily generalized across all central nervous system functioning but may involve specific systems selectively. Much more work needs to be done to examine the possibility that the behavioral problems in methadone infants may not be due to generalized CNS irritability, but may be more differential, being seen in neuromuscular functioning in particular. Interestingly, there is animal research suggesting that chronic exposure to methadone has long-term effects on dopamine receptors and profoundly alters muscular behavior [2, 3].

While in this report we described analyses of only a limited number of behaviors measured with one instrument, it is clear that there is a great need to study how intrauterine exposure to opiates and neonatal abstinence differentially affect CNS functioning. While progress has been made in outlining the more general characteristics of these children, we must now direct our research toward investigating patterns of individual behavior according to specific types of CNS functioning. Such research will require multidimensional data analysis techniques. The results should improve our knowledge of the etiology of problems observed in these children and allow treatment to be more individualized.

REFERENCES

1. Brazelton, T. B. (1973). *Neonatal Behavioral Assessment Scale.* Clinics in Developmental Medicine No. 50. Philadelphia: J. B. Lippincott.
2. Carlson, K. R. and Eibergen, R. D. (1976). Susceptibility to amphetamine-elicited dyskinesias following chronic methadone treatment in monkeys. *Annals of the New York Academy of Science,* 281:336–349.
3. Eibergen, R. D. and Carlson, K. R. (1976). Dyskinesias in monkeys: Interaction of methamphetamine with prior methadone treatment. *Pharmac. Biochem. Behav.,* 5:175–187.
4. Finnegan, L. P., Connaughton, J. F. and Schut, J. (1975). Infants of drug-dependent women: Practical approaches for management. In *Proceedings of the 37th Annual Scientific Meeting of the Committee on Problems of Drug Dependence of the National Research Council.* Washington, D.C.: National Academy of Sciences.
5. Horowitz, F. D., Sullivan, J. W. and Linn, P. (1978). Stability and instability in the newborn infants: The quest for elusive threads. In Organization and stability of newborn behavior: A commentary on the Brazelton Neonatal Behavioral Assessment Scale. A. J. Sameroff, ed. *Monographs of the Society for Research in Child Development,* 43:29–45.
6. Lingoes, J. (1973). *The Guttman-Lingoes Nonmetric Program Series.* Ann Arbor, MI: Mathesis Press.
7. Strauss, M. E., Starr, R. H. Jr., Ostrea, E. M. Jr., Chavez, C. J. and Stryker, J. C. (1976). Behavioral concomitants of prenatal addiction to narcotics. *Journal of Pediatrics,* 89:842–846.
8. Wilson, G. W., Desmond, M. M. and Verniaud, W. M. (1973). Early development of infants of heroin-addicted mothers. *American Journal of Diseases of Children,* 126:457–462.
9. Zvulun, E. (1978). Multidimensional Scalogram Analysis: The method and its application. In *Theory Construction and Data Analysis in the Behavioral Sciences,* S. Shye, ed. San Francisco: Jossey-Bass, pp. 237–264.

31

Children of Methadone-maintained Mothers: Follow-up to 18 Months of Age

Tove S. Rosen and Helen L. Johnson

College of Physicians and Surgeons, Columbia University, New York

Limited information is available on the long-term effects of in utero methadone exposure. This report describes the somatic and neurobehavioral findings of children in the first 18th months of life born to methadone-maintained mothers and to a matched drug-free comparison group of mothers. Findings during the neonatal period were (1) a 75% incidence of moderate-to-severe narcotic abstinence syndrome, (2) a significant incidence of head circumferences below the third percentile, and (3) elevated systolic blood pressure. In follow-up, the methadone children had (1) a significantly higher incidence of otitis media; (2) a significant incidence of head circumferences below the third percentile; (3) neurologic findings of tone discrepancies, developmental delays, and poor fine motor coordination; (4) a high incidence of abnormal eye findings; and (5) significantly lower scores on the Bayley mental and motor developmental indices. These neurobehavioral findings in children of methadone-treated mothers at 18 months of age may be predictors of later learning and behavioral problems.

Reprinted with permission from *The Journal of Pediatrics*, 1982, Vol. 101, No. 2, pp. 191–196. Copyright 1982 by The C. V. Mosby Company.

Supported by National Institute on Drug Abuse Grant No. DA01663.

Abbreviations used: SGA—small for gestational age; MDI—mental developmental index; PDI—psychomotor developmental index.

Methadone maintenance has been used as treatment for heroin addiction for over a decade. When compared to heroin, methadone maintenance is associated with better prenatal care, improved fetal growth and reduced fetal mortality.[1,2] On the other hand, neonatal morbidity is reportedly more severe in the offspring of methadone-maintained mothers[2-5]; however, very few studies are available on the long-term somatic and neurobehavioral outcome of these offspring.[6-9]

Since 1977, we have been conducting a longitudinal follow-up study of somatic and neurobehavioral characteristics of infants born to mothers in methadone maintenance programs during pregnancy. This report will describe some of the medical, neurologic, and behavioral findings during the first 18 months of life in a group of children born to methadone-maintained mothers and in a matched group of children born to drug-free mothers.

METHODS

Subjects

Women maintained on methadone therapy were enrolled in our study through our High Risk Prenatal Clinic and referrals from various methadone programs in New York City after informed consent was obtained. Close contact was established between the methadone-maintained subjects and project staff, as well as with the subjects' methadone-maintenance clinics, to ensure follow-up. Sixty-one mothers on methadone maintenance initially were enrolled in the study. One mother died during pregnancy and three delivered at other institutions, leaving a total of 57 mothers. Five of these mothers had two infants (no multiple births) in the study. The offspring consisted of 30 females and 32 males.

The comparison group of drug-free mothers and their offspring were enrolled from the general ward population within the first 24 hours after birth, and were matched to the methadone subjects for maternal race, socioeconomic class, neonatal sex, birth weight ($\pm$ 250 gm), and gestational age ($\pm$ 2 weeks).[10] The comparison group consisted of 31 mothers and their infants; one mother had two infants in the study. There were 17 males and 15 females.

Procedure

Maternal medical and obstetrical histories were obtained by review of hospital records and study subject interviews. History of drug usage in the methadone-maintained mothers was obtained through interviews and maternal urinary drug screening at each prenatal visit, and at delivery using a TLC Toxi Kit (Analytical Systems, Inc.). Comparison group drug histories were obtained by maternal interview and chart review, and neonatal urinary drug screening. All neonates were examined within the first 24 hours of life by the pediatric nurse practitioner or pediatrician, and all pertinent physical findings were noted. Neurologic evaluations were performed on all neonates at 24 to 48 hours of life. Urine was collected for analysis for drugs of abuse. In the methadone-exposed infants, withdrawal signs and symptoms were evaluated daily until discharge, using a modified version of the narcotic abstinence score of Finnegan et al.[2] Those with severe symptoms were treated with phenobarbital. Blood pressure measurements using a Parks Ultrasonic Doppler were obtained during the first week of life in 20 infants born to methadone-maintained mothers. Blood pressure then was determined weekly until it had fallen to the normal range.

After discharge, both groups were seen in our follow-up clinic at 2, 4, 6, 8, 10, 12, 15, and 18 months of life. Many of the babies born to methadone-maintained mothers were seen more frequently for narcotic abstinence syndrome and other problems. Each follow-up visit consisted of a physical examination including evaluation of growth and development; a neurologic assessment evaluating tone, reflexes, gait, eye movement and developmental milestones; and the Bayley Scales of Infant Development. All subjects received primary medical care, including immunizations and emergency treatment, as well as social service assistance. Hospital charts and project records were reviewed for pertinent information, including the number of clinic and emergency visits and all diagnoses and treatments of each infant.

All data were coded and entered into the computer for analysis. All data are expressed as mean ± 1 SE. Group differences were tested with analysis of variance, chi square analysis, and the Fisher exact test as indicated.[11,12] Correlations among variables also were examined. Analysis of covariance in a regression mode was also employed.[13]

RESULTS

Maternal Data (Table I)

Although the methadone-maintained mothers were significantly older than the comparison mothers ($P < 0.05$), both groups were well within the optimal range for child bearing.[14] The racial distribution was similar

Table I. Maternal data

	Methadone-maintained	Comparison drug-free
Age (M ± SE)	26.8 ± .5	22 ± .9
Race (%)		
White	7.3	3.6
Hispanic	14.5	17.8
Black	78.2	78.6
Prenatal care (%)	77.8	84.6
Obstetrical		
complications (%)	22.2	14.3
Other drug abuse (%)	56	0
Tobacco > 1 pack/day (%)	90	28.6

in both groups; the subjects were predominantly black. The numbers of prenatal clinic visits for the methadone and comparison groups were similar. The methadone-maintained mothers had a higher incidence of obstetrical complications. In the methadone group, the mean number of months on methadone maintenance prior to pregnancy was 34.5 ± 3.2 (range = 2 to 96 months); the mean methadone dose was 42.9 ± 2.6 mg/day. The mean duration of heroin addiction prior to methadone maintenance was 54.7 ± 5.0 months (range = 6 to 180 months). In addition, 56% of the methadone-maintained mothers were multidrug abusers during their pregnancies. The most frequent drugs used, in descending order, were diazepines, opiates, cocaine, barbiturates, amitriptyline, and amphetamines. Moreover, 15.3% of the methadone-maintained mothers had a moderate-to-heavy alcohol intake; none of the comparison mothers did. More methadone-maintained mothers than comparison mothers smoked more than one pack of cigarettes per day.

Neonatal Data (Table II)

In the methadone group, nine babies were premature and seven SGA; in the comparison group, three infants were premature and none SGA. There were no gross congenital anomalies except that one infant of a methadone-maintained mother had signs of the fetal alcohol syndrome. Head circumferences below the third percentile were more frequent among infants of methadone-maintained mothers ($P < 0.001$). Of the infants of methadone-maintained mothers, 75% had moderate-to-severe narcotic withdrawal; 12 were treated with phenobarbital for four to 125 days (17.5 ± 7.4). More infants born to methadone-maintained mothers

Table II. Neonatal data

	Methadone group	Comparison drug-free group
Mean birth weight (gm) (M ± SE)	3,129 ± 192	3,037 ± 101
Premature (28-36 wk)	15.4%	11%
Small for gestational age	13%	3%
Apgar score		
1 min	7.4 ± 0.3	8.1 ± 0.1
5 min	8.5 ± 0.2	9.0 ± 0.1
Withdrawal syndrome	75.1%	—
Mild	24.9%	
Moderate	51.8%	
Severe	23.3% (12 treated with phenobarbital)	
Prolonged hospitalization	28%	11%

required prolonged hospitalization for the treatment of narcotic abstinence syndrome or prematurity than did those in the comparison group.

An additional significant finding in a group of 20 infants of methadone-maintained mothers was elevated arterial pressure. The mean blood pressure was 95.2 ± 56 with a range of 59 to 132 mm Hg. By comparison, the mean blood pressure during the first week of life in healthy newborn infants is 76 ± 11, and at 6 weeks of age, 96 ± 11 mm Hg.[15] The blood pressure elevation occurred irrespective of the severity of narcotic withdrawal and persisted for eight to 12 weeks.

Follow-up Data

Seventeen infants in the methadone group and seven in the comparison group were lost to follow-up. Two study subjects died at 4 and 6 weeks of age, respectively, because of sudden infant death syndrome; the others moved or were lost to follow-up. These dropout rates (27% for methadone, 22% for comparison group) are comparable to attrition rates encountered by other researchers working with this population.[7] The remaining groups consisted of 45 methadone-exposed infants (22 males, 23 females), and 25 comparison infants (12 males, 13 females). The follow-up data are based on study of the above infants and children. The number of subjects assessed varies at each time point because of missing data (caused by erratic attendance), not because of data selection.

No differences were noted in somatic growth of the two groups during the first 18 months of life. We evaluated the number of clinic and emergency room visits for the methadone and comparison groups; no significant difference was present. The numbers of episodes of otitis media per child and the chronicity of otitis were significantly higher in the methadone group than in the comparison group ($P < 0.001$). The most common neurologic abnormalities were tone discrepancies, developmental delays, and eye findings (Table III). Between 6 to 12 months of age tone discrepancies (both hypertonia and hypotonia) still were noted in the infants of methadone-maintained mothers. In addition, delays in sitting and in the development of transfer ability and fine motor coordination were seen. Tone and coordination problems still were present at 18 months and there was no real language development. In addition, at 18 months, 13 of the study children still had strabismus or nystagmus. This finding has been reported by others in young children of methadone-maintained mothers.[16]

Bayley mental and motor scores were corrected for gestational age. The methadone-exposed infants scored lower on the MDI and PDI than

Table III. Neurologic evaluations

	Methadone	Control
6 mo	N = 45	N = 25
Suspect	35.5%	32%
Abnormal	8.8%	4%
12 mo	N = 40*	N = 22
Suspect	14.6%	4.5%
Abnormal	7.3%	0%
18 mo	N = 38†	N = 23
Suspect	7.8%	4.3%
Abnormal	10.5%	0%

*$P < 0.0006$.
†$P < 0.002$.

the comparison infants, although all scores were within normal limits; by 12 months of age this difference was significant ($P < 0.04$) (Table IV). This significant difference was again present at 18 months of age ($P < 0.03$). The gap between the scores of the two groups, especially on the PDI, increased as the subjects became older. The comparison subjects also passed the Bayley language milestone items earlier than the methadone subjects did. At 18 months, there was a significant correlation between the Bayley MDI and PDI and the neurologic evaluations ($P < 0.04$, < 0.02, respectively).

Correlational analyses were run to determine the relation between various parental and neonatal characteristics and developmental out-

Table IV. Bayley Scales of Infant Behavior

Age	Methadone	Comparison
6 mo	n = 41	n = 23
MDI	95 ± 2.52	100.69 ± 4.20
PDI	101.03 ± 2.84	105.13 ± 2.97
12 mo	n = 41	n = 22
MDI	98.37 ± 2.68	107.00 ± 2.81*
PDI	94.93 ± 2.53	102.78 ± 2.30*
18 mo	n = 38	n = 23
MDI	96.00 ± 2.31	106.38 ± 3.56†
PDI	92.62 ± 2.38	105.29 ± 2.21‡

Values expressed as M ± SE.
*$P < 0.04$
†$P < 0.02$.
‡$P < 0.03$.

come.[13] There were no significant correlations between obstetrical complications, prenatal course, length of methadone maintenance, methadone dose, multi-drug abuse, paternal drug history of Apgar scores at one and five minutes, birth weight, gestational age, severity of narcotic withdrawal, and neurobehavioral outcome (neurologic evaluation and Bayley scores) at 18 months. Additionally, an analysis of covariance in a regression mode was used to evaluate the role of obstetrical complications, gestational age, birth weight, Apgar scores, sex, and treatment group (methadone vs comparison) in neurobehavioral performance at 18 months. Treatment group was the only factor significantly related to neurologic outcome and Bayley PDI scores ($P < 0.05$). Both sex and treatment group were significantly related to MDI scores at 18 months (lower scores in methadone vs comparison and male vs female subjects; in both cases, $P < 0.05$).

DISCUSSION

The developmental implications for the infant whose mother received methadone maintenance during pregnancy are complex. During fetal life, the child of a methadone-maintained mother is likely to be exposed to multiple drugs of abuse and to have a paternal history of drug abuse. In the early neonatal period the same infant may experience the narcotic abstinence syndrome and then, during infancy and early childhood, be exposed to poor mothering and poor environment.[17] In addition to these factors, animal data in the rat demonstrate deleterious central nervous system effects as a result of in utero methadone exposure.[18,19] Our own findings at 18 months of age in the children of methadone-maintained mothers point to methadone maintenance and its associated factors as significantly influencing the outcome of these children. Moreover, we have shown that prematurity, intrauterine growth failure, and Apgar scores are not significant determinants of outcome.

Birth weight and gestational age in the methadone subjects were similar to those in other reports.[1-5] A significant number of head circumferences were below the third percentile, which may be an indication of CNS deficit.[20] Rat pups exposed to methadone in utero have shown a decrease in brain weight with reduced DNA, RNA, and protein; by 60 days of age there was no difference in brain weight, but the DNA content was still decreased, reflecting a diminution in cell number. However, the RNA and protein concentrations were increased, reflecting an increase in neural cell size.[18,19] Whether these CNS biochemical findings occur in children of mothers on methadone maintenance is not known. Interestingly, of those infants with head circumferences below the third percentile at birth for whom data at 18 months of age are available, 63% continue to have head sizes below the third percentile.

The neonates of methadone-maintained mothers also had transient elevations of systolic blood pressure. Most commonly, elevated blood pressure in the neonate is secondary to umbilical artery catheterization or renal disease, neither of which was present in this group of infants.[21,22] This transient hypertension may be secondary to dysfunction of the autonomic nervous system caused by in utero narcotic exposure. This possibility is suggested by animal data showing changes in the neurochemical development of cathecholaminergic systems in both central and peripheral nervous tissue in newborn rat pups after in utero methadone exposure.[23]

Our follow-up data revealed a higher incidence, recurrence rate, and chronicity of otitis media in the methadone-exposed children. This finding has not been reported by other investigators,[6-8] and may result from maternal therapeutic noncompliance of infant immune incompetence.[24,25] Recurrent otitis media has been associated with auditory processing deficits which may contribute to subsequent problems in behavior and in learning communicative skills.[26]

The neurobehavioral assessments showed neurologic signs, including strabismus and nystagmus, tone abnormalities, and delays in developmental milestones. Wilson et al.[6] and Strauss et al.[7] have reported similar developmental delays and neurologic findings at 12 months of age.

The Bayley Scales of Infant Behavior showed a widening gap in the scores on mental and psychomotor indices in the methadone versus comparison groups. This was most evident in the PDI scores and may be related to the psychomotor developmental delays. Conflicting evidence has been reported regarding the mental and motor development of children born to methadone-maintained mothers. Some investigators have reported delays in mental development compared to motor development; others have reported delays in motor development, and still others have found no delays in either area.[6,7,27] Lodge et al.[8] reported discrepancies in perceptual, language, and motor abilities.[28] Rats exposed to methadone prenatally have shown developmental delays in certain behaviors as well as a high response output (greater activity).[29-32] Lower Bayley Scales scores can be predictors of developmental difficulties, and there is evidence of a relationship between developmental scores at 8 and 20 months and between IQ at 4 and 10 years in children of low socioeconomic status.[33]

The methadone-exposed neonate enters the world with special needs:

The withdrawal from narcotics leaves him less alert, more irritable, and more difficult to console than normal infants.[7] Many infants born at risk overcome early handicaps and show normal developmental progress by 18 months of age,[34] especially if reared in stable environments which are responsive to their special needs. In the children of methadone-maintained mothers, however, poor environment, family instability, and low socioeconomic background may perpetuate the effects of other risk factors.[26,33] Only further follow-up of these children through school years can determine if any permanent difficulties will be present.

REFERENCES

1. Rementeria, J. L. (ed.) (1977). *Drug Abuse in Pregnancy and the Neonatal Effects*. St. Louis: C. V. Mosby Company.
2. Finnegan, L. P. (1979). Pathophysiological and behavioral effects of the transplacental transfer of narcotic drugs to the foetuses and neonates of narcotic dependent mothers. *Bulletin of Narcotics*, 31:1.
3. Kandall, S. R., Albin, S., Gartner, L. M., Leek, S., Eidelman, A. and Lowman, J. (1979). The narcotic dependent mother: Fetal and neonatal consequences. *Early Human Development*, 1/2:159.
4. Rajegowda, B. K. (1972). Methadone withdrawal in newborn infants. *Journal of Pediatrics*, 81:532.
5. Rothstein, P. and Gould, J. B. (1974). Born with a habit: Infants of drug addicted mothers. Symposium on recent clinical advances. *Pediatric Clinics*, 21:307.
6. Wilson, G. S., Desmond, M. M. and Wait, R. B. (1981). Follow-up of methadone-treated and untreated narcotic dependent women and their infants: Health, developmental and social implications. *Journal of Pediatrics*, 98:716.
7. Strauss, M. E., Starr, R. H., Ostrea, E. M., Chavez, C. J. and Stryker, J. C. (1976). Behavioral concomitants of prenatal addiction to narcotics. *Journal of Pediatrics*, 89:842.
8. Lodge, A., Marcus, M. M. and Panier, C. M. (1976). Brain-behavior correlates associated with perinatal addiction. 9th Annual Winter Conference on Brain Research, Keystone, Colorado.
9. Kallenbach, K., Graziani, L. and Finnegan, L. P. (1978). Development of children born to women who received methadone during pregnancy. *Pediatric Research*, 12:372.
10. Dubowitz, L. M. S., Dubowitz, V. and Goldberg, C. (1970). Clinical assessment of gestational age in the newborn infant. *Journal of Pediatrics*, 77:1.
11. Bruning, J. L. and Kintz, B. L. (1968). *Computational Handbook of Statistics*. Glenview, IL: Scott Foresman & Co.
12. Siegel, S. (1956). Nonparametric statistics for the behavioral sciences. *McGraw Hill Series in Psychology*. New York: McGraw-Hill Book Company.
13. Cohen, J and Cohen, P. (eds.) (1975). *Applied Multiple Regression-Correlation Analyses for the Behavioral Sciences*. Hillsdale, N.J.: Lawrence Erlbaum Ass. Pub.
14. Milunsky, A. (ed.) (1974). *Clinics in Perinatology: Management of the High Risk Infant*. Philadelphia: W. B. Saunders Company.
15. LeSwiet, M., Fayers, P. and Shoneborune, E. A. (1980). Systolic blood pressure in a population of infants in the first year of life. The Bronyrton study. *Pediatrics*, 65:1028.

16. Chavez, C., Ostrea, E. M., Stryker, J. C. and Strauss, M. E. (1979). Ocular abnormalities in infants as sequelae of prenatal drug addiction. *Pediatric Research*, 13:367 (N. 252).

17. Lawson, M. S. and Wilson, G. S. (1979). Addiction and pregnancy: Two lives in crisis. *Social Work in Health Care*, 4:445.

18. Zagon, I. S. and McLaughlin, P. J. (1978). Perinatal methadone exposure and brain development: A biochemical study. *Journal of Neurochemistry*, 31:49.

19. Peters, M. A. (1977). The effect of maternally administered methadone on brain development in the offspring. *Journal of Pharmacology and Experimental Therapeutics*, 203:340.

20. Lipper, E., Lee, K., Gartner, L. M. and Grellong, B. (1981). Determinants of neurobehavioral outcome in low birthweight infants. *Pediatrics*, 67:502.

21. Plummer, L. B., Kaplan, G. W. and Mendoza, S. A. (1976). Hypertension in infants: A complication of umbilical artery catheterization. *Journal of Pediatrics*, 89:802.

22. Rahrman, N., Borneau, F. G. and Lewy, J. E. (1981). Renal failure in the perinatal period. In *Symposium on Perinatal Nephrology. Perinatal Clinics*, 8:241.

23. Lau, C., Bartolome, M. and Slotkin, T. A. (1977). Development of central and peripheral catecholaminergic systems in rats addicted perinatally to methadone. *Neuropharmacology*, 16:473.

24. Scott, G., Mills, E. L., Huff, S. S., Cotes, K. L., Juhn, S. K. and Quie, P. G. (1979). Polymorphonuclear leukocyte dysfunction with recurrent otitis media. *Journal of Pediatrics*, 94:13.

25. Orion, D. K. and Taylor, C. (1977). Epidemiology of recurrent otitis media. *American Journal of Public Health*, 67:472.

26. Gottlieb, M. I., Zinkus, P. W. and Thompson, A. (1979). Chronic middle ear disease and auditory perceptual deficits. *Clinical Pediatrics*, 18:725.

27. Kaltenbach, K., Graziani, L. J. and Finnegan, L. P. (1979). Methadone exposure in utero: Effects upon developmental status at one and two years of age. *Pediatric Research*, 13:332.

28. Ramer, C. M. and Lodge, A. (1975). Clinical and developmental characteristics of mothers on methadone maintenance. *International Journal of the Addictions*, 2:227.

29. Zagon, I. S. and McLaughlin, P. J. (1978). Perinatal methadone exposure and its influence on the behavioral ontogeny of rats. *Pharmacology and Biochemical Behavior*, 9:665.

30. Zagon, I. S., McLaughlin, P. J. and Thompson, C. I. (1979). Development of motor activity in young rats following perinatal methadone exposure. *Pharmacology and Biochemical Behavior*, 10:743.

31. Hutchings, D. E., Towey, J. P., Gorinson, H. S. and Hunt, H. F. (1979). Methadone during pregnancy: Assessment of behavioral effects in the rat offspring. *Journal of Pharmacology and Experimental Therapeutics*, 208:106.

32. Hutchings, D. E., Feraru, E., Gorinson, H. and Golden, R. R. (1979). Effects of prenatal methadone on the rest activity cycle of the preweanling rat. *Neurobehavioral Toxicology*, 1:33.

33. Sameroff, A. J. (1975). Early influences on development: Fact or fancy. *Merrill-Palmer Quarterly*, 21:267.

34. Werner, E., Honzik, M. and Smith, R. (1968). Prediction of intelligence and achievement at 10 years from 20 month pediatric/psychological exams. *Child Development*, 39:1063.

PART VII: FETAL METHADONE AND ALCOHOL
SYNDROMES

32

Development and Psychopathology of Children With the Fetal Alcohol Syndrome

Hans-Christoph Steinhausen, Veronica Nestler, and Hans-Ludwig Spohr

*Department of Child and Adolescent Psychiatry and Neurology,
Free University of Berlin*

Extended psychiatric and pediatric examinations were performed on patients with the fetal alcohol syndrome (FAS). A subgroup of these patients underwent psychological testing to measure intelligence, visual perception, and psycholinguistic abilities. Psychopathology was also studied in a matched control group. The investigation revealed a broad scale of developmental hazards and psychopathologic symptoms indicating the negative long-range effects of alcohol abuse during pregnancy. The extent of morphologic damage was found to be a good predictor of psychopathology and mental impairment. Social environment and socioeconomic status appear less important as predictors.

In recent years, there has been increasing concern about the deleterious effects of alcohol abuse during pregnancy. Beginning with the first mention of the problem in France by Lamache[1] in 1967 and Lemoine[2] in 1968 and the initial description of the fetal alcohol syndrome (FAS) by Jones et al.[3] in the U.S. in 1973, an increasing number of publications

Reprinted with permission from *Developmental and Behavioral Pediatrics*, 1982, Vol. 3, No. 2, 49–54.

have dealt with the numerous physical malformations and developmental hazards associated with FAS. Patients with the syndrome have been identified and documented throughout the world.[4-17] By 1978, more than 400 reports on FAS had been published.

Clarren and Smith[18] recently reviewed a total of 245 reported cases and concluded that the broad variety of symptoms induced by the teratogenicity of alcohol can be classified into four categories. In addition to mental and developmental retardation, present among 85% of the total population reviewed in their survey, Clarren and Smith also encountered reports of retarded growth and a characteristic pattern of facial abnormalities in connection with major and minor malformations. Readers primarily interested in the dysmorphic characteristics of this syndrome are referred to the literature cited above.

Although the vast majority of descriptions of the clinical symptoms emphasize mental retardation as a major feature of FAS, there has been very little detailed reporting on the psychopathology of affected patients. More recently, the literature has begun to deal with such phenomena in greater detail. An interim report of an ongoing study in Sweden[10,11] noted that 19% of the 52 FAS patients examined had IQs lower than 70 and 40% had IQs ranging from 70 to 85. These data are derived from a retrospective analysis; prospective examination of a group of 16 patients revealed a mean IQ of 94 (SD = 11), which was 19 units below the mean score of the control group selected. In addition, the FAS children scored lower in tests involving visual perception and motor development.

A group in Seattle[19] measured the intelligence of 20 FAS patients and recorded a mean IQ of 65, with a range of 16 to 105. Among 60% of these patients, mental functioning was 2 standard deviations below the mean. A close correlation between IQ and severity of the syndrome was established; seriously damaged children had a mean IQ of 55, compared to a mean of 82 among mildly impaired children. During the preschool years, the children in the FAS sample exhibited marked hyperactivity but no serious behavioral disturbances. In school, problems arose mainly due to learning disorders and hyperactivity. Three children displayed both emotional and behavioral disorders, and eating problems during infancy and preschool years were frequent.

Most of the currently available literature reveals significant gaps in reporting and is descriptive in nature. With the exception of IQ tests, psychological parameters have rarely been recorded or measured, and observations on psychopathology remain anecdotal. Finally, there is a lack of studies dealing with the determinants of FAS. It thus seems necessary to direct more of our attention to the factors of social background in addition to problems of morphologic damage.

METHOD

Subjects

The patients were extracted from the patient population of the major pediatric clinics, foster homes, and several private pediatric practices in Berlin, West Germany, over a period of three years (1977–1979). Due to age differences and problems related to availability of patients for examination and of case history data, it was not possible to use all of the methods and techniques with the entire sample. Developmental histories existed for a total of 68 patients, with a mean age of 52.0 months (SD = 34.8; range, 2–186 months). In only 49 cases were we able to examine social history and to perform psychiatric examinations. This reduction in sample size was primarily due to the fact that some of the children were living in foster homes where complete information was not available. Because the psychiatric interview was designed for subjects 3 years of age and older, the sample size was further reduced on this measure. The mean age of this group was 61.0 months (SD = 35.5; range, 36–186 months). Finally, psychological tests could be administered only to a limited age group of 32 patients. This group had a mean age of 75.6 months (SD = 34.1; range, 36–186 months).

To assess the significance of the psychiatric interview findings, a control group of 28 healthy children, matched for age, sex, and socioeconomic status, was also studied. These children were free of pre-, peri- and/or postnatal risks to CNS development or other chronic afflictions. At the time of the examination, the mean age of control subjects was 77.3 months (SD = 30.0; range, 39–133 months).

To offset the possible deleterious effects of living in a setting away from the biological parents (quite frequent in the clinical sample), a similar percentage of healthy children living in foster homes was also included in the control group. Characteristics of the FAS and control subjects who underwent developmental and psychiatric examination are illustrated in Table 1.

Procedure

The diagnosis of FAS was established by a thorough pediatric examination, performed by two experienced pediatricians (V.N. and H.-

TABLE 1. Sample Characteristics of Children Who Received Developmental and Psychiatric Examinations

Variable	FAS		Controls	
	N	%	N	%
Sex				
Male	31	63.3	16	57.1
Female	18	36.7	12	42.9
Social environment				
Biological parents	20	40.9	13	46.0
Foster parents	10	20.3	0	0
Institution	19	38.8	15	53.6
Socioeconomic status				
Unknown	14	28.6	15	53.7
Lower class	19	38.7	6	21.3
Middle class	16	32.7	7	25.0

L.S.), that assessed all malformations and minor anomalies according to a scheme developed by Majewsky[10] and by maternal drinking history. The latter revealed an average daily alcohol consumption of 140 g (SD = 72 g) of alcohol during the critical phase of pregnancy. In addition, the children were given a standardized neurologic examination according to methods developed by Touwen and Prechtl.[20]

Because the available literature contained no precise data on psychiatric morbidity, we decided to use a structured interview covering a wide range of items related to development and psychopathology. Each item was rated on a 3-point scale (0 = none, 1 = mild, 2 = severe). This interview was a modification of an instrument developed by Richman and Graham,[21] which has received several tests of reliability, validity, and applicability in clinical research.[22,23] The psychological test battery was adapted to the age group and was broad enough to cover projected areas of interest. This battery included German versions of several English-language tests: the Columbia Mental Maturity Scale (CMMS) for measuring intelligence, an abbreviated and recently standardized version of the Vineland Social Maturity Scale (VSMS), the Frostig Test of Visual Perception (FTVP), and the Illinois Test of Psycholinguistic Abilities (ITPA).

RESULTS

Our sample is compared with data from the Clarren and Smith survey[18] in Table 2. This table also includes the scores and distributions for

TABLE 2. Comparison of FAS Sample with Previous Literature

Item	Current Study			Clarren and Smith (%)
	Score[a]	N	%	
Pre-/Postnatal growth deficiency	4	58	81.7	> 80
Mental retardation	2/4	66	93.0	> 80
Microcephaly	4	65	91.5	> 80
Hyperactivity	4	51	71.8	> 50
Hypotonia	2	46	64.8	> 50
Epicanthal folds	2	48	67.6	26–50
Blepharophimosis	2	35	49.3	> 80
Ptosis	2	10	14.1	26–50
Strabismus	0	19	26.8	26–50
Short upturned nose	3	37	52.1	> 50
Thinned upper vermilion	1	49	69.0	> 80
Gothic palate	2	30	42.2	26–50
Cleft palate	4	5	7.0	1–25
Hypoplastic teeth	0	22	31.0	1–25
Minor ear anomalies	0	42	59.2	26–50
Retrognathia	2	58	81.7	50
Abnormal palmar creases	3	37	52.1	26–50
Phalangeal anomalies (minor)	1	7	9.9	1–25
Limited joint movement	2	8	11.3	1–25
Cardiac defects	4	24	33.6	26–50
Hemangiomas	0	8	11.3	26–50
Congenital hip dislocation	0	10	14.1	—
Hernias	2	18	25.4	1–25
Minor external genital anomalies	2/4	28	39.4	1–50
Coccygeal fovea	1	42	59.1	—
Renal anomalies	4	6	8.0	1–25
Severity[b]				
Grade 1	10–29	31	43.7	—
Grade 2	30–39	24	33.8	—
Grade 3	40	16	22.5	—

[a] Weighted score for each item, according to Majewski.[10]
[b] Obtained by summing up scores for the individual items of each subject.

each of the individual symptoms. This comparison reveals that our patients had the same classic pattern of FAS described in the international literature.

It was found that, compared to the control group, the FAS children (1) had mothers who were older at time of birth (mean = 26.0 years vs. 37.7; t = 4.09, df = 87.4, p < .001), (2) weighed less at birth (mean = 3137 vs. 2310 g; t = −3.83, df = 44.7, p < .001), (3) had higher sibling ranks (mean = 1.5 vs. 3.0; t = 4.29, df = 91.7, p < .001) and (4) were born into larger families (mean number of siblings = 1.0 vs. 2.6; t = 3.97, df = 91, p < .001). Figure 1 compares the early histories of the two groups; only those items which significantly distinguished the two groups (by chi-square analysis) are included. The FAS mothers' abuse of alcohol was accompanied by nicotine abuse also. Paternal alcohol abuse was also quite frequent. Children suffering from FAS had high rates of complications during the neonatal period, such as feeding problems, failure to thrive, and a significantly higher susceptibility to serious illnesses during the first 2 years of life. In addition, separation from the mother was more frequent among the children suffering from FAS, although fewer of these mothers than control mothers were continuously

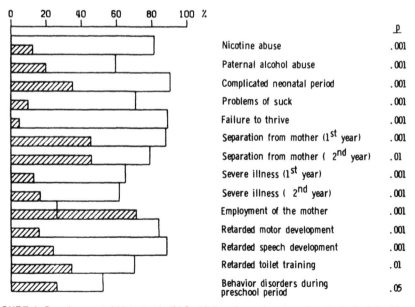

FIGURE 1. Developmental histories in FAS children (open bars) and controls (hatched bars).

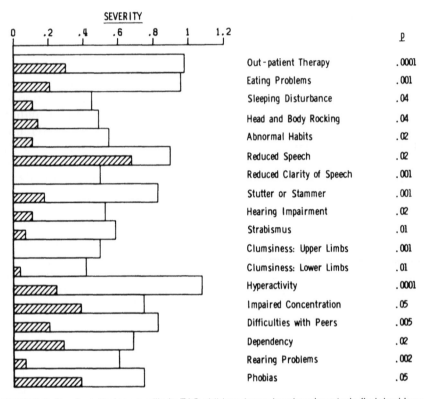

FIGURE 2. Psychopathology profile in FAS children (open bars) and controls (hatched bars

employed. Typical milestones of motor and speech development and toilet training were more often retarded among the FAS children. Finally, the older FAS children more often had behavioral problems during the preschool period.

From a total of 60 items in the psychiatric interview, 18 emerged as indicators of significant differences between the two samples ($p < .05$, chi-square). All of these items were rated on either a frequency or an intensity scale; mean profiles are presented in Figure 2 for the two groups. Compared to controls, the FAS children had greater frequencies of outpatient therapy, eating and sleeping problems, head and body rocking, stereotyped habits (e.g., facial tics, nail biting, hair plucking), reduced vocabulary and clarity of speech, speech impairment (stammering and/or stuttering), hearing impairments, and strabismus. The FAS children were also more susceptible to general clumsiness, hyperactivity, and inattentiveness. Finally, the FAS children had more diffi-culties in peer relationships, tended to be more generally dependent, and had more problems with management and phobias in general. In addition to these statistically significant differences, a number of other items tended to distinguish the two groups (p = .10), indicating more frequent encopresis, enuresis, and temper tantrums among the FAS children.

Psychological testing also revealed indications of functional impair-ments among the FAS patients. Because psychological testing could not be done with the control group, analysis was restricted to comparisons with standard data by computation of standardized scores and confi-dence intervals. Mean (T) scores were 42.5 for intelligence and 31.4 for social maturity. Both scores are significantly lower (p < .05) than the population norm on both scales. (Transformed into the standard IQ scale, the mean IQ would be 89; mean social maturity = 71). The mean score for visual perception (37.8 on the percentile scale) was also statis-tically lower (p < .05) than the population mean. A broad pattern of psycholinguistic impairment was also found (T = 42.8 compared to the population norm of 50, p. < .05).

In an effort to gauge the impact of morphologic damage on the psy-chopathology of the FAS children, several indices of physical and psy-chological impairment were correlated. From the standardized neurologic examination, we calculated indices of focal deficits and coordination problems. Pediatric assessment of dysmorphic signs led to the devel-opment of an index of severity of malformations (Table 2). Data on levels of alcohol consumption and birth weights were also incorporated into the analyses. These indices were correlated with IQ and with a

TABLE 3. Predictors of IQ and Psychopathology*

Predictor	IQ		Index of Psycho-pathology	
	r	N	r	N
Focal deficits	−.40[a]	25	−.05	26
Coordination problems	−.47[b]	25	−.01	26
Severity of FAS	−.35[a]	32	−.35[a]	49
Maternal alcohol consumption	−.68[a]	8	−.10	17
Birth weight	−.33[a]	29	−.09	45

* Spearman correlation coefficients.
[a] p < .05.
[b] p < .01.

TABLE 4. Relations of FAS Severity and Psychological
Variables (Mean Ranks, Mann-Whitney U Test)

Variable	Grade 1 (Mild)	Grade 2 or 3 (Severe)	U	p
Eye-motor coordination	15.8	7.9	103.0	.003
Figure-ground relation-ships	15.6	8.0	101.5	.004
Constancy of forms	14.1	9.3	86.5	.08
Position in space	13.4	9.9	79.5	N.S.
Spatial relationships	15.0	8.5	95.5	.01
Total score	15.9	9.0	104.0	.01
Social maturity	22.4	16.4	223.0	.09

further index of psychopathology comprised of the total sum of symptom scores. The findings are illustrated in Table 3. Intelligence was negatively correlated with neurologic damage, severity of the syndrome, and level of alcohol consumption, and positively correlated with birth weight. The index of psychopathology was significantly correlated only with severity of FAS. Similar analyses correlating FAS severity with psychological test data revealed poorer performance in the areas of visual perception and social maturity for children suffering from severe FAS (Table 4).

In separate analyses of variance, we studied the effects of sex, age, socioeconomic status, and social environment on the total score for psychopathologic symptoms. (The social environment factor was introduced to differentiate between children who lived with their biological parents and those who lived with foster parents or had been raised in children's homes.) It was found that boys had higher scores than girls ($F = 8.29$, $df = 1, 43$, $p. = .005$) and older children tended to have significantly lower scores ($F = 3.50$, $df = 1, 43$, $p = .06$) for psychopathologic symptoms. By contrast, both socioeconomic status and social environment appeared to have no effect on the psychiatric status of the children ($F = .98$ and 1.12, respectively).

DISCUSSION

This study of the development and psychological functioning of children with the fetal alcohol syndrome revealed that several problems occurred more frequently in this group than among matched controls. The differences observed may be attributable primarily to prenatal maternal alcohol consumption, inasmuch as the potentially detrimental effects of being raised in a foster home were controlled. In addition to maternal alcohol abuse, high rates of nicotine abuse correlated positively with reduced birth weight and retarded intrauterine growth, as has been reported by others.[24–26] Paternal alcohol abuse was also frequent. Thus, these children may have suffered from a combination of teratogenic and genetic factors from conception.

Postnatal development and life events then involved a chain of detrimental circumstances, including feeding problems, failure to thrive, and repeated hospitalization in the neonatal and infancy periods. In addition, the FAS children tended to experience higher rates of separation from their parents, a factor generally believed to be deleterious to development in this age group. It is possible that these children have also suffered from disturbances in bonding and other deficits in the mother-child relationship. Developmental retardation was evident in the areas of motor functions, speech, and toilet training. Data collected retrospectively indicated that behavioral problems (temper tantrums, hyperactivity, and dependency) were apparent in the preschool period, a finding which contrasts to some extent with results of a previous study.[19]

Detailed psychiatric examination revealed a broad pattern of characteristic symptoms manifested more often among the FAS children than among the matched controls. The data indicate that it is not sufficient to search for indicators of mental retardation or impaired psychological functioning alone. We must expect numerous psychiatric symptoms in FAS children, which can lead to further problems. In the present study, we recorded high rates of eating and sleeping problems, head and body rocking, stereotyped habits, speech and hearing impairment, strabismus, general clumsiness, hyperactivity, and inattentiveness. Several of these psychiatric symptoms may be clearly traced to prenatal morphologic damage. Symptoms such as hyperactivity may have been genetically transmitted; there is some limited evidence that the hyperkinetic syndrome is genetically linked to alcoholism, at least in some cases.[27,28]

However, we must exert great caution in attempting to explain the symptoms observed here solely on the basis of organic or genetic factors. Multiple interactions are a more probable exploratory framework in that many of the recorded symptoms can also be linked to poor environments. Disturbances in peer relationships and the high rates of dependency and difficulties encountered in upbringing imply problems in social interaction which can lead to further difficulties for the FAS child.

Psychological testing demonstrated that social maturity, visual perception, and psycholinguistic abilities, as well as intelligence, were negatively affected in the FAS children. Again, some of these findings reflect the severity of prenatal brain damage. It becomes apparent from these findings that the children with FAS require remedial training and therapy to promote and develop social skills, psychomotor functions, visual perceptions, and speech facilities.

This study clearly documented that the amount of neurologic damage is a good predictor of psychopathology and mental impairment. Intellectual capacities can be predicted on the basis of neurologic assessment, as well as knowledge of prenatal maternal alcohol consumption and birth weight. Given the scope of psychopathology seen and the multiplicity of causal factors, it is remarkable that amount of morphologic damage was the only good predictor of the number of psychiatric symptoms. We found little indication that socioeconomic background had a comparable effect. Age and sex tended to correlate with psychopathologic status, but socioeconomic status and social environment did not. It thus appears that prenatal morphologic damage is the key determinant of development and psychopathology. It must be noted that our study model did not provide an adequate means of dealing with the reciprocal effects of intrauterine exposure to alcohol and general socialization. This issue requires further longitudinal analysis.

To conclude, a multidimensional interdisciplinary approach provided substantial evidence that children suffering from the fetal alcohol syndrome are susceptible to a wide variety of developmental hazards that are related to the severity of morphologic damage. It remains to be seen whether these handicaps will persist or diminish during the course of maturation and development. It is probable that seriously affected children will endure some lasting retardation and handicaps that will not respond to rehabilitative measures. On the other hand, many FAS children deserve and would benefit from remedial training and therapy.

REFERENCES

1. Lamache, A. M. (1967). Reflexion sur la descendance des alcooliques. *Bulletin of the Academy of National Medicine*, 151:517.
2. Lemoine, P., Harousseau, H., Boteyru, J. P. et al. (1968). Les enfants de parents alcooliques. Anomalies observées à propos de 127 cas. *Quest. Med.*, 25:477.
3. Jones, K. L., Smith, D. M., Ulleland, C. et al. (1973). Pattern of malformation in offspring of chronic alcoholic mothers. *Lancet*, 1:1267–1271.
4. Jones, K. L., Smith, D. W., Streissguth, A. P. et al. (1974). Outcome in offspring of chronic alcoholic women. *Lancet*, 1:1076–1078.
5. Jones, K. L. and Smith, D. W. (1975). The fetal alcohol syndrome. *Teratology*, 12:1–10.

6. Hanson, J. W., Jones, K. L. and Smith, D. W. (1976). Fetal alcohol syndrome. Experience with 41 patients. *Journal of the American Medical Association*, 235:1458–1460.
7. Bierich, J. R., Majewski, F., Michaelis, R. et al. (1976). Das embryofetale Alkoholsyndrom. *European Journal of Pediatrics*, 121:151–157.
8. Samaille-Villette, C. and Samaille, P. P. Le syndrome d'alcoolisme foetal. A propos de 47 observations. Medical Thesis, University of Lille.
9. Shurygin, G. I. (1974). Ob osobennostiiakh psikhickeskogo razvitiia detel ot materel stradaiushchikh khronicheskim alkoholizmom. *Pediatriia*, 11:71–73.
10. Majewski, F. (1978). Uber schädigende Einflüsse des Alkohols auf die Nachkommen. *Nervenarzt.*, 49:410–416.
11. Fiocchi, A., Colombini, A. and Codara, L. (1978). La embriopatia alcoolica. Rassegna della letteratura e contributo personale. *Minerva Pediat.*, 30:9–28.
12. Clarren, S. K., Alvord, E. C., Sumi, S. M. et al. (1978). Brain malformations related to prenatal exposure to ethanol. *Journal of Pediatrics*, 92:64–67.
13. Hayden, M. R. and Nelson, M. M. (1979). The fetal alcohol syndrome. *South Africa Medical Journal*, 54:571–574.
14. Kyllerman, M., Aronsson, A., Karlberg, E. et al. (1979). Epidemiologic and neuropediatric aspects of the fetal alcohol syndrome. *Neuropädiatrie*, 10 (Suppl):435–436.
15. Olegard, R., Sabel, K.-G., Aronsson, M. et al. (1979). Effects on the child of alcohol abuse during pregnancy. *Acta Paediatrica Scandinavica* (Suppl), 275:112–121.
16. Scianaro, L., Prusek, W. and Loiodice, G. (1979). La sindrome del feto alcolizzato. Observazione cliniche. *Minerva Pediat.*, 30:1585–1588.
17. Puespoeky, G. (1979). Embryopathia alcoholica. *Orv. Hetil.*, 120:775–777.
18. Clarren, S. K. and Smith, D. W. (1978). The fetal alcohol syndrome. Experience with 65 patients and a review of the world literature. *New England Journal of Medicine*, 298:1063-1067.
19. Streissguth, A. P., Herman, C. S. and Smith, D. W. (1978). Intelligence, behavior and dysmorphogenesis in the fetal alcohol syndrome: A report on 20 patients. *Journal of Pediatrics*, 92:363–367.
20. Touwen, B. L. and Prechtl, N. F. R. (1970). *The Neurological Examination of the Child with Minor Nervous Dysfunction*. London: Heinemann Medical.
21. Richman, N. and Graham, P. J. (1971). A behavioral screening questionnaire for use with three-year-old children. Preliminary findings. *Journal of Child Psychology and Psychiatry*, 12:5–33.
22. Richman, N. (1977). Is a behaviour checklist for pre-school children useful? In *Epidemiological Approaches in Child Psychiatry*, P. J. Graham, ed. London: Academic Press.
23. Richman, N. Short-term outcome of behavioural problems in three year old children. *Ibid.*
24. Rantakallio, P. (1979). Social background of mothers who smoke during pregnancy and influence of these factors on the offspring. *Soc. Sci. Med.—Med. Psychol. Soc.*, 13:423–429.
25. Fielding, J. E. and Yankauer, A. (1978). The pregnant smoker. *American Journal of Public Health*, 68:835–836.
26. Persson, R.-H., Grennert, L., Gennser, G. et al. (1978). A study of smoking and pregnancy with special reference to fetal growth. *Acta Obstet. Gynecol. Scand.* (Suppl), 78:33–39.
27. Goodwin, D. W., Schulsinger, F., Hermansen, L. et al. (1975). Alcoholism and the hyperactive child syndrome. *Journal of Nervous and Mental Disease*, 160:349–353.
28. Morrison, J. R. and Stewart, M. A. (1973). Evidence for polygenetic inheritance in the hyperactive child syndrome. *American Journal of Psychiatry*, 130:791–792.

Part VIII

ETHICAL AND LEGAL ISSUES

One of the broad social movements of the past few decades has been the challenge to the traditional biases which restricted the civil rights of women, minority groups, and the mentally ill. This has now been extended to children, with a new serious look at the rationale for the disenfranchisement of children because of their "immaturity."

Gaylin takes up this question of the competence of children, and explores most thoughtfully its moral, ethical, and psychological implications. His subtitle, "No Longer All or None" provides the theme of his exposition. Simplistic legalistic formulas are not possible, considering the interplay of the child's own viewpoint, the responsibility of the parents, the needs of society, and the competence of the child to evaluate the immediate and long-term consequences of his or her decision. Gaylin identifies the dilemmas and hard choices that the researcher and clinician face in many situations. General principles are necessary, but the decisions still have to weigh all the pertinent factors in individual cases.

Knitzer focuses on the legal issues of the children's rights movement. She provides a historical survey and reviews the most important questions, illustrated by well-selected cases. Like Gaylin, she emphasizes the complexities of the issues involved, as reflected in her subtitle "Dilemmas and Realities." She is especially concerned with the necessity for the struggle for the rights of children who are poor or handicapped, who are members of minority groups, or who have grown up without the benefit of any real parents.

The final paper, by Ilfeld and co-workers, reports a study of a large series of custody cases, the results of which suggest that joint custody is a more beneficial arrangement in terms of reduced parental conflict. The authors are aware of the limitations of their study because of the nature of their sample, but their report does highlight the importance of this question for the welfare of the children of divorced parents.

505

ETHICAL AND LEGAL ISSUES

33

The "Competence" of Children: No Longer All or None

Willard Gaylin

College of Physicians and Surgeons, Columbia University, New York

Traditionally, under a fixed age set by the state, the child existed as an essentially disenfranchised member of the community. Current developments are demanding a variability in our assignment of autonomous rights, forcing a concept of "variable" competency. The courts increasingly require guidance as to "maturity" and "judgment" of children in their capacity to speak for themselves. This paper attempts to define some of the general conditions that limit competence and begins the process of establishing some general guidelines to help in deciding when we ought to allow children to enter into the decision-making process in important areas concerning their lives and futures.

FROM ARBITRARY TO VARIABLE COMPETENCE

On the day before one's 18th birthday (21st in some states), an individual under law traditionally existed as an essentially disenfranchised member of the state. He lived according to laws set by others, governed

Reprinted with permission from the *Journal of the American Academy of Child Psychiatry*, 1982, Vol. 21, No. 2, 153–162. Copyright 1982 by the American Academy of Child Psychiatry.

Dr. Gaylin is Clinical Professor of Psychiatry, College of Physicians & Surgeons, and President of The Hastings Center, Institute of Society, Ethics and the Life Sciences.

A modified version of this paper will appear in Who Speaks for the Child: The Problems of Proxy Consent, Plenum Press, 1982.

The material was prepared with the joint support of the National Science Foundation, grant No. 0SS74-12745, and the National Endowment for the Humanities.

by leaders in whose selection he had no part, and with little or no control over his estates and fortune. One day later that same individual was miraculously transformed, and was welcomed into the decision-making apparatus of his country.

It is patent that one 18-year-old differs from another. Nonetheless, we ignored distinctions in intelligence, wisdom, impulsiveness, maturity, emotional stability, balance of selfishness and greed, conscience, and public service.

We preferred a fixed definition for competence—with full awareness that in the "real" world there would be marked variability in true competence—over the greater accuracy of individual judgment, with its unwieldiness, subjectivity, and unlimited potential for corruptibility.

Increasingly, however, the insistence on a fixed age of competence is being undermined. Not just because case law is operating on an *ad hoc* basis to destroy that position, but also because the conditions of the new technology (e.g., safe abortion techniques) and the new decisions they require—in addition to the temper of the times—mitigate against it.

To the argument that one cannot determine maturity, the answer is now being presented that, to an extent, we always automatically had. The decision to use 18 years instead of 18 months was, after all, not an arbitrary one. There is obviously an easy distinction between an 18-year-old and an 18-month-old. There are, as well, distinctions between an 18-year-old and a 14-year-old, but here the distinguishing factors are much less evident.

However, even if one concurred that an arbitrary age determinant might in the long run be more secure from abuse, or more "just," the current pressures from society at large, particularly in the areas of medical research and treatment, are demanding a variability in our assignment of autonomous rights, and forcing a concept of variable competence.

Some of the reasons for adopting a concept of variable competence that were suggested in a previous article (Gaylin, 1979) are worth reexamining. We live in a society that has elevated individual rights beyond any example, with the possible exception of our own country in the late 19th century. We are emotionally committed to autonomy, and we assume the state somehow survives despite our emphasis on liberty and the rights of individual decision-making.

Currently we are going beyond even this; we are raising the individual and his rights to a higher position of power in relationship to the other institutions of social life that traditionally had been perceived as benevolent, and therefore less threatening to autonomy than the state. The power of the individual in relationship to the caring professions—and the rights of self-determination in medical treatment—has certainly been extended. In addition, we are now questioning the power of the individual within (and against) the family, even when the individual is *legally* still a child.

Concern about the disenfranchised and the disadvantaged in our country has led to an increase in the casting of moral arguments in terms of the language of rights; we are only just beginning to see a return to respectability of the concept of "responsibility." Responsibility, obligation, and duty imply to too many (unfortunately) a paternalism that has been in disrepute in our modern, liberal time. No better spokesman for this distress exists than that quintessential, liberal humanist Lionel Trilling (1950): "Some paradox of our nature leads us," he states, "when once we have made our fellow man the object of our pity, then of our wisdom, ultimately of our coercion."

This belief in the ultimate corruptibility of power—even when in the hands of the benevolent institutions of our society—has led to such extreme arguments as Thomas Szasz's defense of the rights of suicide even for an individual who is temporarily delusional due to toxicity; or pressing the rights of the mentally retarded, even to the point of permitting physical parenthood when actual child-rearing is impossible.

It is to prevent the corruption of benevolence, "the most ironic and tragic that man knows" (Trilling, 1950) that has led us to distrust all paternalism and demand its exclusion from a role in our social system.

But there is one place where paternalism cannot be abandoned, and that is in the relationship of parent to child. Here an abandonment of parental authority would be an act of immorality, as well as a failure in nurturing. The good parents do not just nurture to a point of maturation; they are expected to inhibit self-destructive impulses; they are expected to substitute their superior judgment for the short vision of the child; they are expected to use education, persuasion, seduction, and even force and coercion when necessary in the service of producing a healthy and independent adult.

The distrust of paternalism has not, however, stopped at the borders of the family. As a result, the expanding claims of individual rights are now in conflict with two other ideals that have also traditionally been highly valued: one is the principle of paternal authority, i.e., the acceptance of paternalism at least within the family; and second, the concept of family autonomy, that is that just as there are certain rights vested in the individual (as against the state), there have been traditional powers vested in the family, which have been deemed to be independent of state interest. Obviously, at its limits—as in enforced blood transfusions of the

Jehovah's Witnesses' children—we have consistently been prepared to invade family autonomy. But the very nature of the invasion and the use of the courts to do so has implicitly recognized that, for the most part, the decision-making apparatus must abide with the family. Only in extremis do we intrude. Now, however, we are intruding increasingly more as we expand our concepts of rights of self-determination even for those of limited competence. One thinks of the legal right of the 12-year-old girl to an abortion without the knowledge or consent of her parents (although she still requires her parents' permission to be released from classes).

The problem then remains to define some of the conditions that limit competence; and some of the border areas where those limitations may not be so great as once had been thought, and where we may begin to allow the individual of limited competence to enter into the decision-making process concerning important elements of his or her life and future.

LIMITING CONDITIONS TO COMPETENCE

Competent, at its most basic definition, means capable. Competence as it is used in this paper, however, refers to the legal acknowledgment by the state of one's capability, by the granting of autonomous rights. First, it might help to examine conditions that limit "actual" competence. I shall examine the conditions that limit one's capability to take charge of one's life—to make the decisions which are normally considered one's decisions to make. The limiting conditions may be divided into the following categories: (1) limits of consciousness, (2) limits of intelligence, (3) limits of rationality, (4) limits of perception, (5) limits of experience, and (6) limits of age.

Limits of Consciousness

As with most questions that relate to mental functioning, the normal limits occur along a spectrum from the extremes. One obvious extreme, and in that sense perhaps the easiest case, is the unconscious patient. The fact that he may be an intact perceptual being—only in a transient state of incapacity—is beside the point. During the state of unconsciousness there is absolutely no way for him to communicate what his desires might be, and he is, therefore, totally incompetent.

Even at the extreme of unconsciousness, however, there are conditions which ought to alter our attitudes. The rules for usurping a person's

autonomous rights will vary depending on the length of time we anticipate he will remain unconscious. With the permanently unconscious we
feel free to intervene for minor decisions, because we are obliged to
make *all* decisions. With the temporarily unconscious we may even take
risks, close to the point of survival, to avoid decision, with the acknowledgment that only a matter of hours (or minutes) may free the individual
to participate in the decision-making himself. Therefore, even with a
seemingly easy case of the unconscious individual there is a spectrum
of judgment and doubt.

Limits of Intelligence

When we move away from absolute incommunicability as represented
by the unconscious person, we enter into that more complex spectrum
of issues that plague the competent/incompetent polarity. At the most
extreme end of the spectrum, the severely retarded person, although
conscious, is demonstrably not competent by nature of his or her limited
intelligence to make important decisions. At that level of retardation,
speech is, of course, not present, but a severely retarded person's limitation is not just one of communication, which would link him to the
unconscious, but rather his inability to assess or determine his own best
interests. Even were he capable of communicating by grunting or nod-
ding, most of us would not honor his decision not to take a health-
preserving medication.

As we move up the level of retardation, we will again come to a border
area where the intelligence of the retarded will need to be weighed
against the seriousness of the decision and multiple other variables involving dignity, social well-being, and the like, complicating our decision
in advocating autonomy.

Limits of Rationality

If the severely retarded person is not competent, neither is the gifted
toddler. He is not competent either because he has not reached the age
of communication or, having reached that age, his perception of his
world and his place in it, or his grasp of the problems of the world and
their implications, is too limited. Or it may be that he still lacks moral
and psychological development. This entire classification could be broken down into a number of specific variables, but many of them can be
lumped together under the heading of rationality—our suspicion of the
reasonableness of his decision. Here our doubts arise not because he is

not intelligent, but because we recognize that there are many more components to reason than simple ability to learn.

Limits of Knowledge and Perception

Examples from the field of mental health are particularly suited to explore the bridge between the concepts of rationality and perception. But here, too, it may be better to step back from a controversial category such as mental health, and first examine a physical example. If a blind man is about to walk into a busy thoroughfare, without knowing it he may be hit by an object he does not perceive or, indeed, see, and we are free to knock him down without being accused of an assault. In this case we recognize that the limits of his perception modify the nature of his behavior, so as to seriously bring into question whether his behavior is serving his purposes. We have a right to nullify his decision because we recognize that the end of his behavior is to get to the other side of the street, not to be squashed under the wheels of a truck.

There are emotional conditions that limit one's "perceptions" as severely as do sensory deficiencies. The phobic overreacts to certain harmless things because of the symbolic value with which he endows them and can be made to jump out of a window to protect himself from that which realistically is no threat to his survival. Our knowledge or assumption that the individual is attempting to avoid danger would justify our "restricting his liberty" by barring him from the window, at least until the imagined threat could be eliminated.

Another limit of perception would involve areas where the absence of factual knowledge raises questions about whether the person's behavior coincides with his purpose. Those ignorant of explosives or firearms should be protected from their limits of knowledge which border on limits of perception. It is easy to see that with this fourth category we are now entering areas more and more controversial, with a wider spread, and a greater potential for corruptibility.

Limits of Experience

It was William James who wisely distinguished between knowledge of something and knowing about something. Surely, part of what goes into our abridgment of autonomy of the child is the recognition that while he might be conscious, intelligent, rational, and probably quite perceptive, the nature of his experience has distorted his capacity for sound judgment. An adolescent might well value ambulation over life. To ask a 12-year-old for permission to amputate a leg to save his life is to prematurely impose judgments on the value of life that demand more "living" (i.e., more knowledge of life) than can be condensed into 12 years. A mere examination of the precipitating factors in suicide attempts of adolescents indicates the degree to which factors that will seem trivial in later life can tip the balance for a teenager: the failure to be elected to public office in a high school, being dropped from an athletic team, a low SAT score, a disappointment in a love affair.

It will be argued that experience and maturity vary with normal adults, which of course they do, and I am not prepared to say that we must give a test of experience to each adult. We can, however, depend—as we do in all rule-setting—on a statistical average which justifies the rule. Generally, one sees "maturity" increasing with age, at least to a limited point.

Limits of Age

Here we have returned to the comfortable and arbitrary origin of the original rule of competence. Age, in many ways, is seen as the summation of intelligence, rationality, perception and experience. We assume a coming together and a maturation of these faculties at a certain time when we, the society, are willing to take the risk of allowing the child into the moral community and the world's political decision-making. In the past, we had been prepared to say that statistically the balance tips for freedom and away from paternalism at a specific age. Our current dissatisfaction with a specific arbitrary test of competence is related to the complexity of decisions which we now face, and the incredible consequences of many of them. It is for this reason that we must begin the examination of the evidence of competence to establish a variable grid, establishing competence at differing ages, for different decisions.

We are in that difficult area of defining what is a child and when does he leave childhood. By Peters' (1972) definition, children are seen to "finally pass to the level of autonomy when they appreciate that rules are alterable, that they can be criticized and should be accepted or rejected on a basis of reciprocity and fairness. The emergence of rational reflections about rules . . . central to the Kantian conception of autonomy, is the main feature of the final level of moral development."

On the other hand, the age of autonomy would never be achieved if we were to use the decision of Judge S. Lee Vavuris in a 1977 case involving five members, aged 21 to 26, of the church of the Reverend Sun Myung Moon. Judge Vavuris awarded these "children" to their parents under a conservatorship law usually reserved for senile adults who are incompetent. "We are talking about the essence of civilization—mother, father, and children. There is nothing like it. I know of no greater love than parents' for their children, and I'm sure they would not submit their children to harm. The child is the child, even though a parent may be 19 and the child, 60" (Ledbetter, 1977).

It is part of the complication of the English language that with all its richness (3 times as many words as German or French) we seem to use only the word "child" to denote both the progeny and the young. It may be a reflection of the fact that we tend to respond to *our* children always as though they *were* children (incomplete and dependent). But surely, even Judge Vavuris would not have us bind the 20-year-old, let alone the 60-year-old, to complete economic and sociological dependence on his parents. "The search for a single test of competency is a search for a Holy Grail. Unless it is recognized that there is no magical definition of competency to make decisions about treatment, the search for an acceptable test will never end. Getting the words just right is only part of the problem. In practice, judgments of competency go beyond semantics or straightforward applications of legal rules; such judgments reflect social considerations and societal biases as much as they reflect matters of law and medicine" (Roth et al., 1977).

If this is true for competence, it is exquisitely so when we begin to adjust definitions of competency to accommodate special cases—when we move from an absolute to a variable concept of competence.

VARIABLE COMPETENCE

What is necessary at this point is the establishment of a grid—crude though it may be—that sets some limits and identifies some principles upon which we can begin to fill in the specifics of variable competence. This ought to be done before we are forced to conclude, let us say, that at age 11 a child should have the right to decide to have an abortion or, indeed, to carry to term without parental guidance or permission; or that a 13-year-old will be free to consent to sex, as has recently been proposed in the State of New Jersey. At this stage, what is most urgently needed is an outline of principles, which others may modify according to their value systems and in terms of the specific situations of different cases. It should be explicitly understood from the start that this first attempt will be acknowledgedly crude. It is hoped that the argument here will start a process that can lead to a refinement of the ideas presented.

In its peculiar way, the law does not view competence as indigenous to the person, but rather as something with which one is vested by society. It is a judgment of maturity. At age 13 the Jewish child shall be permitted to be a full participant in the house of God. In some states of our country a child does not become an adult, in terms of the privilege of determining his representatives in government, until age 18—in others at age 21. Many states allow a 16-year-old woman the right to determine whether she shall have sexual intercourse; under 16, her agreement has no standing in law. Even were she to seduce a "mature" (over 16) man, *he* will be guilty of the charge of statutory rape. At age 14, at age 15, at age 18, at age 21 (there are certain trusts and estates that can limit control until age 35, 45, and 60), the law will arbitrarily invest a person with competence to make his or her own decisions.

How should we judge? How can we bring some order, some sensibility to the chaotic and contradictory code that emerges when these decisions are left to case law?

To simplify matters in this thicket of variables, I have decided to focus on "medical" procedures, recognizing that even the definition of what is, or is not, a medical procedure is an arbitrary and elusive one.

Before reducing the data to a grid, it is best to understand the way the terms will be used. There are at least five major variables:

Risk

Risk as it is used here means risk to the individual involved, that is, risk to the subject of the decision to be made. It is not used to mean risk to the family or risk to society.

Gain

Similarly, gain is used exclusively in terms of the individual. I am well aware that in both these categories the decision of what is high risk or high gain is itself dependent on personal values. For the most part, therefore, I will try to give examples that would fall within the *general* standards of society. For example, I will place an extraordinarily high value on survival. This will, of course, do disservice to those religious groups who view life on earth as an ephemeral and unimportant transition point to an eternal and better life somewhere else. But since we are dealing with policy, not theology, it seems best to adopt the standards of our culture—wrongly or rightly—that life on earth is a central value, rarely transcended by others.

Risk-Gain Ratio

It will soon be seen that the definitions of risk and gain will be altered in a peculiar way when they are viewed as a ratio rather than independently.

Social Benefits or Costs

In the most individualistic of states, we must still be aware that we are all part of a complex society, and that there will inevitably be times where transcendent rights of the society will force a limitation of individual rights. Biologists since Aristotle have been reminding us, even when the philosophers and social scientists have forgotten, that man is a social animal by design, not by choice, and that even his *individual* needs require respect for the community on which he is dependent. A commitment to individual liberty is meaningless if the social matrix that supports all freedom is allowed to be destroyed.

The Nature of the Decision

It is evident that, depending on the decision to be made, even such specifics as "risk," "gain," and "social benefits" begin to have different definitions and meanings. I am limiting my examples to medical ones. But those who would extend this grid beyond that purpose will immediately recognize that there are assumptions that arise out of the medical model, which are quite different from those that would surface with an economic, sociological, or pedagogical frame of reference. For example, one need only think about our abhorrence of pain inflicted for political purposes, which is defined as torture, and the legitimacy of pain inflicted for medical purposes. This is not simply a distinction between individual and state purposes. Even when only the individual and his family are involved, we draw crucial distinctions. We will allow painful methods to be inflicted on a child if it is necessary for ambulation. Yet I suspect we would not allow whipping or other painful methods to be used if it were necessary for a child to learn to read, or simply to learn. It is not because reading is less important than ambulation, but rather that under the medical model we are protected in the assumption (often false) that only the good of the individual is concerned, while with the pedagogical model we are frightened that we may slip from serving the individual's needs into serving society, at which point the pain would be morally unacceptable. At any rate, it is a fact that the nature of the case will shift our relative values on the grid.

Other terms that will be used as variables are "generous" and "limited." Since I have defined competence as that which we (the state) are conferring on and endow the individual with, "generous" means that we should indeed be liberal in our allowance, even at times beyond our logical evolution of "true" competence. When I say "generous," then, I mean we should be relatively free in granting the right of autonomy to the human being involved. When I say "limited," we should be careful in our readiness to certify competence. "Generous" and "limited," therefore, refer to the attitude of the state in granting competence.

Here again, another set of variables must be introduced, and that is whether what is being granted is the right to elect to do something, or the right to refuse. As we get to the specific examples, it will be seen that often the state's generosity in certifying competence will be polar in these conditions. Where we are generous in granting a right to refuse, we will often limit the right to volunteer.

Since we are using the medical model, it is important to understand the meaning of therapeutic and nontherapeutic experimentation or procedure. A therapeutic procedure is one that is done as "therapy." It is a treatment for the individual, and presumed to serve his purposes and welfare. A therapeutic experiment involves the use of a procedure that is not yet proven, but is used in this specific case to test its efficacy on the condition of the individual. To gove someone penicillin for his pneumonia is a therapeutic procedure today; to have given someone with pneumonia penicillin in the early days before the proven risks and benefits of the drug were established would have been an experimental procedure, but a *therapeutic experiment.* To give someone penicillin who did *not* have pneumonia to test the effects of the drug on a healthy physiological system is a *nontherapeutic experiment.*

Whenever we are involved with certifying the competence of a child, the assumption will be that when he or she is certified as noncompetent, the decision-making, out of respect for family autonomy, rests with the family. However, since we are aware that the family is not a totally trustworthy instrument, but only the safest of instruments, we acknowledge the rights of society to intervene in family autonomy when it is felt that the family violates its primary charge to sustain, nurture, and protect the individual. The intrusion on family autonomy will be cast in terms of the state's right to intervene. Let us now look at our four major categories.

Category 1: High Risk/Low Gain

The obvious example of this category is the classic yellow fever experiment where Walter Reed and his colleagues risked their lives to serve society at large. Despite the fact that they need not have been exposed to yellow fever, they ran the risk of the experimental procedure. Many more modern examples can be anticipated. Herpes virus has been implicated as a possible source of cervical cancer. Supposing a live-virus vaccination has been developed and is now in stage 3 testing. The marketing drug company is looking for healthy volunteers on whom to test the vaccine. Since the potential subject does *not* have the disease, but does have a chance of developing a herpes infection or a herpes-caused cervical cancer, the gain is low and the risk is high. Common sense indicates that a young child ought not be permitted to volunteer for such hazards before an age of understanding. Her right to refuse should be highly respected. Therefore, in this case, it would seem that our equation should be: autonomous right to volunteer—limited; autonomous right to refuse—generous.

When the prospective volunteer is a child, we are faced with the secondary question of whether the state has a right to intervene when permission or refusal is given by a surrogate, i.e., a parent. Obviously, in cases where there is no social value, the state never has a right to intervene, but the two examples given above are both examples of high social value. The principle here at its extreme seems simple: on a high risk/low gain nontherapeutic procedure (the risk of a child to serve others is a prototype example), the state has the right to intervene to forbid the procedure, and has extremely limited rights to intervene demanding the procedure.

Category 2: Low Risk/High Gain

The classic example here is a Jehovah's Witness' refusal to authorize a blood transfusion (a limited risk procedure) to save a life (a high gain). In granting the autonomous right to elect the procedure in this situation, we obviously should be generous; the autonomous right to refuse should be limited. Even a young child would seem competent to decide to save his life when there is no risk to him involved. Similarly, we must wait until the absolute date of maturity (or even beyond that, some would argue) to allow someone to refuse such a procedure.

The state's position in this type of case is an interesting one. Although no social purpose might be served directly, there is a social commitment to the high value on life. Here, one would expect state intervention. The state, therefore, should overcome the presumption of family autonomy in such cases. Indeed, such was the decision of Judge Murphy for the Superior Court for the District of Columbia *In Re Pogue* (1974). Judge

Murphy intervened and overruled the parents, allowing a blood transfusion for a healthy, newborn baby who would have died without the
transfusion.

This is a case of particular interet because at the same time Judge
Murphy recognized the rights of the *mother* to refuse a blood transfusion
for herself, even if refusing to intervene meant her death. In the case
of the infant, however, the judge as a surrogate decided to protect the
child's right to live to the age of majority, when he would be entitled to
make such life-and-death decisions for himself. In so doing, the judge
implicitly found the mother temporarily *incompetent* to decide for the
child, while at the very same time he acknowledged her *competence* by
declining to use her refusal of blood, despite its obvious danger, as a
basis for declaring her incompetent.

There is an interesting subheading in this category that tends to modify
our attitudes about the relative respect we give to family autonomy. At
the extremes of life, when we are dealing with a fetus or a senescent old
man, we tend to *increase* the degree of family autonomy, that is, decrease
the state's right to intervene. Most people are prepared to accept a
difference between a first-trimester fetus and a child, and the law has
already acknowledged that much. We will allow the fetus to be destroyed
by parental authority. Some would even argue the case for non-thera-
peutic experimentation on the about-to-be-destroyed fetus. It may well
be that at the ends of life the state should also place a lesser value on
the comatose old man irreversibly deteriorating into death, and allow
a greater degree of family autonomy in weighing the potential value of
the experimental procedure for society as a whole, as against the specific
value of the life at risk. Here the arguments are complex, and the slope
particularly slippery.

Category 3: High Risk/High Gain

Here the prime examples would be where the risk is life and the gain
is life. As an example: a child with a severe cardiac impairment and the
need for an experimental operative procedure to correct it; the child's
life is at risk because of the cardiac insufficiency, and yet the high mortality rate of the operation is also an awesome risk. It seems clear here
that since both the risk and the benefit involve that which is valued
highly by the state, i.e., life, the rights of the state are cancelled by the
balance, and the state ought to abandon its power of intervention. When
we talk about certifying competence here, it is balancing the right of the
child as a decision-maker against the right of the parent.

Should the child have any say in such decisions? I think we have been remiss in the past in totally ignoring the child, and I would press for some moderately generous certification of competence both for the right to refuse and the right to elect. In a state where the age of competence is 18, it seems inconceivable that a decision to operate on a 16-year-old can now be made independent of his feelings or judgments. I am prepared here to be moderately generous in the application of competence. Even when we are aware of living parents, there is something inappropriate for the individual whose life is at risk to be totally on the sidelines in such a decision. Participation need not mean complete autonomy. In either case, we must decide how much participation, and at what age. To exclude him completely, to acknowledge no autonomy and no competence, seems most unreasonable.

High risk/high gain, however, does not mean simply life versus life; certainly it can mean life versus capacity to work, life versus ambulation, etc. Here too, I would press for a moderately generous lowering of the age of competence. Consider an operative procedure which would remove an individual from a state of permanent invalidism but which represented a significant risk to his life. Here too, common sense would demand some consideration of the judgment of the person to whom the risk or gain is most germane.

It becomes clear that as one moves farther and farther away from life-saving, the pressure to include the individual in the decision-making becomes less. With work and ambulation, it will often be the case that were his parents to refuse the operation, the patient could reverse them when he reaches the age of maturity. On the other hand, there will be examples where the operative procedure must be done at a certain age or it cannot be done at all. In those cases I would insist that we be generous in allowing the child the role as a competent judge of the future life he is about to lead.

Category 4: Low Risk/Low Gain

Here we must subdivide into two categories, depending on whether the experimentation or procedure is (a) of low social value, or (b) of high social value. Let us first consider category 4(a), where there is low risk, low gain, and low social value. In this case, with low social value, there is an automatic assumption that the state has little or no right to intervene, particularly since the child is not at risk. Once again, if we allow the child competence, the autonomy we are granting is specifically in relationship to the parent. Here, in seeking an example, I am obliged to leave the medical arena, because there is no medical experimentation that is proposed that is not thought to have some social value—if only in the mind of the experimenter himself. Let us therefore take the example of a movie screening. The producer has completed a picture for children; he wants to test audience reaction. There is little to be gained by the child and little to be risked. The automatic right to refuse (vs. the parents), it seems to me, should be extremely limited. Some might argue that, since no risks are involved, whether the parent volunteers the child or not, a child at a very early age ought to be able to decide that he simply "doesn't want to"; similarly, an automatic right to volunteer should also be generous—a child ought to be able to make such decisions at a very young age. I take the contrary position—not because I think a child should not be free to make these decisions, but in this case out of respect for family integrity as distinguished from family autonomy, I would not want to make it a *right*. Even while I would hope that sensible parents would allow the child to make such decisions, I would not want to elevate this to a point of *rights*. It seems to me we ought not encourage family discord over trivial matters.

Category 4(b) is low risk/low gain with a high social value. Here, it seems to me, is a case where the state has a strong right to intervene.

If a parent has no sense of moral obligation to the community at large, it may be to the good of the child as well as the community for the state to instruct the parent as well as the child on his or her social responsibility. Take for example an epidemiological study where urine is collected as it is transmitted through the urinals in school. This would assume no particular exposure of the child; the child, indeed, would be unaware that he was part of an experiment. The risk, therefore, is zero to him. On the other hand, the epidemiological purposes could be significant. If we were looking for base lines of certain trace elements excreted through the urine to determine the impact of environmental pollution, this is the kind of data we would need, and the child might someday benefit. But even if there were a case where no possible gain to the child would accrue, I would allow state intervention. Refusal of permission for such experimental involvement would be trivial, arbitrary, and ungenerous. There are limits to family autonomy. Here, the autonomous right of the individual to refuse would be extremely limited, and the autonomous right to volunteer extremely generous.

This category introduces another violation of a principle dearly held by many. For years I have felt that nontherapeutic experimentation ought not be allowed via *proxy* consent. It was one of the few basic principles which it seemed could be established in an unconditional way. My reasoning was that while it was a noble and generous act for someone to offer himself at risk for the good of the community or science, it is somewhat less generous, noble, or courageous for one person to offer another person. I was forced to make one exception to that rule when I began to examine the problem of fetal experimentation. That argument has already been fully developed (Gaylin and Lappé, 1975). But another example offered to me by a friend further shook my confidence in the inviolability of this principle. He described a scene in an office where he had taken his 9- or 10-year-old son for a physical examination. The doctor, after having completed the examination, turned to the child in a formal manner and asked for permission to take a small sample of blood for an epidemiological research that he was doing on a major disease of childhood. As the father related the story, the doctor in a somewhat precious way explained to the child that this was not a part of his examination but would help some "other little boys." Johnny asked the doctor, "Will it hurt?" The doctor answered "A little—like a pinprick." Johnny said "I don't want it," whereupon the father said to his son "Listen, young man, you just get your hand up on that table and let the doctor take the blood." Johnny, recognizing the note of authority in his father's voice, immediately complied, whereupon the doctor, forgetting the formalism of his original consent proceedings, gladly took the sample.

In explaining the situation to me, the father said that it was not just an expression of authoritarianism, or paternalism if you will, but his moral obligation to teach his child there are certain things one does, even if it causes a small amount of pain, to the service or benefit of others. "This is my child. I was less concerned with the research involved than with the kind of boy I was raising. I'll be damned if I was going to allow my child, because of some idiot concept of children's rights, to assume that he was entitled to be a selfish, narcissistic little bastard."

Paternalism by a parent in relationship to a young child is not, this father would offer, patronizing or "paternalistic." The instillation of a set of values is the moral responsibility of a parent, and the failure to do so is a grievous abdication of responsibility. I tend to agree with the father, and while my method of approach might have been different from his, each parent has the right to his or her own style within the limits of decency. I accept this as another category where proxy consent may be suitable in a nontherapeutic experimentation. The benefit to this child at this time is zero (i.e., it is a nontherapeutic procedure), but the cost is very low and the social gain may be very high. In such cases a parent may "volunteer" his child for a nontherapeutic experiment.

All of these principles can now be summarized as shown in Table 1.

Table 1

Summary of Principles of Variable Competence

Category	Family Autonomy	Rules Certifying Competence	Individual Autonomy
1. High risk/low gain, example given: life-risking, nontherapeutic experiment	State has right to intervene (forbidding)		Autonomous right to refuse: generous Autonomous right to elect: limited
2. Low risk/high gain, example: blood transfusion to save life	State has right to intervene (demanding)		Autonomous right to refuse: limited Autonomous right to elect: generous
3. High risk/high gain, examples given: —life vs. life —life vs. work —life vs. ambulation	State has no right to intervene		Autonomous right to refuse: moderately generous Autonomous right to elect: moderately generous (Here vs. parents, since State has no authority)
4a. Low risk/low gain-low social value, example: movie screening	State has no right to intervene		Autonomous right vs. parents to refuse: extremely limited Autonomous right vs. parents to elect: extremely limited
4b. Low risk/low gain, high social value, example: urinalysis for epidemiological purposes	State has right to intervene		Autonomous right vs. State to refuse: extremely limited Autonomous right vs. State to volunteer: generous

The second column indicates family autonomy, and will set the limits for state intervention and intrapersonal decision-making; the third column indicates the state's readiness to certify competence (grant legal autonomy) at variable ages.

What Table 1 represents is a crude and tentative set of principles. It is a primitive grid composed of a structured set of principles on which we can begin to locate the specific case, rather than simply depending on an individual, situational approach, which inevitably leads to the inequities inherent in any *ad hoc* system.

Even with the tentative principles presented, certain complications are already apparent. I have alluded (in category 2) to one of them, i.e., the tendency to extrapolate assumptions and recommendations for the end of life (the elderly dying) from conclusions drawn at the beginnings of life (the damaged newborn). More mischief has been created by equating the moral decisions about life-saving and the termination of treatments at these two extremes. There are very few generalizations that hold one to the other.

Even in the intervals in between we are aware that the age of the individual alters our attitudes, not just about the capacity for autonomy, but also about the relative importance of the area of decision-making. Let me offer one example: suppose that the situation we are dealing with is the permission to withdraw from a life-saving treatment such as a dialysis machine. If the legal age of maturity in the state is 18, I for one would want to be extremely ungenerous in lowering that age of permission to discontinue treatment. Even acknowledging the fact that the 16-year-old—by almost every set of variables—is close to maturity, one recognizes that a certain level of *consciousness* is different at that age from what may exist at 30—let alone 50. By "consciousness" I mean a sense, not just of one's own identity, but of one's own purposes; the relationship of the sense of self not only to the environment but beyond that to a concept of one's future. The mere appreciation of time varies between the 15-year-old to whom the 3 months before his graduation seems like an eternity, as compared with the 65-year-old, whose 40 years of productive work seems like a single yesterday. From a distance, we can know that 2 years is not that great a time to wait before allowing a 16-year-old to sacrifice a potential 30 to 50 more years of living.

Can this decision be defended on logical grounds? I doubt it. It is, by every definition, paternalistic. But it seems to me the state might well want to be paternalistic at this point when what is at risk is a future life of unknown and unlimited potential. I grant that at 18 the same bias might still be there, but one presumes that age brings a certain solidification of values, and 18 may be 2 years more balanced a time than 16.

Similarly, we may be aware that a 72-year-old man on the same dialysis machine may have, over the years, arteriosclerotic deterioration and brain damage of a sort that clearly indicates, by objective and measurable criteria, that he is no longer the rational human being he once was. If we compare the 16-year-old and the 72-year-old in an adversarial position in a court of law, I have no doubt that the 16-year-old would win hands down against all variables introduced as determinants of competence. Nonetheless, I would allow the 72-year-old to be "deemed competent," even when he is beyond the limits of certain objective criteria of competence, i.e., when there are beginning signs of impairment of memory, judgment, and the like.

What I am suggesting therefore is that, as in many other moral issues, there is not a direct correlation between "is" and "ought." We may deprive the younger person of certain privileges of autonomy out of respect for the person he might become, and out of fear that his own vision of this future may be too limited to allow, even himself, proper respect for its value. Whereas with the older person we must honor a lifetime of feelings, achievement, experiencing, relating, and simply being; we must measure his limited future against the residuals of his past; and we must respect his right to protect his own dignity, which is in such short supply in older age. The old man is often less concerned with his potential for the future than with the preservation of his past; the future he is sacrificing may be only a short period of pain and deterioration. With the adolescent, we have a right to be concerned about where he is going, and with the elderly, where he came from. A person is, after all, not only what he is, but also what he was.

It seems to me therefore that even were we capable of absolutely judging "true" competence (which we never will be), there would be psychological, social and moral reason for allocating competence independent of the actual fact. There are certain illusions which ought to be maintained out of respect for the simple biological life cycle. In my scheme I would propose that even as we begin to accumulate more knowledge about moral decision-making, we maintain a distinction between "true" competence and the state's acknowledgment of competence. In other words, I propose the comparison shown in Figure 1 between competence as it might indeed be, and competence as it ought to be allocated.

I offer this as an example of my personal value system and to point the way in which others might wish to modify moral judgments independent of the facts of development. In my system, I am more than

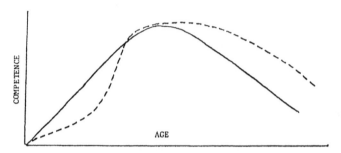

FIG. 1. Decision-making competence and age: ———, true competence
(what is); - - - -, allocated competence (what ought to be granted).

prepared to limit the autonomy of the child beyond my intellectual
recognition of its presence. I am prepared to allow him to suffer the
humiliation, or the loss of pride, that comes with limited autonomy,
secure in the knowledge that he will shortly achieve an age in which it
will automatically be awarded him, and that this short delay will do little
harm to his self-image or the values of our society. I propose that we
compensate this young person for this deprivation by granting him, in
his senescence, a more liberal allocation of autonomy (a more generous
judgment of competence) than he deserves.

This, then, is simply one example of a form of value analysis—a mechanism of negotiation, analysis, and arbitration—that will be necessary to
establish some sound underpinnings to a concept as complex as variable
competence.

REFERENCES

Gaylin, W. (1979). Who speaks for the helpless. *This Journal,* 18:419–436.
——— & Lappé, M. (1975). Fetal politics. *Atlantic,* 235:66–71.
Ledbetter, L. (1977). Parents win custody of 5 members of Moon's church. *The New York
Times,* March 25, pp. 1 and 9.
Peters, R. S. (1972). In *Education and the Development of Reason,* R. F. Dearden, ed. London:
Routledge & Kegan Paul, p. 130.
In re POGUE. (1974). *Washington Post,* C. at 1., col. 1, November 14 (No. M-18-74, Super.
Ct., D.C.).
Roth, L. H., Meisel, A. and Lidz, C. W. (1977). Tests of competency to consent to treatment.
American Journal of Psychiatry, 134:283.
Trilling, L. (1950). In *The Liberal Imagination.* Garden City, N.Y.: Doubleday Anchor Books,
p. 215.

34

Children's Rights in the Family and Society: Dilemmas and Realities

Jane Knitzer

Institute for Child and
Youth Policy Studies
Rochester, New York

This paper seeks to examine and place in perspective recent legal activities on behalf of children, focusing both on efforts to define, expand, and clarify the rights of children and parents as family members, and on efforts to enforce the obligations of broader social institutions, such as education and child welfare, to children and their families.

During the past two decades, legal activity on behalf of children and adolescents has increasingly centered on efforts to define, expand, and enforce their rights both in relation to families and in relation to broader social systems. Such legal advocacy has been welcomed by some, and stridently challenged by others. Seeking to provide some perspective on the controversy, this paper will define the scope of legal activities affecting children in both a familial and a nonfamilial context; examine some of the major dilemmas and criticisms such activities have engendered; assess the impact of the legal rights movement on children and families, professionals, and public policy; and, finally, speculate about the future of the children's rights movement.

Reprinted with permission from the *American Journal of Orthopsychiatry*, 1982, Vol. 52, No. 3, 481–495. Copyright 1982 by the American Orthopsychiatric Association, Inc.

RIGHTS OF CHILDREN IN A FAMILIAL CONTEXT

Scope of Legal Activities

Recent litigation involving children in a familial context has addressed at least four central and difficult sets of questions: 1) Under what conditions should children have access to independent legal representation? 2) What should be the legal grounds for removing children from their families, terminating irrevocably the rights of natural parents to their children, and ensuring children permanence? 3) Under what circumstances should there be oversight by the courts of parental decisions about children? 4) In what circumstances should minors be permitted to make decisions independently of their parents? First, the nature of the legal activity surrounding each of the questions will be considered briefly, then the nature of the dilemmas that they raise will be addressed.

Legal counsel.—Perhaps the most fundamental tenet of the legal system is that when judicial decisions are made, the subject of those decisions has the opportunity, through counsel, to be heard. Children historically have not had this opportunity. Under traditional legal doctrine either the parents have virtually unlimited authority over their children or, in instances of egregious action by the parents, the state under the doctrine of *parens patrie* assumes comparable parental authority. In either situation, children have had no say in legal decisions affecting their status as a family member.

Legal advocates have argued that this approach leaves the child virtually unprotected from the predictable conflict-of-interest situations that sometimes make it impossible for parents or agencies to act solely on behalf of the child, or even to ascertain what the child needs. Advocates argue that in these situations, which typically involve children with disrupted or nonexistent families, the children should have either independent counsel or at least a guardian *ad litem*;[5] that is, an advocate (although not necessarily a lawyer) charged to represent the child's interests. Thus, there have been numerous challenges of the failure to appoint counsel for children facing removal from home because of alleged abuse or neglect, for children who are the subject of petitions to terminate parental rights, for children who are the object of custody battles between divorcing parents, and for children who have no parents but the state.

Changing legal grounds for removal/termination.—The effort to ensure children access to counsel is a due process issue, reflecting a concern with procedural fairness. Children in vulnerable family situations have also been the foci of a debate about their substantive rights regarding the grounds for judicial intervention into family life. Backed by empirical studies which show the states have overused the power to remove children from homes, and underused their authority to terminate parental rights after real psychological parent ties have ended,[11,14,23] lawyers and other children's rights advocates have turned the spotlight on the prevailing legal grounds for making such decisions and typically have found them either too vague or too broad. This in turn has stimulatd efforts to modify existing state statutory criteria and to develop new standards for both removal and termination. Exactly what those grounds should be is the subject of debate among lawyers and others. With regard to removal from homes, some, like Goldstein, Freud and Solnit,[6] have argued for extremely narrow grounds and made no demands on the state for the provision of services prior to removal, primarily because they are skeptical that any effective services can be delivered. Others[23] have suggested slightly broader grounds for removal (including, for instance, emotional as well as physical abuse) but have urged that whatever the grounds, there be evidence that the questionable parental behavior results in definable harms to the child. Still others have emphasized the affirmative obligation of the state to provide services to keep a family together except in the most dangerous circumstances, and have cautioned against premature removal.

Similarly, consensus as to the appropriate grounds for termination of parental rights is also nonexistent. Statutes that make classes of parents (i.e., retarded or mentally ill parents) liable to termination are especially suspect in the eyes of many children's rights proponents because these statutes do not also require specific evidence that the parental impairment results in clear harm to the child.[8] However, legal decisions have not been uniform as to whether or not such specific evidence should be required. Further, there is no consensus as to whether the state has an obligation to provide reunification services, how its failure to do so should be weighed, or how long such efforts should be required. And, finally, there is no consensus as to the emphasis that should be put on balancing evidence about the past or future parenting capacity of the natural parents with the current psychological needs and realities of the child, who very often has established strong psychological bonds to foster or adoptive parents.

Limits of parental decision-making.—The third theme that has emerged in litigation involving children in a family context has to do with defining which, if any, parental decisions about children should be subjected to judicial or other quasilegal scrutiny. This question has been raised, for example, around whether parents have the right to decide, without court acquiescence, whether one sibling can donate an organ to another or whether parents can permit, without court involvement, the sterilization of a retarded minor. It has also been raised regarding whether parents have a right to commit a minor to a psychiatric hospital in the absence of due process protections. In these situations, the children's rights proponents generally argue that the consequences of the proposed action are so significant for the child that parental judgment alone is not a sufficient protection, and that some additional mechanism for weighing the pros and cons (and, in some instances, seeking alternatives) is required.

Granting children independent decision-making authority.—Finally, the fourth question that has shaped the debate about children vs. parents has to do with the nature of the decisions children should legally be allowed to make, the extent to which parental knowledge of these decisions is required, and the possible role of the state in overseeing the decision-making process. These questions have been raised primarily in relation to activities of older adolescents and involve such issues as abortion, emancipation, and access to health and mental health services in non-life-threatening situations. As such, notwithstanding the image held by the public (and sometimes the press) of youth being given unchecked powers to make decisions independent of parents, the legal debate about the boundaries of parental authority has involved primarily older adolescents, in very circumscribed areas. In these arenas, the courts have moved slowly and ambivalently in extending the rights of minors. So, for instance, with regard to abortion, they have sought for the most part to define roles for both parents and minors, not to totally exclude one or the other from the decision-making process.

Dilemmas, Criticisms, and Realities

Efforts to use the court as a forum for resolving these difficult legal and often psychologically complex issues concerning parent-child relationships have met with considerable resistance, and have generated much empty rhetoric as well as serious professional and legal debate. Basically the criticisms center around three concerns. The first and perhaps most widespread criticism is that efforts to expand the rights of children represent an undesirable challenge to notions of the supremacy of parental or family autonomy. At its most simplistic level the argument is made that extending rights to children in at-risk situations (primarily by ensuring them independent counsel) will lead to the extension of such rights in all situations, and thus will undermine the integrity of the family. The fear is perhaps best captured by the cartoons that show a child taking a parent to court because she could not watch a favorite television program or go to summer camp. One critic passionately declared that the most basic right of a child is not to be abandoned to his rights.[7]

While it makes for good sloganeering, this domino theory of children's rights romanticizes the "autonomy of the family"[18] and ignores evidence of substantial abuses inflicted on too many children by either families or the state in its role as surrogate family.

At the same time it is clear that trying to correct an imbalance between the rights of children and families is a very difficult task, fraught with potentially undesirable as well as desirable consequences. So, for example, Uviller,[20] in her capacity as Director of the Children's Rights Project of the American Civil Liberties Union, cautioned that, since children are, after all, dependent beings, expanding their rights in relation to parents may only result in the substitution of state for parental authority, a troubling outcome for civil libertarians as well as many others.

The fact is that in the area of parent-child relationships, not only is legal precedent either minimal or murky, so too often are hard psychological data to back up legal positions. For example, there is no research examining systematically the parenting strengths or weaknesses of retarded parents, or the immediate or long-range consequences of returning children after a long absence to natural parents as opposed to permitting them to remain in foster care or ensuring their adoption. Further, psychological data cast doubt on the ability of either clinicians or researchers to predict future outcomes or future behavior of either parents (for instance, abusive parents) or children. As a result, there is no clear framework from which to generate appropriate legal standards when a question of parent-child relationship is confronted. Yet, surfacing the issues and forcing professional/legal debate about the "realities" of childhood (realities that exist with or without the "children's rights movement") may eventually lead to clearer notions of family rights and responsibilities as well as of children's rights.

The second major criticism that has been expressed about the consequences of the children's rights movement is that family matters are being over-legalized and that a legal "due process" decision-making model is being imposed in inappropriate circumstances. This charge has surfaced particularly (although not exclusively) with regard to the boundaries of independent decision-making authority of children and parents. Burt,[3] for example, has been a vocal critic of efforts to seek judicial scrutiny of family decisions about minors (including those around psychiatric hospitalization). He has argued that while there may be abuses, for the most part families can and should make such decisions, that the emotional bonds between parents and child are a positive rather than a negative factor, and that the courts have no superior wisdom to enable them to make better decisions. While compelling, this argument overlooks the possibility that a judicial forum can serve, as Rothman[18] has noted, purposes other than undermining parent-child relationships—for example, ensuring that alternatives to psychiatric hospitalization for a minor have been considered.

Others, recognizing the fundamental legitimacy of protecting children's rights, nonetheless take the position that the more lawyers, the harder it is to resolve family disputes. Recent efforts to develop nonlegal mediation strategies to resolve custody disputes reflect this concern. Similarly, social workers and others involved in child abuse and neglect cases often complain that tension between foster parents and natural parents is exacerbated by lawyers who will not let the parents communicate informally. As a result, some have evolved what is essentially a "counsel as a last resort" philosophy. So, for example, Goldstein, Freud and Solnit[6] have argued that until there has been an adjudication of abuse in an abuse proceeding, the child should be considered part of a family, and not independently represented, although they recognize that once an adjudication of abuse is made, the child should have a right to independent counsel.

The third criticism that has been raised in relation to parent vs. child litigation is in many ways the most difficult to counter. Sometimes, for individual children and families, legal action may be hurtful rather than helpful. Too often, representation is pro forma. Moreover, legal proceedings even in individual cases take a very long time. This is particularly true around contested termination cases, and often leads to potentially tragic consequences for the psychological health of both younger and older children. Solnit,[19] for example, recently described a case that illustrates many of the psychological risks to the child and dilemmas for mental health professionals such cases can engender. In that case, despite the interest of the foster mother (black, single, and in her forties) in adopting a two-year-old interracial child who had been placed with her since shortly after birth, the child welfare agency, with judicial concurrence, removed the child and placed her in a white adoptive home. The foster mother protested the placement and an evaluation of the child was done. It showed that she had deteriorated in her developmental progress and was somewhat distant from her new mother. The court, however, upheld the agency decision to keep her with the adoptive parents. The lawyers for the foster mother appealed. By this time, the child was now over three, and had been away from the foster home for thirteen months. The clinicians, with obvious anguish, recommended leaving the child in the adoptive home. As Solnit noted, "It was a difficult decision because it meant submitting to a wrong decision for the child made a year earlier."

It is of course not difficult to see why mental health professionals (and others) who encounter such judicial decisions express skepticism about the benefits of the children's rights movement to children. On the other hand, there has been no systematic monitoring of such decisions; we hear little of judicial interventions that work well for children, and lack an overall sense of how frequently bad decisions occur. Moreover, taking a case-by-case perspective, it is too easy to lose sight of the well-documented, widespread evidence that countless children in placement have been harmed by the absence of any decision-making at all about their family status. The increased use of the legal arena is a direct response to past systemic neglect of children in out-of-home placement. Lawyers and other children's rights proponents have not created the problems, but are seeking to stimulate a better response to them.

This attempt to provide a perspective on legal efforts to expand the rights of children in a familial context would not be complete, however, without raising two additional issues that for the most part have been ignored by the critics. The fact is that the children's rights movement has not been exclusively concerned with extending children's rights. It has also sought to equalize parental power against the state, particularly for parents facing the temporary or permanent loss of their children. For these parents, notwithstanding pro-family, pro-parent rhetoric, do not have automatic access to counsel. Indeed, a recent analysis[11] of statutory provisions regarding neglect/abuse and termination proceedings found that nine states do not mention a right to counsel for either parents or children in neglect proceedings and eight do not in termination proceedings. Even more startling and disturbing for those who worry about either family autonomy or a just legal system is the fact that the Supreme Court in a recent decision (*Lassiter v Department of Social Services of Durham Co., N.C.*, 1981) took the position that the due process clause of the Constitution did not require that parents facing the threat of termination of parental rights have appointed counsel. In other words, they argued that the potential irrevocable loss of a child was not a deprivation of such magnitude as to require the state to pay for the parent to have legal representation, although they supported the current practice of discretionary appointment by the judge. This is, of course, in sharp contrast to decisions affecting criminals in which states are required to provide counsel.

Secondly, it is also important to note that while the legal spotlight on children and parents has had a significant role in airing the difficult and long-ignored issues involved in protecting children in questionable family situations or in out-of-home care, it has also served to mask issues in other areas. So, for example, the debate about the appropriate commitment procedures for children facing hospitalization consumed an inordinate amount of psychiatric and legal energies. Supposedly the issue pitted parents against children; in reality the real issue was which set of professionals, legal or mental health, should make the final decision. But more importantly, the debate has been dysfunctional for both children and parents because it has reinforced the tendency within the so-called children's mental health system to avoid grappling with the reality that, regardless of parental or professional wisdom, significant percentages of children are hospitalized by default, because no less restrictive alternatives are actively sought or because none exist. And further, the debate (and the landmark legal decision in *Parham*) has consistently underplayed the fact that at least one-third, and in some places more, of the children committed to psychiatric hospitals are not even in the care of the parents, but in the custody of the state.[12]

The picture, then, regarding children and their rights in and to families is extraordinarily complex. The lack of consensus reflected in the debate is not surprising given the rapid changes in family constellations and life styles[1] and in the role of socializing institutions.[9] Thoughtful observers[18] have noted that the global debate about whether or not children should have rights in families reflects a fundamental tension between those who view the family in a romantic, sentimental light and those who view it as an arena in which potential excesses of power can occur. For the former, extending rights to children is both inappropriate and unnecessary. For the latter, the family becomes a legitimate arena to apply legal checks and balances. It also reflects a fundamental tension between those who view all government interventions as unnecessary and inappropriate, and those who would seek to end excessive governmental intrusion into families, but recognize governmental intervention can also be supportive of families. One thing is clear. Because of the complexity surrounding attempts to clarify children's rights in relation to parental rights, it is unlikely there will be a clear resolution for the children or the parents for a long time.

RIGHTS OF CHILDREN IN A NONFAMILIAL CONTEXT

Scope of Legal Activities

Because the so-called children vs. parents aspect of the children's rights movement has generated so much attention and controversy, it has obscured other legal efforts on behalf of children. As a result, the body of litigation (particularly class action litigation) that has challenged either abusive state practices toward large numbers of children, or the failure of states to carry out mandated responsibility to them has received relatively little attention and its cumulative impact has been little understood. This section, therefore, discusses the scope and goals of such litigation, its impact, and the criticisms and dilemmas it has engendered.

Children vs. systems: due process protections.—The earliest litigation to challenge the response of a public system to children involved juvenile justice. It sought to establish the principle that juveniles charged with a delinquency offense were entitled to a range of due process protections including counsel. The *Gault* case reached the Supreme Court in 1967, and the court handed down the now-famous decision that a minor charged with a juvenile offense was entitled to representation by counsel and to certain other due process rights. In so doing, it sounded one of the major themes reflected in subsequent legal activity on behalf of minors[17]—the effort to extend to juveniles without any consideration of their special dependent status the rights accorded to adults. This is reflected not only in challenges to delinquency proceedings,[21] but also to those (as discussed earlier) involving parents and children in conflict. Moreover, the effort to extend procedural protections to children in non-court settings, such as schools, can also be traced in part to the *Gault* challenge.

Children vs. systems: protection against abuses.—In addition to cases involving the extension of due process protections to minors, early legal challenges also involved substantive as well as due process grounds. One such early case, *Morales v Turman* (1974), challenged abuses and excesses in the care and treatment accorded to children incarcerated in Texas training schools, and detailed specific service system changes desired as a remedy.[21] The initial decision in that case (subsequently modified substantially through the appeals process) did in fact mandate widespread changes in the training school system.

Morales v. Turman marked one of the first of a series of class action lawsuits, brought on behalf of children institutionalized in juvenile justice or retardation facilities. These suits challenged abusive or egregiously harmful practices, such as excessive confinement, absence of educational programming, and censorship in the institutions. At least one major lawsuit also challenged, albeit unsuccessfully, abuses within the public schools, specifically the use of corporal punishment. That case, *Ingraham v Wright* (1977), brought on behalf of two Florida youth who had been so severely beaten that they required medical care, argued that the Constitutional right of the youth to be free from excessive punishment had been violated. The court disagreed and instead took the position that the Constitutional protection did not extend to schools because schools are "open" institutions. In a variant of litigation focusing on abuses of children, litigation has also challenged the use of children, particularly institutionalized children, as research subjects in either grossly unethical projects or projects of questionable benefit to the child.

Children vs. systems: seeking appropriate care.—Still other litigation has challenged the failure of public agencies to provide appropriate education, treatment, or placement for children or to monitor the delivery of those services (often in conjunction with specific abuses). Such lawsuits go beyond efforts to define procedural rights or to stop abuses, but seek to define the affirmative obligations of the state, and of specific service delivery systems to their child clients. So, for example, early in the 1970s a group of parents challenged their handicapped children's exclusion from Pennsylvania schools. As a result of the lawsuit (*Pennsylvania Association for Retarded Children vs. Commonwealth of Pennsylvania*, 1971) the state was required to ensure appropriate identification of and programming for handicapped children, and reallocate its educational resources.[2] PARC signaled the beginning of a widespread, continuing effort through class action, system-focused litigation to challenge educational practices and policies harmful to children and, equally significantly, to seek remedies involving specific changes in policies, administrative and clinical practices, and resource allocation.

Similarly, children at risk of or in out-of-home placement have been the focus of a significant body of class action litigation designed to address often noted, but long uncorrected, systemic problems. For example, *Gary W. v Cherry* (1976), brought by the Children's Defense Fund in conjunction with local counsel, challenged the Louisiana practice of placing handicapped children far from their own homes in Texas facilities, many of which were marginally if not egregiously inadequate. As a result, the state was required to evaluate and implement an appropriate treatment/service plan for each of the children in the class. Further, the court ruled that each child placed in Texas facilities had the right to care, education, and medical and personal treatment suited to his or her characteristics and ordered the state to spend as much money on in-state as had been spent on out-of-state care. Implementation of that decree has not always been smooth. Indeed, it is now five years after the initial order was filed, and the state is still not in full compliance. However, the lawsuit has prodded the state to begin to try to create some locally based services, and it did establish, in principle, the child's right to an appropriate placement. Further, since the plaintiffs who were sent out of state were disproportionately black, the lawsuit also challenged and forced the state to respond to some clearly discriminatory practices in its child-placing systems. And it called attention not only in Louisiana but elsewhere as well to the harms to children and families of out-of-state placements, stimulating both additional litigation and administrative challenges elsewhere.

Other lawsuits in the child placement area have also sought, with various degrees of success, to prod the responsible jurisdiction into modifying other harmful placement practices and policies. So, for example, a long-drawn-out lawsuit in New York City challenged placement practices which allegedly resulted in discriminatory treatment of minority children. Another class action lawsuit, this one in Washington, D.C., *Bobby D. v Barry*, challenged the practice of placing handicapped, neglected, and dependent children in long-term medical facilities and keeping them long after medical needs had ceased, simply because the city made no attempt to develop the kind of specialized but less restrictive settings that would be more appropriate for these children. More recently, reflecting the legacy of those early suits, litigation is now in process in North Carolina, *Willie M. v Hunt* (1980), challenging the failure of the state to respond to the needs of violent or multiply handicapped, emotionally disturbed children and adolescents. As a remedy, that lawsuit seeks the development of a system of care for the class, including a range of community-based placements designed to eliminate inappropriate institutionalization of the children as well as require individualized evaluation of and treatment planning for all members of the class.

As is true regarding educational litigation, lawsuits like these identify gaps both in services and in the capacity of the public systems to monitor the care and progress of individual children. And they highlight one other little heeded aspect of children's rights litigation—the role of parents in challenging the state on behalf of their children. For in many of these broad-based, class action lawsuits, parents have either been involved as plaintiffs (*Gary W., PARC*) or court testimony has documented, with sometimes excruciating poignancy, the ways in which educational and placement systems have ignored parental efforts to seek services and to participate in decisions about their children.

Children vs. systems: enforcing existing mandates.—Finally, it should be noted that class action litigation has also been used on behalf of children to seek compliance with statutory mandates that are not properly implemented. The most dramatic example of this can be seen in the extensive legal efforts to ensure compliance with the EPSDT (Early Periodic Screening, Diagnosis and Treatment) Program, the Medicaid-related program designed to ensure that the health problems of all Medicaid-eligible children are identified and treated. The legislation was enacted in 1967. However, it took litigation to force the HEW to issue regulations, and subsequent legal challenges in a number of states to ensure even minimal compliance with those regulations. (Indeed, by 1980, nationally the program was still serving only a small percentage of its potential clients and many of them not very well.[4])

Dilemmas, Criticisms, and Realities

In sum, during the past decades, legal efforts to compel a more adequate state (public) response to children have sought the elimination of abusive practices, the application of procedures to guard against capricious decision-making, and the provision of services of at least minimal quality to children. At their most ambitious, they have also sought to use the court (through the development of broad-ranging remedies) to restructure often sluggish and unaccountable service delivery systems.

Comprehensive class action lawsuits have affected both directly and indirectly far greater numbers of children than have lawsuits involving real or potential parent-child conflicts. They have also been far less controversial for professionals and the public at large (except perhaps within the jurisdiction in which the lawsuit occurs). Two general types of criticisms have been made. First, it has been argued that class action lawsuits consume service system time and resources that could be better spent on delivery services. However, this ignores the reality that such litigation has only been brought in the face of carefully documented evidence about long-standing and repeated acts of commission or omission by public agencies.

Second, there has been concern about the "overlegalization" of decision-making about children. (This is a variant of the theme discussed earlier.) Legal critics themselves have noted that because the legal decision-making model relies so heavily on "procedures," it can be seductive, creating the illusion that rational, constructive decision-making is going on when this is not necessarily true. Those who work in service delivery systems (particularly schools) have expressed a similar concern. Some, in fact, have argued that an overemphasis on due process creates passive professionals, less willing to take risks on behalf of individual children and less willing to engage in creative programming, unless compelled through fair hearing procedures or litigation. There has also been concern about substituting legal or judicial wisdom for professional expertise. (This, too, parallels the concern about moving family matters into the legal arena, described earlier.)

So, for example, social workers have argued that increasing oversight of the child welfare system, as seen in efforts to encourage periodic case reviews of a child's progress by courts (or by citizen review bodies), diffuses responsibility for children and places it in uninformed hands. Some of these arguments have validity. But they also ignore the well-documented reality that, regardless of who makes them, decisions about children are often shaped by pressures other than a child's needs or are made by staff with limited relevant expertise or training.

Notwithstanding such criticisms, however, it is also important to note, particularly in view of the disproportionate attention accorded the parent vs. child aspect of the children's rights movement, the litigation involving children in nonfamilial contexts appears to have had a far greater impact on public policies affecting children than has child vs. parents litigation. Such a legacy, for example, is dramatically clear in both *PL 94–142*, the Education for All Handicapped Children's Act, and *PL 96–272*, the Adoption Assistance and Child Welfare Act of 1980. Both of these laws embody principles established in litigation. They require due process safeguards for both the children and their parents; they address the affirmative obligation of the service system to meet the individual needs of their child clients by providing appropriate services; and they specify opportunities for redress when this does not happen. Similar instances of the policy translation of legal decisions can also be found in state statutes. Moreover, in general, even in the absence of specific litigation, new expectations have gained currency about the kind of services public agencies must provide to children, the kind of planning and monitoring they must engage in for individual children and groups of children, and the kind of public scrutiny they must tolerate.

Litigation, in short, has opened the way for a serious examination of the quality of services to children and of the dimensions of public responsibility to them. Although at times painful, such scrutiny serves children for whom public agencies have substantial responsibility better than simplistic acceptance of the assumption that those who serve children can automatically be trusted to act in "the children's best interests."

At the same time, there are signs that maximizing the policy and service delivery gains of class action litigation may in the future be more difficult. First, courts appear to be increasingly wary of mandating broad-scale remedies. Secondly, past experience has shown that even if court decisions are favorable, that is only a first step; implementing the decision involves an often long-drawn-out process that in turn requires both new legal strategies and political ones as well, since ultimately the implementation of remedies involves either reallocating or increasing resources committed to an issue. In times of limited resources, this obviously means public priorities will be more carefully reviewed by those who have fiscal authority, such as state legislatures, making the task of ensuring compliance with mandates resulting from lawsuits even harder.

THE IMPACT OF THE CHILDREN'S RIGHTS MOVEMENT

Any overall assessment of the legal efforts on behalf of children, given the range of those efforts and the complexity of the issues they address, is at best difficult. Clearly, legal advocacy on behalf of children has taken on a form and shape of its own. In 1974, Rodham,[17] in a thoughtful overview article, called children's rights "a slogan in search of a definition." Since then it has become evident that the children's rights movement has generated a new threshold of awareness about the kind of psychological and legal complexities and dilemmas that are embedded in problematic parent-child relationships and, although to a lesser extent, in problematic transactions among children, families, and broader publicly supported socializing institutions. The sweep of this effort has been broad, and as yet there have been few careful evaluations of any subset of litigation (class action or individual) within it. However, even in the absence of such evaluations, some conclusions about how it has affected children and families, professionals, and public policy do seem justified.

First, with regard to the impact of children's rights litigation on individual children and families, the results are mixed. Litigation around parent vs. children issues sometimes benefits the children, sometimes the parents, and sometimes both. No data exist to sort out exactly how the proportions work out either within jurisdictions or nationally, or more importantly what the long-term consequences to the children are. On the other hand, the broader children's rights movement has also led to an increased use of legal challenges on behalf of individual children to ensure them appropriate services from responsible agencies. This is, of course, most obvious around educational issues although it is also evident with regard to other children's services. Indeed, it might even be said that the children's rights movement has had a significant impact in raising the consciousness of service providers about the importance to children of individualized age and stage appropriate care and treatment, a tenet long espoused by developmental psychologists, clinicians, and others, but one not so easily realized.

With regard to the impact of the children's rights litigation on professionals, two clear patterns emerge. On the one hand, there is no question that "helping professionals" accustomed to defining, without much outside questioning, what is in the child's best interests have come in for some uncomfortable scrutiny, particularly those who have been directly involved as defendants or experts for defendants in class action lawsuits; and, by extension, many others as well. In so doing, it has also created a new set of dilemmas for professionals about the limits of their roles, and made highly visible some of their hitherto underplayed potential for harming children.[16] This, in turn, has led to some thoughtful reassessment of traditional roles, and an examination of the implications of the children's rights movement for professionals.[13,15]

Perhaps most interesting, the children's rights litigation and its sequelae have resulted in a very promising and positive interactive relationship among lawyers, helping professionals, and social scientists, one that is all too rarely acknowledged. Often psychological data have played a vital role in convincing the court that in the light of psychological knowledge, there ought to be reassessment of what rights/protections children should have. For instance, psychological evidence maintaining that any child was capable of learning was instrumental in persuading the court in PARC that mentally retarded children should have access to an education. Similarly, psychological evidence about a child's need for stability and permanence has often (although not always) been determinative in dispositional decisions in termination and adoption cases.

Beyond contributing evidence, once new rights have been established (particularly within the educational arena), professionals have turned their attention to the diagnostic and programmatic needs of the affected class of children. This has led to the development at times of new program intervention strategies and research related to making the legal victories (and their policy ramifications) meaningful for individual children.

With regard to the impact of the children's rights movement on broad public policy for children, the influence has been, as noted earlier, dramatic. In specific areas, particularly education and child welfare, litigation has served as the catalyst that has resulted in the reshaping of national expectations and policy. It has also forced public agencies to rethink the nature of public responsibility to children for whom they have significant responsibility, and to face scrutiny of the adequacy of bureaucratic and professional checks and balances to protect children. And litigation along with other nonlegal advocacy efforts[10] has stimulated address to long-standing, easily ignored problems such as institutional abuse and public neglect of children.

Beyond the relatively specific ramifications of children's rights litigation just described, it is also important to note that the term "children's rights" itself has taken on in the public eye a symbolic and pejorative life of its own. Opponents of children's rights have, in fact, extended the scope of the effort beyond any conceivable grounds for legal intervention and used the argument that any public effort on behalf of families is a threat to parental autonomy, and therefore suspect, even if families voluntarily seek services and services are offered in a noncoercive fashion.

This view, as the analysis in this paper suggests, bears little relationship to either legitimate criticisms of legal actions on behalf of children or a close analysis of those activities. Yet it has gained considerable political and ideological currency and represents a serious threat to continued efforts to respond to children's needs and rights. For instance, various versions of a so-called Family Protection Act have already been introduced in Congress. One version would have eliminated all federal funding for child abuse programs. Other versions have expressly prohibited any federal definition of either child abuse or corporal punishment and required explicit state legislated authority for the expenditures of federal funds for programs in these areas. Thus, clearly, the generalized view that any state action threatens families is a potent factor that legal and other child advocates will have to confront.

CONCLUSIONS

Litigation on behalf of children is not a cure-all. For individual children, sometimes it makes a positive difference and sometimes it makes a negative one. Further, some problems are not immediately responsive to litigation. So, for example, there are countless instances in which lawsuits have sought to establish the principle of treatment or placement in the least restrictive setting appropriate to a child's (and, indeed, an adult's) needs. But in fact, since this has not led to any significant change in funding patterns, which still in the main provide reimbursement primarily for more restrictive settings, these principles have not been translated widely back into service system changes. (This is particularly true regarding the mental health service system.)

At the same time, notwithstanding such limitations, it is also clear that the effort to move beyond rhetorical proclamations of children's rights and into the arena of enforceable rights[20,22] has focused a new level of attention on specific harmful situations (both familial and nonfamilial) that can deprive children of developmental opportunities, and on the need to think through individual and systemic protections to guard against such situations. This has been particularly significant because many of the children who have been the concern of this legal focus are particularly vulnerable children, children who are poor, children who are handicapped, children who are members of minority groups, and children of the state who have grown up without the benefit of any real parents. In short, legal advocacy of the past decade and a half has focused on the children who are otherwise most likely to be ignored. In so doing, it has also, along with legal and nonlegal advocacy on behalf of other disenfranchised groups, called attention to our ambivalent feelings about what society owes such groups.

In the face of current legal, psychological, and political realities, the future of the children's rights movement is uncertain. Within the legal arena, the complexity of the legal and psychological issues in litigation involving children in family contexts, and the emerging judicial reluctance to mandate broad, systemic remedies in class action litigation, both of which in a way attest to the past success of legal activity, may also now slow down future gains. Further, there is no question that the current salience of conservative political and ideological forces is likely to have a negative and perhaps chilling effect on the capacity to maintain the policy gains of the children's rights movement. So, for example, although *PL 94–142* and *PL 96–272* remained intact during the first part of the 97th Congress, efforts are already underway to seek their repeal in future Congressional action; even if they survive, the political will to implement them has been undermined.

At the same time, the core of committed lawyers and their colleagues who have brought so many legal challenges will not go away; nor, predictably, will the abuses and excesses the litigation challenges. While the way will be harder, the children's rights movement can remain a significant force as we seek to refine, in the face of ongoing legal and psychological ambiguities and new political realities, the shape of a responsive social policy to children.

REFERENCES

1. Bane, M. (1976). *Here to Stay: American Families in the Twentieth Century.* New York: Basic Books.
2. Bersoff, D. (1982). From courthouse to schoolhouse: Using the legal system to secure the right to an appropriate education. *American Journal of Orthopsychiatry,* 52(3):506–517.
3. Burt, R. (1979). Children as victims. In *Contemporary Perspectives on Children's Rights,* P. Varden and I. Brody, eds. New York: Teachers College Press.
4. Children's Defense Fund. (1977), *EPSDT: Does It Spell Health Care for Poor Children?* Washington, D.C.: Children's Defense Fund.
5. Davidson, H. (1981). The guardian ad litem: An important approach to the protection of children. *Children Today,* 10:20–23.
6. Goldstein, J., Freud, A. and Solnit, A. (1979). *Before the Best Interests of the Child.* New York: Free Press.
7. Hafen, B. (1976). Children's liberation and the new equalitarianism: Some reservations about abandoning youth to their "rights." *Brigham Young University Law Review,* 605–658.
8. Horowitz, R. (1980). Mental incapacity—parents—state intervention: How the courts have put them together. *Legal Response: Child Advocacy and Protection,* 2(2):1; 7–10.
9. Keniston, K. (1977). *All Our Children: The American Family Under Pressure.* New York: Harcourt Brace, Jovanovich.
10. Knitzer, J. (1976). Child advocacy: A perspective. *American Journal of Orthopsychiatry,* 46(2):200–216.
11. Knitzer, J., McGowan, B. and Allen, M. (1978). *Children Without Homes: An Examination of Public Responsibility to Children in Out-Of-Home Care.* Washington, D.C.: Children's Defense Fund.
12. Knitzer, J. (In press). *Unclaimed Children: The Failure of Public Responsibility to Children in Need of Mental Health Services.* Washington, D.C.: Children's Defense Fund.
13. Koocher, G. (ed.) (1976). *Children's Rights and the Mental Health Professions.* New York: John Wiley.
14. Levine, R. (1973). Caveat parens: A demystification of the child protection system. *University of Pittsburgh Law Review,* 35:1–52.
15. Mearig, J. et al. (1978). *Working for Children: Ethical Issues Beyond Professional Guidelines.* San Francisco: Jossey-Bass.
16. Polier, J. (1975). Professional abuse of children: Responsibility for the delivery of services. *American Journal of Orthopsychiatry,* 45(3):357–362.
17. Rodham, H. (1973). Children under the law. *Harvard Educational Review,* 43(4):487–514.
18. Rothman, D. and Rothman, S. (1980). *Putting Parham in Perspective.* Hastings Center Report. Hastings, N.Y.: Institute for Ethics and the Life Sciences.
19. Solnit, A. (1980). Three times in two years. *Zero to Three,* 2:4, 5, 9.
20. Uviller, R. (1979). Children versus parents: Perplexing policy questions for the ACLU. In *Having Children,* O. O'Neill and W. Ruddick, eds. New York: Oxford University Press.
21. Wald, P. (1980). Introduction to the juvenile justice process: The rights of children and the rites of passage. In *Child Psychiatry and the Law,* D. Schetky and E. Benedek, eds. New York: Brunner/Mazel.
22. Wald, M. (1979). Children's rights: A framework for analysis. *UCD Law Review,* 12(2):255–282.
23. Wald, M. (1976). State intervention on behalf of "neglected" children: Standards for the removal of children from their homes, monitoring the status of children in foster care, and termination of parental rights. *Stanford Law Review,* 28:623–706.

35

Does Joint Custody Work? A First Look at Outcome Data of Relitigation

Frederic W. Ilfeld, Jr., Holly Zingale Ilfeld, and John R. Alexander

University of California at Davis School of Medicine and the West District of the California Superior Court for Los Angeles Country

Joint custody, with both divorced parents sharing childrearing functions, is a recent and controversial phenomenon. To the authors' knowledge there have been no published quantitative outcome studies establishing its efficacy. The authors present data on 414 consecutive custody cases in a Los Angeles court over a 2-year period, comparing relitigation rates (indicative of postdivorce parental conflict) of exclusive and joint custody. In those cases which were returns to court, the p.oportion of relitigation for joint custody families was one-half that of exclusive custody families, suggesting that joint custody is a more beneficial arrangement in terms of reduced parental conflict.

Joint custody has been proposed as a partial solution for the deleterious effects on children of the high number of divorces (1–3). However, others have felt that effective child rearing is compromised by joint custody and that there are critical flaws in shared parenting (4, 5). A great deal of controversy exists on this issue, but one thing that all investigators agree on is that there is a lack of empirical data about the effects of joint custody on which to base their arguments. The need for information is especially acute because social policy is now at issue in many states; although joint custody currently represents a small per-

Reprinted with permission from the *American Journal of Psychiatry*, 1982, Vol. 139, No. 1, 62–66. Copyright 1982 by the American Psychiatric Association.

centage of divorce outcomes, this arrangement is being considered as an option by a number of state legislatures. Already, family welfare in California is being decided daily under the new law of 1980 with its consideration that joint custody is in the best interests of a minor child (Section 4600 of the California Civil Code and reference 6).

Fortunately, the West District (Santa Monica) of the Los Angeles County Superior Court has collected data on its awards of joint and exclusive custody over a 2-year period, from fall 1978 through fall 1980. In this paper we will present these data, which compare the outcome, as defined by relitigation after an initial custody award, for both exclusive custody (276 families) and joint custody (138 families). To our knowledge, such quantitative information contrasting joint and exclusive custody has not been published before.

What exactly is joint custody? The definition used for the cases in this paper is embodied in California law, which states in part that "custody should be awarded in the following order of preference, according to the best interests of the child: to both parents jointly . . . or to either parent" (Section 4600[b] of the California Civil Code). The law proceeds to define joint custody as "an order awarding custody of the minor child or children to both parents, and providing that physical custody shall be shared by the parents in such a way as to assure the child or children of frequent and continuing contact with both parents" (Section 4600.5[c] of the Civil Code). Among nonlegal authors writing on this subject there is moderate consensus as to the meaning and definition of joint custody. One definition that is representative of most authors as well as being congruent with California's new law is that offered by Woolley (3), who defined shared parenting as "any form of custody or visitation arrangement which allows both parents to have lots of normal, day-by-day interaction with the off-spring and provides that each adult participates in both the responsibilities and the rewards of child raising" (p. 13). The reader should note that under California law as well as under this definition, there is no precise delineation of how much time the child should spend with each parent. Practice has shown that the time-sharing arrangements vary highly according to the particular needs of each set of children and parents.

What existing data might speak to the effects of joint custody? Several authors (2, 7) have traced the historical trend of custody changing from the father to the mother around the turn of the century and moving recently toward more equalization in custody. The authors pointed out that current opinions opposed to shared custody are based not on documented evidence but rather on social custom and tradition that have solidified over the years. Despite a lack of data comparing different custody arrangements, Goldstein and associates (4) recommended placing the child with one parent only and advocated that the custodial parent, not courts or the noncustodial parent, should retain the right to determine when and if visitation will occur. Benedek and Benedek (5) have suggested there might be some benefits to joint custody, but without citing any evidence they cautioned about several presumed risks of joint parenting.

Several longitudinal clinical studies have looked at children of divorce and arrived at conclusions supportive of joint custody. In a 5-year study of 60 families with 130 children in Marin County (California), Wallerstein and Kelly (8) found that divorce might be beneficial for the adults but not for the children. The psychological relationship between the child and each of his original parents did not diminish in emotional importance to the child over the 5-year study, regardless of the degree of visitation of the noncustodial parent. Their findings pointed to the desirability of the child's continuing relationship with both parents during the postdivorce years whereby each parent would be responsible for and genuinely concerned with the child's well-being. They felt that the major hazard which divorce posed to the psychological health of the children was in the disruptive or diminished parenting that might be consolidated within the postdivorce family arrangements, such as a functional absence of one parent and an overburdening of responsibility on the custodial parent. Thus the postdivorce arrangements of continuing contact between the children and both parents seemed to be most important for the long-term outcome of the children. Both Wallerstein and Kelly (8) and Heatherington and associates (9) have further acknowledged the economic, social, and psychological vulnerability of the typical family in which divorce has occurred, i.e., a family with one custodial parent and one noncustodial parent.

Another source of data has been case histories of those pioneering families who have developed joint custody. These couples have done this largely against familial and legal opposition and were few in number before the California law of 1980. Several authors (1, 3, 10–12) have taken an in-depth look at the arrangements these families have made and the effects on the children. Of these studies Steinman's (12) is the most extensive. She examined the experience and impact of living in a joint custody situation for children and parents of 24 San Francisco Bay area families. On the basis of two clinical semistructured interviews with each family member, she explored issues of parental relationships, time-sharing, finances, loyalty to each parent, confusion of the children, problems of geographical distance, and school and friendships. She concluded that these children had access to both parents and felt that both parents loved and wanted them. However, about one-third of the children felt overburdened by the demands and requirements of two homes and the need to maintain a strong presence in both homes. A major drawback to Steinman's study is that there has been no parallel assessment of exclusive custody families. It is difficult to judge the degree of success of joint custody without a comparison of exclusive custody families. Moreover, none of these studies included joint custody families in which both parents did *not* agree to the joint arrangement, so the question of feasibility for unconsented joint custody remains unanswered.

Within the past few months Pojman has made available his data demonstrating the superiority in emotional adjustment of boys in joint custody over boys in exclusive custody (E. Pojman, unpublished doctoral dissertation, 1981, California Graduate Institute, 1100 Glendon Ave., Los Angeles, Calif. 90024). His quasiexperimental study compared four groups of 20 boys each (age range, 5–13 years) living in the following situations: joint and exclusive custody arrangements and intact families with happy and unhappy marriages. Three different tools were used to assess the boys: the Louisville Behavior Checklist (parent's rating), the Inferred Self-Concept Scale (teacher's rating), and the California Test of Personality (child's rating). Boys of joint custody were significantly better emotionally adjusted than boys of exclusive custody and of the unhappily married group on the security scale of the Louisville Behavior Checklist (p < .05) and on the Inferred Self-Concept Scale (p < .01, one-way analysis of variance). Joint custody boys had higher personal adjustment scores on the California Test of Personality than did exclusive custody boys, but the difference between the two groups fell just short of statistical significance at the .05 level. In a comparison between boys of exclusive custody and boys living in intact families with unhappy marriages, Pojman found no significant differences on any of the three tests.

Comparing the outcomes of several different types of custody will be the task of this paper, for we have unique, systematically collected data on parental conflict and subsequent relitigation among both joint and exclusive custody families. We assume that relitigation of custody means that parents are in conflict with one another and that parental conflict strong enough to bring them to the courts has adverse effects on the children. In short, postdivorce parental conflict implies trouble for the children. While we realize that relitigation is only one indicator of whether custody works well for the children, it does seem to be an objective measure closely reflecting parental conflicts. In this regard our findings show a clear superiority of joint custody over exclusive custody. A subset of our sample (18 cases) is a rather controversial group—those families who have been awarded joint custody *without* the consent of both parents. Although small in number, this subsample is an important group, for it speaks to the question of whether joint custody can work even when one of the parents has this form of custody forced on him or her by court mandate. Even in this subsample we found the amount of postdivorce conflict to be no greater than that in the exclusive custody cases.

STUDY DESIGN

In searching for an answer to the feasibility of joint custody, one of the coauthors (J.R.A.) began collecting data for a firsthand study of consecutive custody cases on the court calendar in Department West J of the Los Angeles County Superior Court. The study ran from the fall of 1978 through September 30, 1980, thus covering a period of about 2 years, the last 9 months of which were after January 1, 1980, the effective date of the new joint custody legislation in California. The 414 consecutive cases covered by the study (276 exclusive and 138 joint custody) included both permanent awards and relitigation cases.

Altogether, 91% of the exclusive custody awards and 86% of the joint custody awards were based on agreement between parents. The awards of joint custody were given in line with the previously cited definition provided by California's Civil Code, but the court made many variations concerning time-sharing of the children between the parents. We have not attempted to delineate the specific types of arrangements made between the parents concerning visitation, time-sharing between the two homes, or style of decision-making. Obtaining that information would have entailed expensive, time-consuming research investigating official court files along with home interviews.

RESULTS

Table 1 compares relitigation for exclusive and joint custody cases over four time points. One may question whether relitigation of joint custody cases was artificially low because the bulk of the joint custody awards may have been granted late in the study, after the inception of California's new law. The data show this not to be the case, since the joint custody awards occurred in substantial numbers throughout the

TABLE 1. Relitigation in Exclusive and Joint Custody Cases, Fall 1978 to Fall 1980

| Item | Cases Cumulative to | | | |
	8/31/79	11/30/79	5/31/80	9/30/80
Total number of cases	108	161	306	414
Awards of exclusive custody				
Number	76	118	216	276
Percent	70	73	71	67
Awards of joint custody				
Number	32	43	90	138
Percent	30	27	29	33
Cases of relitigation of prior exclusive custody awards				
Number	22	31	64	87
Percent[a]	29	26	30	32
Cases of relitigation of prior joint custody awards				
Number	5	9	15	22
Percent[b]	16	21	17	16

[a]The percent of relitigation for exclusive custody was determined by dividing the number of relitigated cases arising out of prior exclusive custody awards by the total awards of exclusive custody.

[b]The percent of relitigation for joint custody was determined by dividing the number of relitigated cases arising out of prior joint custody awards by the total awards of joint custody.

entire period of study. Also, notice that the percent of joint custody relitigation did not increase over the four time periods; rather, at the end of the 2-year period it stood at a low of 16%. These facts again speak to the concern of possible bias that joint custody cases were not in the study long enough to have been involved in relitigation. If there were such a bias, the percent of joint relitigation should have increased over time, which it did not.

Before turning to our main findings, we will examine another potential source of bias. Are noncustodial parents returning to court in dispro-portionate numbers, trying to obtain joint custody because of the 1980 change in California's custody law? This phenomenon could account for a heightened rate of relitigation in exclusive custody cases. However, further examination of the reasons for relitigation in each case shows that this is not so. Only 6 of 69 relitigated exclusive custody cases were requesting joint custody. (Data on the purpose of the relitigation were not sufficiently clear or complete in 18 of the 87 cases.) The remaining 63 cases arose mainly from requests to change exclusive custody from one parent to the other, from requests to modify visitation schedules or conditions, or from contempt-of-court charges due to violation of conditions of visitation. We conclude that the rate of relitigation in exclusive custody cases was not artificially increased because of the 1980 law.

We will now turn to the main results of the 2-year tabulation (see data for 9/30/80 in Table 1). There were half as many relitigations in joint custody cases (16%) as there were in exclusive custody cases (32%). These proportions are significantly different (z = −3.9, p < .001) and suggest that joint custody results in less parental conflict and, implicitly, in lower child distress than exclusive custody.

But what about the custody group at presumably highest risk for later conflict—the subsample of 18 in which joint custody was awarded without the consent of one parent? Even though this is a small number, it is an important group to examine because so many judges, lawyers, and mental health professionals feel that both parents must have a commitment to joint custody for the arrangement to work (5). This common belief questions whether both parents can work together if they do not agree on custody arrangements. However, only 6 (33%) of the 18 cases have been on the court calendar for later adversary proceedings. This percentage of relitigation is virtually the same as that for our total exclusive custody sample (32%), suggesting (tentatively, due to the small sample size) that unconsented joint custody is no more disruptive in terms of parental conflict than exclusive custody. Furthermore, of the 6 relitigations, 2 were settled out of court by agreement of the parties involved.

DISCUSSION

Over a period of 2 years the West District Department J of the Los Angeles County Superior Court had 414 consecutive custody cases, two-thirds involving exclusive custody and one-third joint custody. In those cases which were returns to court, the proportion of relitigation for joint custody families was one-half that of exclusive custody families. From our preliminary study (including a small subsample in which joint custody was decreed without the consent of one of the parents), we conclude that the custody arrangement most beneficial in terms of lack of subsequent parental conflict is joint custody. (Of course, time-sharing and other specific arrangements will vary according to the circumstances of each family.)

An alternative interpretation of our findings is that the courts awarded joint custody to those parents who appeared more able to cooperate without court supervision, thus predisposing to a lower relitigation rate for joint custody. Since the precise basis of the court's decision is not known, we cannot directly test this interpretation. However, our data, which show that a higher proportion of exclusive custody awards were based on parental agreement than was the case for joint custody awards (91% versus 86%), do not support this interpretation.

We make two assumptions in drawing conclusions from these data. First, following evidence from Wallerstein and Kelly (8), we assume that problems with children's adjustment after divorce are due more to the postdivorce arrangement and amount of conflict than to the divorce itself. Second, we assume that relitigation over a custody issue represents moderate to severe parental conflict that adversely affects the children. Given these assumptions, our findings and those of Pojman carry suggestions for future research and perhaps for social policy and family law. Considering that the best interests of the children are foremost, all professionals should recognize a strong, positive indication for joint custody. Unless future data persuasively contradict our and Pojman's findings, the burden of proof that joint custody would not be in a child's best interests should be on the parent requesting sole custody.

In addition to our relatively short follow-up period, other limitations of the data point the way for future investigations. To begin with, we have not examined the children firsthand. Furthermore, we have no information on how each family put the custody order into practice. For instance, how did joint custody families allocate time-sharing between the two homes? How much visitation with the noncustodial parent occurred in the exclusive custody families? Were both parents involved in major decision-making more in joint custody than exclusive custody arrangements? To what extent was a written plan formulated and made a part of the court mandate? Such information would be important in determining the components of joint custody that make it more workable than exclusive custody.

Beyond the specific arrangements made by each family, other factors, such as level of income; race or ethnicity; ages, sex, and number of children; and geographic proximity of the parents, may well influence the success of a particular custody arrangement. In future studies such factors as these need to be taken into account in assessing outcome. In addition, any future study should extend at least 2 years beyond the initial custody decision to ensure adequate time for follow-up. We plan to continue monitoring the present sample of custody cases if they reappear in the Santa Monica court to see whether the trends reported herein continue to hold, and we hope to have a future report on such long-term, follow-up data. We hope that other investigators will collect comparative data on different custody arrangements and that future social policy and family law will be based on such factual information rather than on historical precedent, social bias, hypothetical speculation, or the adversarial milieu of the legal system.

Further research needs to document the effects of joint custody on parenting practices and on the children. As for which factors of a joint custody arrangement might lead to a successful outcome, we have our own hypotheses based on others' and our own clinical experience, which might be tested in future studies. First, we hypothesize that the more equal the time-sharing between the parents, the better the chance for successful outcome for the children. Second, we anticipate that having a mandated written plan covering the common issues faced in joint decision-making, such as that suggested by Galper (1), should prove more beneficial than leaving such guidelines unstated. A part of such a plan might include, for example, defined actions following such listed contingencies as cohabitation, remarriage, or one parent's move from the area. Third, the children should do better the closer the parents live to one another, especially if they are in the same school district. Last, we hypothesize that those joint custody families should do better who have agreed to (or had mandated by the court) a process of mediation and arbitration specified for major decisions when family consensus cannot be reached. This last point suggests a changing role for mental health professionals in custody decisions and deserves further comment.

Until now mental health professionals have participated in the custody process as expert consultants (13). In the adversarial arena of the legal system we have had to assess the family and recommend a choice between the two parents. With no-fault decisions, in which custody is retained functionally by both father and mother, we may lose this role of court consultant and evaluator. (An important exception occurs when one or both parents may be abusive to the child.) However, we may gain several new functions. First, we can help the separating family to develop a joint custody arrangement that meets that family's needs. Outside of the win/lose atmosphere of the courts, a divorcing couple should find it easier to work through the details of a custody plan when assisted by the skilled collaboration of counselors and lawyers. Several multidisciplinary clinics oriented to this primary prevention function of counseling for divorce and custody have already started in California. A second potential function for mental health professionals is that of mediator and arbitrator when the parents and children in a joint custody arrangement cannot agree on major decisions. Whether an arbitration clause is agreed to by both parents and/or mandated by court judgment, this measure will provide a partial way to resolve parental conflict without returning to the court system, which drains economic resources and fosters more conflict. New roles such as these need to be explored and developed as mental health professionals act to sustain the well-being of children and parents during the stressful transition of family breakup.

REFERENCES

1. Galper, M. (1978). *Co-parenting: A Source Book for the Separated or Divorced Family.* Philadelphia: Running Press.
2. Roman, M. and Haddad, W. (1978). *The Disposable Parent: The Case for Joint Custody.* New York: Holt, Rinehart and Winston.
3. Woolley, P. (1979). *The Custody Handbook.* New York: Summit Books.
4. Goldstein, J., Freud, A. and Solnit, A. (1979). *Beyond the Best Interests of the Child.* New York: Free Press.
5. Benedek, E. P. and Benedek, R. S. (1979). Joint custody: Solution or illusion? *American Journal of Psychiatry,* 136:1540–1544.
6. Cook, J. (1980). Joint custody, sole custody: A new statute reflects a new perspective. *Conciliation Courts Review,* 18(June):1–14.
7. Derdeyn, A. P. (1976). Child custody contests in historical perspective. *American Journal of Psychiatry,* 133:1369–1376.
8. Wallerstein, J. and Kelly, J. (1980). *Surviving the Break-Up: How Children and Parents Cope with Divorce.* New York: Basic Books.
9. Heatherington, E., Cox, M. and Cox R. (1976). Divorced fathers. *Family Coordinator,* 25:417–428.
10. Greif, J. (1979). Fathers, children, and joint custody. *American Journal of Orthopsychiatry,* 49:311–319.
11. Abarbanel, A. (1979). Shared parenting after separation and divorce: A study of joint custody. *American Journal of Orthopsychiatry,* 49:320–329.
12. Steinman, S. (1981). The experience of children in a joint custody arrangement: A report of a study. *American Journal of Orthopsychiatry,* 51:403–414.
13. Derdeyn, A. (1975). Child custody consultation. *American Journal of Orthopsychiatry,* 45:791–801.